A NEW DEAL FOR AMERICAN HEALTH CARE:

HOW REFORM WILL RESHAPE HEALTH CARE DELIVERY AND PAYMENT FOR A NEW CENTURY

A NEW DEAL FOR AMERICAN HEALTH CARE:

HOW REFORM WILL RESHAPE HEALTH CARE DELIVERY AND PAYMENT FOR A NEW CENTURY

by Richard M. Sorian
and the Editors of the
Healthcare Information Center

Introduction by Robert J. Blendon, Sc.D.

F&G FAULKNER & GRAY
THOMSON PROFESSIONAL PUBLISHING

Faulkner & Gray, Inc., New York
Healthcare Information Center, Washington DC

A New Deal for American Health Care: How Reform Will Reshape Health Care Delivery and Payment for a New Century

ISBN 1-881-393-20-8

The sponsoring editor was Luci S. Koizumi; production director was Susan Namovicz-Peat; project editor was Virginia Vitzthum; printed by McArdle Printing Co.

Published by Faulkner & Gray's Healthcare Information Center

1133 Fifteenth Street, NW
Washington DC 20005

PRINTED IN THE UNITED STATES OF AMERICA

THE AUTHORS

Richard Sorian
Writer and Journalist

Richard Sorian is a veteran observer and reporter on U.S. health policy. He is the former editor of Faulkner & Gray's *Journal of American Health Policy* and *Medicine & Health*. Mr. Sorian is also the author of *The Bitter Pill: Tough Choices in America's Health Policy* (McGraw-Hill, 1988).

Healthcare Information Center

Janet Firshein
Editor
Medicine & Health

Janet Firshein is editor of Faulkner & Gray's *Medicine & Health* and former editor of *Health Legislation*. She has also been Washington bureau chief for *Hospitals* and a staff writer for the American Hospital Association.

Cathy Tokarski
Editor
Journal of American Health Policy

Cathy Tokarski is the editor of the *Journal of American Health Policy*. Before joining Faulkner & Gray in 1990, she was Washington editor for *Modern Healthcare*.

Daniel B. Moskowitz
Senior Editor
Faulkner & Gray

Daniel B. Moskowitz writes regularly about health law issues for the Faulkner & Gray publications *Health Business* and the *Journal of American Health Policy*. His articles on trends in legal affairs have appeared frequently in the *Washington Post*, *BusinessWeek*, and *Medical World News*. Mr. Moskowitz has won three awards in the American Bar Association's annual Silver Gavel journalism competition.

Karen J. Migdail
Editor
Long Term Care Management

Karen J. Migdail is editor of *Long Term Care Management* and serves as Washington correspondent for Faulkner & Gray's *Medical Outcomes & Guidelines Alert*. She is co-editor of the forthcoming 1994-1995 edition of the *Medical Outcomes and Guidelines Sourcebook*. Previously, Ms. Migdail was a policy analyst with the American Health Care Association.

David Strickland
Editor
Medical Outcomes & Guidelines Alert

David Strickland is editor of Faulkner & Gray's *Medical Outcomes & Guidelines Alert* and co-editor of the forthcoming *Medical Outcomes & Guidelines Sourcebook*. He is the former editor of *Outcomes Measurement & Management* and *Quality Pathways* and was a staff reporter for *Medical World News*.

Allan Holmes
Assistant Editor
Journal of American Health Policy

Allan Holmes is assistant editor for Faulkner & Gray's *Journal of American Health Policy*. Previously, he was associate editor for *Triangle Business Journal* in Raleigh NC. Mr. Holmes also has reported for *U.S. News & World Report*, *Time Magazine*, and the *New York Times*.

Harvard School of Public Health

Robert J. Blendon, Sc.D.
Roger I. Lee Professor and Chairman
Department of Health Policy and Management
Harvard School of Public Health

Robert J. Blendon is Roger I. Lee Professor and Chairman of the Department of Health Policy and Management of the Harvard School of Public Health. Prior to his Harvard appointment, Dr. Blendon was senior vice president at the Robert Wood Johnson Foundation, where he worked for 15 years. He is best known for his research on access to health care, satisfaction with national health care systems, AIDS and discrimination, and public opinion on health care.

Tracey Stelzer Hyams, J.D., M.P.H.
Deputy Director
Program on the Future of Health Care
Harvard School of Public Health

Tracey Hyams is deputy director of the Harvard Program on the Future of Health Care at the Harvard School of Public Health. Her research efforts focus on health care reform initiatives at the national and state levels, including the politics of reform, the role of special interest groups, and the impact of public opinion on the health care reform debate. In her work in the health care field she has drafted hospital finance legislation, developed course materials on pharmaceutical policy, and analyzed malpractice claims for hospital risk management programs.

John M. Benson, M.A.
Deputy Director
Harvard Program on Public Opinion and Health Care
Harvard School of Public Health

John Benson is deputy director of the Harvard Program on Public Opinion and Health Care at the Harvard School of Public Health. He analyzes survey data to identify key trends in public opinion and helps design surveys conducted by the program. His work focuses on the role public and leadership opinion plays in the formation of the nation's agenda on health. Previously, Mr. Benson was senior opinion analyst at the Roper Center for Public Opinion Research and associate editor of *The Public Perspective*.

Mollyann Brodie, M.S.
Assistant Director
Harvard Program on the Future of Health Care
Harvard School of Public Health

Mollyann Brodie is assistant director of the Harvard Program on the Future of Health Care at the Harvard School of Public Health. She is also a Fellow in Health Policy at Harvard University. Her research efforts focus on the political economy of health care and the role of political institutions in health policy. Previously Ms. Brodie worked as a health policy analyst for the U.S. Department of Health and Human Services in the Office of Evaluation and Inspection, performed research at the RAND Corporation, and served as an intern for Rep. Henry Waxman (D-CA).

Contributing Authors

Richard A. Knox
Reporter
The Boston Globe

Richard A. Knox is an award-winning, nationally syndicated reporter for the Boston Globe who has specialized in medicine and health care since 1969. Knox has held academic fellowships at Stanford University and the Harvard School of Public Health. While a Harvard Fellow in Advanced Public Health Studies in 1990-1991, he travelled in Germany on a Commonwealth Fund grant. He is the author of Faulkner & Gray's *Germany's Health System: One Nation United With Health Care for All*. Knox's writing has also appeared in *Science*, the *Journal of the American Medical Association*, and *Health Affairs*.

Diane Rowland, Sc.D.
Senior Vice President, The Henry J. Kaiser Family Foundation and
Executive Director, Kaiser Commission on the Future of Medicaid

Dr. Rowland is senior vice president of the Henry J. Kaiser Family Foundation and executive director of the Kaiser Commission on the Future of Medicaid. She also holds an appointment as associate professor in the Department of Health Policy and Management at the School of Hygiene and Public Health of the Johns Hopkins University. She has published numerous books and articles on health care for low-income and elderly Americans as well as comparative international studies of health care policy.

Lois Simon
Policy Analyst
Kaiser Commission on the Future of Medicaid

Lois Simon is a policy analyst at the Kaiser Commission on the Future of Medicaid. Previously she was a research associate for James Bell Associates. Ms. Simon is working toward a Master of Health Science in Health Policy at the School of Hygiene and Public Health at the Johns Hopkins University.

Roy Bredder, J.D.
Associate
Janet L. Kuhn and Associates

Roy Bredder is an associate with the law firm of Janet L. Kuhn and Associates, Vienna, Virginia. A contributing Editor of Faulkner & Gray's *Health Legislation and Regulation* newsletter, he has tracked health-related legislation since 1974, and writes the weekly legislative and regulatory summaries.

TABLE OF CONTENTS

Introduction

Robert J. Blendon
with Tracey Stelzer Hyams, John M. Benson, and Mollyann Brodie

For the fourth time since World War II, Congress is engaged in a major debate over reforming the nation's health care system. While each past campaign for health care reform centered on a unique policy proposal, there are common features between the current debate and the contests of the past. Prior to the introduction of each bill, there existed strong public interest in and expectation for reform. And after each plan was introduced, interest groups spent millions of dollars convincing the public that enactment of the proposal would result in a health care delivery system even worse than the status quo. Examining these past contests provides important lessons on the role of public opinion and interest group activity in determining the outcome of the national health care reform debate.

Almost 50 years ago, President Truman proposed a comprehensive prepaid national health insurance plan to be financed through the social security tax program. Initially, Truman's proposal had the support of an impressive array of legislators and organizations, prompting political analysts to predict that passage of the plan would proceed smoothly. But special interests mounted a public relations campaign unprecedented in scope and unparalleled in term of campaign expenditures spent fighting the plan.[1] Unable to match their resources, President Truman ultimately lost out to the interest groups' exaggerated claims regarding the details of his plan, and his proposal failed to attract sufficient public or legislative support. In fact, Gallup polls from the outset of the campaign showed the public evenly divided in its support for Truman's plan. By the end of the campaign, Americans were two to one against its enactment (see Table I-1).[2-4]

National health insurance was again hotly debated after President Johnson's election to office in 1964. Three distinct proposals were being floated: one from the Johnson Administration, one the product of the Republican party, and one from the proponents of health care for the poor. Strategically merging these three plans, House Ways and Means Chair Wilbur Mills created a comprehensive program that resulted in the 1965 enactment of Medicare and Medicaid.[5] While this reform covered only the nation's poor and elderly citizens, proponents of universal national health insurance supported these programs as a necessary first step towards achieving their ultimate goals.[6]

In 1974, the Nixon White House proposed a more extensive national health program called the Comprehensive Health Insurance Program (CHIP). This program mandated health insurance coverage for workers through their employers, and provided a separate program to cover the unemployed.[7] Given the similarities between the Nixon bill and the Democratic proposal sponsored by Mills and Sen. Edward Kennedy (D-MA), compromise seemed likely. However, the Watergate scandal significantly reduced the President's influence with the Congress and the American public, and dominated the political agenda at a time when health care reform might otherwise have been achieved.[8]

Table I-1

Public Support for the Truman Health Reform Plan

	Among those who heard of the plan		
	March 1949	Nov.-Dec. 1949	Nov. 1950
For	38%	33%	29%
Against	38	47	60
No opinion	25	20	11

Source: Gallup Poll.

Today, the U.S. again faces major questions regarding health care reform, with the introduction of President Clinton's plan and a variety of additional proposals, both Democratic and Republican, being debated in Congress. Once again a new Administration is proposing comprehensive national health reform, including health insurance coverage for every American citizen.

To those outside the health field, the reasons underlying the current surge of interest in health reform are not immediately apparent. Some believe that the issue is high on our national agenda because the health care system has reached a state of crisis: A large number of Americans are either uninsured or underinsured, and many are threatened by high health costs. If these conditions were the sole drivers of reform, however, then a national health insurance bill should have been enacted in Truman's day, when a far greater percentage of Americans were uninsured, and far more were seriously threatened by high medical costs.

At the time President Truman introduced his bill for national health insurance, 55 percent of Americans were without health coverage, and surveys showed that 80 percent of American families could not afford to meet the costs of a major illness (see Figure I-1). Servicemen returning from World War II had recently experienced free medical care for the first time and saw how it could benefit their

Figure I-1

Percentage of Americans Without Health Insurance During Prior Debates About National Health Insurance

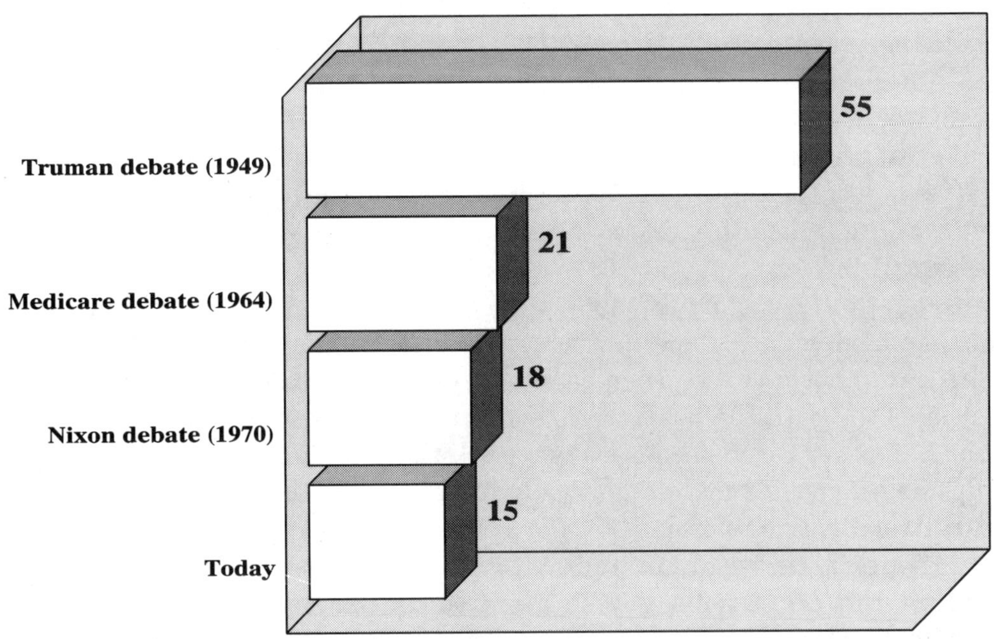

lives. More recent debates over Medicare and President Nixon's bill occurred at times when the percentage of Americans without health coverage had steadily decreased. By the time Medicare was proposed in 1964, only 20 percent of the nation lacked health insurance, and at the time of President Nixon's proposal, this figure had decreased to 18 percent.[9-13]

Thus, the national debate over health insurance has never been a reflection of the aggregate problem. With only 15 percent of Americans lacking health insurance today, and with Medicare and Medicaid covering many of the nation's poor and elderly citizens, today's campaign is largely being driven by something else: *middle-class anxieties over the security of their health insurance coverage.*

Anxiety about health insurance extends far beyond the ranks of the uninsured. The inability of the U.S. to control sharply rising medical costs has created a situation where health coverage is beginning to disintegrate for average working families. Sixty-four percent of Americans are worried that their health insurance will become too expensive to afford, 52 percent fear that very large medical bills will not be covered, 52 percent are concerned that their health benefits will be cut, and 31 percent of Americans worry that their family will lose health insurance coverage (see Figure I-2).[14]

These anxieties are based on real problems Americans experience. One in four lose their health insurance during any two year period.[15] Nearly one-half of employed Americans have had their health benefits cut during the last two years.[16] One in eight households has someone locked into a job for health insurance reasons,[14] and one in five households has had someone denied coverage for a pre-existing medical condition.[16] Surveys show that 20 percent of Americans have had a problem paying medical bills in the past year.[17] Similarly, 10 percent of Americans report that there was a time in the past year when they needed medical care, but did not get it for economic reasons (see Figure I-3).[14]

It is not surprising, therefore, that health care is near the top of the national political agenda. According to a 1990 survey conducted in 10 industrialized countries, Americans are the least likely to say that their own country's health care system works pretty well (see Table I-2).[18] Voters in the 1992 Presidential election cited health care as the third most important issue, with 19 percent of voters naming it as one of the top two issues in deciding how they voted. Among those who voted for Clinton, health care was the number two issue, second only to the economy (see Table I-3).[19]

Given this level of public anxiety and interest, it would seem that enactment of a major health plan is now inevitable. But history tells us that public support for health care reform can be fragile. While Americans express strong opinions on what is wrong with the health care system, there are four key reasons why the public has never reached consensus on health care reform. In the past, interest groups have appealed to these uniquely American values in their efforts to defeat national health care reform.

1. Americans want the federal government to solve the health care problem, but don't trust government to do things right. Americans differ from citizens of most other industrialized countries in their views about the role of

Figure I-2

Public Anxiety About Coverage, 1993

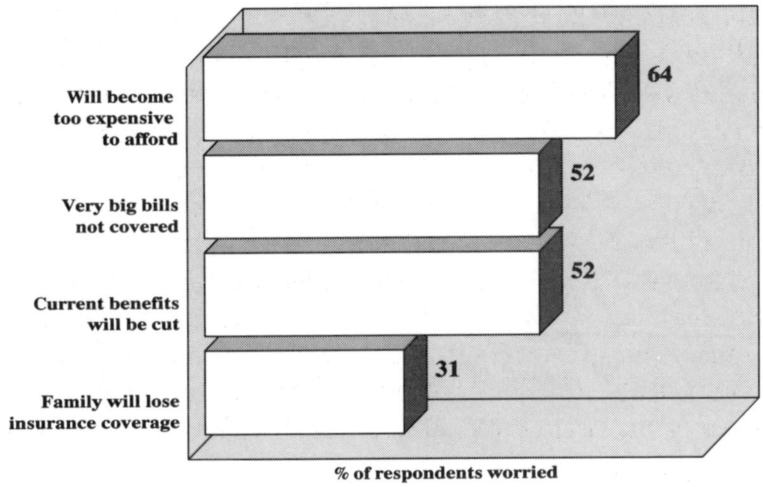

Source: Kaiser/Commonwealth/Harris, 1993.

Figure I-3

Was There a Time When You Needed Medical Care But Did Not Get It for Economic Reasons?

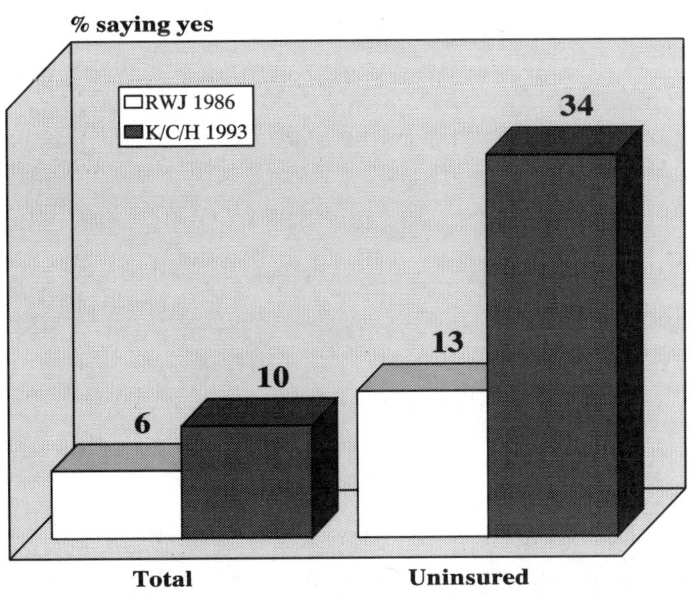

Source: Robert Wood Johnson, 1986; Kaiser/Commonwealth/Harris, 1993.

Figure I-4

Americans' Trust in the Federal Government To Do the Right Thing, 1958-1993

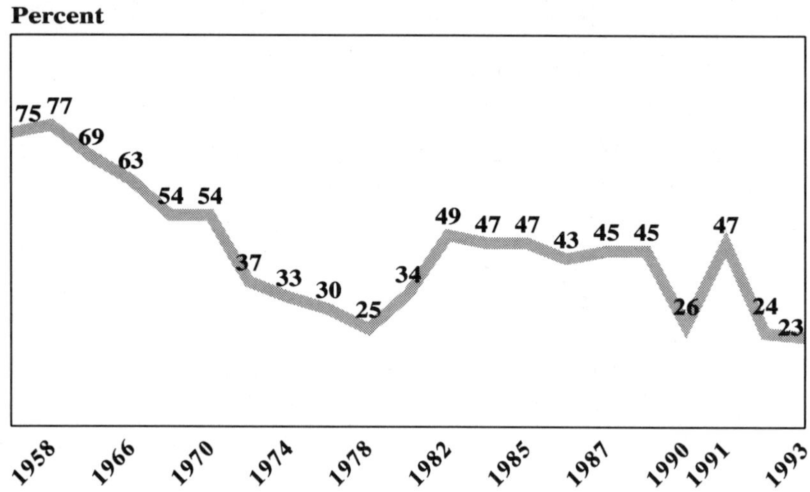

Source: Center for Public Studies; CBS News/New York Times, 1993.

government in solving society's problems — the U.S. has a stronger tradition of reliance on private sector action. In a multi-national survey conducted in 1985, only 36 percent of Americans said it should definitely be the government's responsibility to care for the sick, compared to 87 percent in Italy, 86 percent in Great Britain, and 54 percent in West Germany.[20]

Additionally, Americans' trust in the federal government has never completely recovered from the cynicism of the Watergate era. In the late 1950s, three-quarters of Americans said they trusted the government in Washington to do the right thing;[21] in 1993, fewer than one in four (23 percent) expressed such trust[22] (see Figure I-4). Between 1972 and 1974, Americans' trust in the federal government dropped from 54 percent to 37 percent.[21] Similarly, President Nixon's approval ratings fell from 67 percent in January 1973[23] to 24 percent shortly before his resignation in 1974,[24] likely contributing to the defeat of his national health reform plan.

2. There has never been a consensus among the American people regarding an acceptable approach to health care reform. While Americans are willing to applaud the goal of national health reform, they do not agree on the means of achieving that goal. In a 1945 survey, 82 percent said that something should be done "to make it easier for people to pay for doctor and hospital care." When asked whether each of three different plans (group insurance through an insurance company, the federal government plan as part of Social Security, and a doctors' organization plan) was a good, fair, or poor idea, a plurality of Americans

Table I-2

The Public's View of Their Health Care System in Ten Nations

	Works pretty well/ needs only minor changes	Fundamental changes needed	Completely rebuild system
Canada	56	38	5
Netherlands	47	46	5
West Germany	41	35	13
France	41	42	10
Australia	34	43	17
Sweden	32	58	6
Japan	29	47	6
United Kingdom	27	52	17
Italy	12	46	40
United States	10	60	29

Source: Harvard/Harris/ITF, 1990 Ten-Nation Survey.

Table I-3

Top Five Issues in the 1992 Presidential Election

Rank	
1	Economy and jobs (43%)
2	Deficit (21%)
3	Health care (19%)
4	Family values (15%)
5	Taxes (14%)

Source: Voter Research and Surveys, National Election Day Exit Poll, 1992.

rated each plan as good, and at least two-thirds rated each plan as good or fair. But when asked to choose among the three plans, none came close to achieving majority support. The government option was preferred by only a third (34 percent) of the public (see Table I-4).[25]

Similarly, during the debate over the Nixon health reform plan, 66 percent of Americans agreed that "we need a new nationwide federal health insurance plan."[26] But when asked whether they preferred to receive health insurance from a private insurance company or through the government, the public was split almost evenly.[26,27,28]

Again in the current debate, there seems at first glance to be strong support for a national health insurance program. Fifty-nine percent of Americans say they favor "national health insurance, which would be financed by tax money, paying for most forms of health care."[16] Yet by more than a two-to-one margin (57 to 26 percent), Americans believe that private industry can do a better job managing health care than the government.[29] Similarly, when offered a choice among the three principal reform options, the public has consistently been divided almost evenly: 32 percent preferred a plan similar to President Clinton's; 32 percent opted for a tax credit plan such as the Republican proposal; and 28 percent preferred a single payer system like that proposed by Rep. Jim McDermott (D-WA) and Sen. Paul Wellstone (D-MN) (see Figure I-5).[14] Thus, no matter which of the three options is actually being promoted, two-thirds of the American public will always believe that there could have been a better plan proposed.

Each of these examples suggests that caution is necessary in interpreting the public's will. First, agreement on a goal does not necessarily imply agreement on the means to achieve that goal. Additionally, where opinions on the means to achieve

Table I-4

Support for Three Health Reform Plans, 1945

	% saying "good or fair idea"	Preferred in three-way choice
Insurance company plan	88%	39%
Federal government plan	72	34
Doctor organization plan	69	12

Source: Opinion Research Corporation Poll, 1945, cited in S. Payne, Some Opinion Research Principles Developed Through Studies of Social Medicine, *Public Opinion Quarterly*, 1946.

Figure I-5

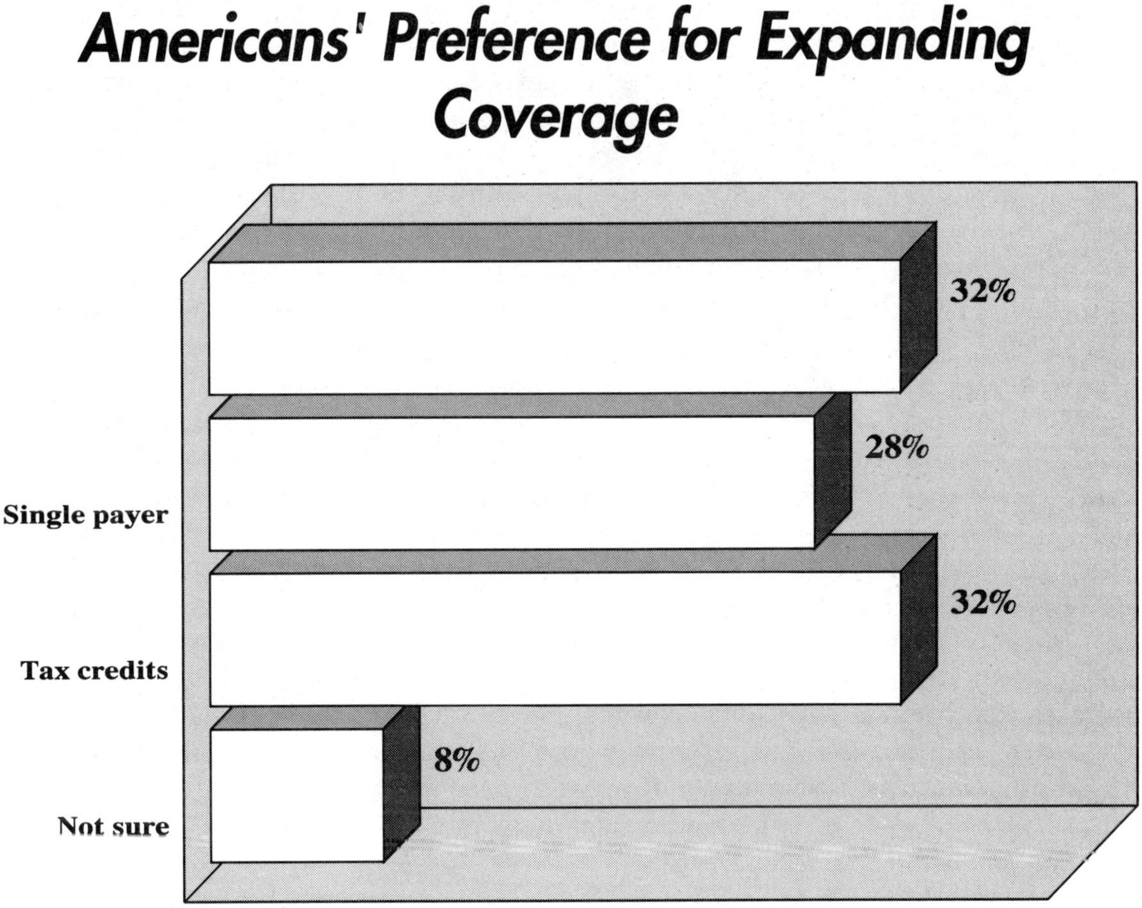

Source: Kaiser/Commonwealth/Harris, 1993.

a goal are not strongly held, an idea presented alone receives higher approval than when it is presented along with alternative proposals.

3. While Americans are willing to spend a lot of money on health care, they have strong reservations about doing it through the tax system. The longest continuous trend measuring public opinion on health spending shows that Americans consistently believe the U.S. is spending too little, not too much on health.[30] However, support for health spending does not necessarily translate into support for increased taxes. This pattern is evident as far back as 1944, when 68 percent of the public said they thought it would be a good idea for Social Security to cover doctor and hospital care. Support for the plan dropped to 41 percent, however, when respondents who opposed a payroll tax increase and respondents who preferred a private sector plan were removed from the approval rating.[25]

In the months immediately after the 1992 election, Americans expressed some willingness to pay additional taxes dedicated to a national health reform plan. A March 1993 survey found 65 percent of Americans willing to pay either increased taxes or higher premiums for "a national health care program that would provide every American with access to health care." At the same time, only 40 percent were willing to pay as much as $30 a month more.[31] And this willingness to pay even a small tax increase is on the decline. By late September 1993, support for higher taxes fell to 48 percent,[32] and by early October 1993, just 40 percent supported an increase in taxes to help pay for President Clinton's health reform plan.[33]

4. While Americans are dissatisfied with the health care system overall, they are quite satisfied with the quality of their own health care. Americans have consistently rejected significant health care reform because while they believe there may be problems with the aggregate system, they are highly satisfied with the care they personally receive. In 1993, 71 percent of Americans reported being satisfied with the quality of their medical care;[34] at the same time, 73 percent believed that our health care system is fundamentally unsound.[35] This disparity makes it possible for opponents of health reform to advance the argument that changes made to the aggregate health care system might adversely affect the patient's own health care arrangements.

Even as far back as the 1940s, interest groups have been able to rally Americans against health reform by claiming that the quality of their own medical care would be worse under a reformed system. Political advertisements attacking President Truman's health insurance plan contrasted Norman Rockwell images of the personal medical relationships so valued by the public with the threat of government bureaucrats interfering with the sacred doctor-patient relationship. The interest groups' campaign played on public anxieties by questioning whether in the future patients would be able to freely choose their own physicians (which was guaranteed by the Truman plan) with slogans such as, "Your Doctor, or Doctor X?"[36]

Taken together, these four key public attitudes toward health care reform have historically served as constraints on policymakers' ability to restructure the U.S. health care system. The paramount lesson they provide for those interested in promoting health care reform is that early public support for health reform ultimately may not translate into major change in the health care system.

In today's campaign for health reform, President and Mrs. Clinton have wisely made specific policy choices in an effort to reduce the divisiveness seen in previous debates. For example, in contrast to Truman's all-government plan, the Clinton proposal incorporates a deliberately moderate approach designed to appeal to a broad coalition of supporters. Like President Nixon's bill, the Clinton plan relies heavily on employer mandates and health maintenance organizations (or managed care), preserves the private insurance industry, and emphasizes the role of the states. Additionally, while the general public is almost evenly split between government regulation and private competition as approaches to containing health care costs, business groups and physicians view competition as the clear winner. Thus, the Clinton plan emphasizes increased competition, with government policing the private sector to guard against abuse.

The Clinton proposal also incorporates specific measures designed to garner the general public's support. The bill strongly emphasizes patients' freedom to choose their own health providers and to enroll in fee-for-service health plans. Additionally, its financing mechanisms are structured so as to avoid imposing significant new taxes — for much of the American public, new benefits are provided almost for free.

Despite these measures, however, the Clintons have reason to be wary. History shows us that the success of any initiative depends in part on the popularity of the President. President Clinton was elected with only 43 percent of the popular vote, and his approval ratings have proven somewhat volatile. The continuing popularity of both the President and Mrs. Clinton can be expected to play a large role in determining the extent to which their health reform proposal is ultimately implemented.

In closing, it is essential that the reader not mistake the enactment of health reform legislation, whatever the final version, as the end of this debate. Our final history lesson is that enactment does not guarantee implementation, but represents only the beginning of a new era of politics in which opponents of the bill work toward a watered-down version or even repeal.

In 1988, for example, the Congress enacted the Medicare Catastrophic Coverage Act, which provided the largest expansion of Medicare benefits since the program's inception. However, the bill's financing provisions, including the requirement that beneficiaries pay the entire cost of the expanded coverage through tax increases levied even before receiving any benefits, led to an outcry for repeal by the nation's middle- and upper-income elderly. Congress was ultimately forced to repeal the legislation the following year.[37] Similarly, in 1988, Massachusetts became one of only two states (with Hawaii) to have enacted legislation designed to provide universal access to health insurance. The bill was to phase in coverage over a four-year period. Before the phase-in began, however, new legislation was enacted to delay implementation of the major provisions of the bill, including the threat of ultimate repeal of the universal access law.

Legislation can often be broadly interpreted to support a variety of goals, and is particularly vulnerable when subject to a long, phased-in implementation period. There is every reason to believe that both President Clinton and key congressional leaders will face strong challenges in coming elections, significantly weakening the coalitions promoting health reform legislation. We therefore expect to see the debate over a national health plan continue to evolve for many years to come.

In preparation for today's deliberations, a number of issues of overriding importance are examined in this volume. The book begins with a discussion of the forces behind the health care reform debate and the risks of maintaining the status quo. Chapter 2 presents an overview of President and Mrs. Clinton's health care reform bill, analyzing and critiquing the major components of this proposal. Chapters 3 and 4 address the two principal issues facing policymakers with regard to health care reform — universal access to care and skyrocketing health care costs -- evaluating the various approaches to resolving these critical problems. The legal ramifications of health care reform, including malpractice and antitrust issues, will be included in any reform plan; these are examined in Chapter 5. The next two chapters explore specific issues that will likely receive increasing attention as the health reform debate enters a second phase — long term care and outcomes measurement. Chapters 8 and 9 present lessons from individual states and from other countries in their efforts toward achieving high-quality medical care for all citizens at reasonable cost. The book concludes with three chapters explicitly detailing the role of politics in the health care reform debate. Chapter 10 examines the roles of lobbying, political influence, and interest group agendas on the outcome of the reform movement. Chapter 11 examines Congress, analyzing the legislative process and delineating the key players. The authors close by predicting how the politics of health care reform will play out in the fight ahead, and speculating about what is likely to be enacted by the 1994 Congress.

This book, the third in a series on the Future of American Health Care, is a groundbreaking resource that provides comprehensive guidance on the issues, players, and protocols that will shape the next phase of the reform debate.

REFERENCES

1. Starr P. *The Social Transformation of American Medicine*. Basic Books, 1982.
2. Gallup Poll. Roper Center for Public Opinion Research, March 1949.
3. Gallup Poll. Roper Center for Public Opinion Research, November-December 1949.
4. Gallup Poll. Roper Center for Public Opinion Research, November 1950.
5. Marmor TR. *The Politics of Medicare*. Aldine Publishing Co., 1973.
6. Fein R. *Medical Care, Medical Costs: The Search for a Health Insurance Policy*. Harvard University Press, 1989.
7. Thompson MC, ed. *Health Policy: The Legislative Agenda*. Congressional Quarterly, 1980.
8. Peterson MA. *Leading Our Way to Health: Entrepreneurship and Leadership in the Health Care Reform Debate*. Center for American Political Studies, Occasional Paper 92-6. Center for American Political Studies, 1992.
9. U.S. Bureau of the Census. *Statistical Abstract of the United States: 1973*. U.S. Bureau of the Census, 1974.
10. *Medical Care Financing and Administration*. U.S. Department of Health, Education, and Welfare. Health Economics Series 1-A. Publication (PHS)947-1A, February 1969.
11. *Basic Facts on the Health Industry*. U.S. House Committee on Ways and Means. Government Printing Office, June 28, 1971.
12. Richardson E. *Towards a Comprehensive Health Policy for the 1970s*. U.S. Department of Health, Education, and Welfare, 1971.
13. Piacentini JS and JD Foley. *EBRI Databook on Employee Benefits*. Second Edition. Employee Benefit Research Institute, 1992.

14. Henry J. Kaiser Family Foundation/Commonwealth Fund/Louis Harris & Associates Poll. Roper Center for Public Opinion Research, September 1993.

15. U.S. Bureau of the Census. *Current Population Survey*. U.S. Bureau of the Census, March 1992.

16. CBS News/*New York Times* Poll. Roper Center for Public Opinion Research, March 1993.

17. Henry J. Kaiser Family Foundation/Harvard School of Public Health/National Opinion Research Center. Low Income Study. Unpublished, 1993.

18. Blendon RJ, R Leitman, I Morrison, and K Donelan. Satisfaction with Health Systems in Ten Nations. *Health Affairs*. 9 (2), 1990: 185-92.

19. Voter Research and Surveys National Election Day Survey. Roper Center for Public Opinion Research, November 1992.

20. International Social Survey Program Poll. Roper Center for Public Opinion Research, 1985.

21. Opinion Roundup: The State of the Nation. *Public Opinion*. 8 (4), 1985: 21-40.

22. CBS News/*New York Times* Poll. Roper Center for Public Opinion Research, January 1993.

23. Gallup Poll. Roper Center for Public Opinion Research, January 1973.

24. Gallup Poll. Roper Center for Public Opinion Research, August 1974.

25. Payne S. Some Opinion Research Principles Developed Through Studies of Social Medicine. *Public Opinion Quarterly* 10 (1), 1946: 93-98.

26. Opinion Research Corporation Poll. Roper Center for Public Opinion Research, January 1972.

27. Opinion Research Corporation Poll. Roper Center for Public Opinion Research, March 1971.

28. Roper Organization Poll. Roper Center for Public Opinion Research, February 1974.

29. Fact Finders/Novalis Corporation Poll. Roper Center for Public Opinion Research, January 1993.

30. Davis JA and TW Smith. *General Social Surveys, 1972-1993: Cumulative Codebook*. Roper Center for Public Opinion Research, 1993.

31. Harvard School of Public Health/Marttila & Kiley/Robert Wood Johnson Foundation Poll. Roper Center for Public Opinion Research, March 1993.

32. Princeton Survey Research Associates/*Newsweek* Poll. Roper Center for Public Opinion Research, September 1993.

33. ABC News/*Washington Post* Poll. Roper Center for Public Opinion Research, October 1993.

34. CBS News/*New York Times* Poll. Roper Center for Public Opinion Research, September 1993.

35. Gallup/CNN/*USA Today* Poll. Roper Center for Public Opinion Research, September 1993.

36. Kelley S. *Professional Public Relations and Political Power*. Johns Hopkins Press, 1956.

37. Holstein M and M Minkler. The Short Life and Painful Death of the Medicare Catastrophic Coverage Act. *International Journal of Health Services* 21 (1), 1991: 1-16.

CHAPTER 1

Converging on Reform

Richard M. Sorian

As the great national debate over health reform begins, the broad outline of the discussion has been sketched, and everyone is trying to visualize the finished work. Policymakers, providers, and pundits are trying to predict how a reformed health care system will look and what its impact will be on everything from routine podiatry to the United States' stature as a superpower.

It is only natural that the pending debate over health reform has many people agitated. Some have high hopes for universal coverage, hoping that it will wipe away the inequities between rich and poor, black and white, urban and rural. Others fear that tight cost controls will undermine the entrepreneurial spirit that has propelled the American health care system to excellence.

The anxiety is understandable. Reforming health care, after all, involves changing one-seventh of the U.S. economy and affects virtually all elements of society — manufacturing and service industries, doctors and hospitals, makers of pharmaceuticals and medical devices, insurance agents and marketing companies, federal, state and local government, employers, and ultimately every citizen.

If done right, health reform could revitalize the American economy. Freed from the onerous burden of finding and retaining affordable health insurance, business could turn its attention to what it knows best — producing goods and services and competing not only with the company down the street but with the company across the ocean. Freed from the need to defend existing health insurance benefits, labor unions could improve wages undistracted by the fear of diminishing coverage. And, with access now available for the formerly uninsured, doctors and hospitals could turn their attention to what they do best — caring for patients — instead of what they do worst — struggling to cope with a highly bureaucratic patchwork system that requires the 85 percent of Americans who have insurance to pay for the 15 percent who don't.

If done wrong, however, health reform could wreak havoc not only on the health care system but on the national economy, small and medium-sized businesses, and on the political future of more than a few members of Congress (not to mention one very ambitious President).

CHANGES IN THE INDUSTRY

What is certain is that health reform will significantly alter the medical landscape. Today in the United States, there are approximately 6,000 acute-care hospitals[1]. Each of these employs hundreds and, in many cases, thousands of individuals — everyone from doctors and nurses to security guards and janitors. But many of those facilities are vastly underutilized. The average occupancy rate of American hospitals is 60 percent. In hospitals in New York City or Atlanta, where interns patrol emergency room hallways to tend to patients waiting for beds, it's hard to conceive of overcapacity, but many suburban and rural hospitals are half empty. Health reform is almost certain to result in fewer acute care hospital beds. Experts predict that as many as 1,000 hospitals could be closed by the end of the 1990s, and many others will have converted their excess acute care beds into "subacute," long term care, and rehabilitation beds. Those hospitals that remain will be forced into efficiency and participation in health care networks.

American-style medicine has provided a good standard of living for the nearly 600,000 physicians — nearly 2.3 per 1,000 population — now working in the U.S.[2] . The average net income of an American physician was $171,000 in 1992, placing doctors in the top tier of earners. For specialists, the current system has been very profitable; some of them make more than $1 million a year. Even the "underpaid" family doctor earns an average of $110,000 a year. Health reform will certainly mean a change for physicians. Highly paid specialists will be forced more than ever into managed care arrangements in order to retain the volume of patients they now see. Income will grow more slowly and, for some, could even decline. Managed care will mean less autonomy but also less responsibility for complying with "hassle factor" rules and regulations. Primary care physicians will become more sought-after as the new system emphasizes their use as case managers or "gatekeepers." Reform probably will reduce the pay differential between specialists and primary care doctors and give the latter greater authority over referrals. New physicians may feel the greatest pressure, as the government makes a concerted effort to push them into primary care practices and managed care settings. Some mid-career specialists may even resort to retraining themselves as primary care providers.

Insurance companies certainly will feel the impact of health reform. The current system, which permits insurers to pick young healthy enrollees and reject older, sicker applicants, has indeed been profitable. With the likelihood of insurance reform quite high (it is the one topic on which nearly every policymaker agrees), the number of insurers is sure to drop dramatically from 1,500 today to as few as 300 plans by decade's end. Many of the smaller plans won't simply go away, they'll be bought up by the larger companies. Large insurers, especially those that are already well-invested in managed care, stand to do very well under the new system. Insurance agents could very well be an endangered species. The new system envisions a much smaller role for employers in selecting insurance plans and a much greater role for individuals. Insurance products will be marketed more like the other products sold by Madison Avenue. The number of television and radio ads promoting health insurance has been on the rise in recent years, and it could double or even triple. Insurers may be able to replace some of their lost business by tapping new markets for long term care insurance (which may become tax-exempt) and wrap-around policies for upper-income individuals who want more coverage than is likely to be offered in the basic benefit package.

Pharmaceutical manufacturers are rightly worried about the prospect of further government involvement in their pricing system. However, the great promise of reform for them is the introduction of millions of new insured customers into the pharmaceutical market, which will push drug industry revenue sharply higher. The selling of drugs also is expected to change, with less marketing to physicians (who now make the choice of which drug to order) and more to health plan managers (who will dictate, through the plan's formulary, which drugs will be available for doctors to prescribe).

THE BIG PICTURE

Reform will be felt beyond the medical community. First, in this extended period of public distrust of government officials, health reform provides a true opportunity for Congress to deliver meaningful change; health reform would be tangible evidence of lawmakers' ability to deliver. Those who were elected in 1992 on a platform of change will be held accountable by the voters in 1994. When incumbents running for reelection are asked "What have you done for me lately?" they will be able to point toward reform. The post-reform period also could be beneficial to federal officials, who could be freed of the nearly annual demand for temporary savings in programs like Medicare and Medicaid.

At the state level, reform holds great promise and the potential for great rancor as well. By giving governors and state legislators a major stake in implementing reform, the federal government avoids some of the disruption that a preemptive federal effort would have caused. But the responsibility of implementation will carry a very tight timetable that puts state leaders on the spot if the program is delayed. Reform also could greatly enlarge the size of state government. If Congress adopts the concept of powerful purchasing alliances to collect and distribute nearly all health premiums paid in the U.S., those bodies may handle an amount of money greater than most state budgets. And, finally, greater control over health spending would free state lawmakers to invest greater amounts of tax revenues in education, job training, and infrastructure repairs.

Business has borne the burden of the American health care system for nearly 50 years. Under reform, that burden will grow heavier but be more evenly distributed. Some businesses will have to start buying insurance for their workers; some others will have to pay more for health insurance than they do now. But many will pay considerably less — including the small firms that now struggle to maintain such benefits. Despite contention over who wins and who loses, it is now generally estimated that 60 percent of Americans now insured will pay the same or less for benefits that are about equal to what they have now. Another 25 percent will pay somewhat more for coverage that will be considerably better than their current plan. And another 15 percent will pay more for coverage that is about the same as they now enjoy.

Finally, reform will demand change of American families and individuals. For those who have, by choice or by chance, been outside the insurance system, reform will require participation. But for some, it will mean a financial burden that, until now, has been easily avoided. Young, healthy Americans have been able to gamble with their health; reform places new obligations on such people, and they will pay the price. On the other hand, it's hard to quantify peace of mind — the notion that health insurance is something permanent that "can't be taken away." But that is perhaps the greatest gift reform can give individuals, families, and businesses. Changes in health status and employment will no longer determine insurability. Illness and injury are inevitable facts of life, but reform can remove the financial threat inherent in the current American system.

HIGH STAKES

Health reform is America's great unfinished business. Bill Clinton's predecessors have been cowed by the prospect of overhauling the nation's health care system, and as each decade has gone by, the price of reform has risen exponentially. In 1935, when FDR rejected adding health care reform to his landmark Social Security proposal, the United States spent $2.9 billion on health care. In 1940, the nation spent $4 billion on its health care; by 1950, spending reached $12.7 billion. In 1965, when President Johnson signed into law Medicare and Medicaid, moving the country only a small step closer to a national system, spending hit $41.6 billion.[3]

By 1973, when President Nixon became the first Republican Chief Executive to propose employer-sponsored national health insurance, health spending totaled $102.5 billion. In 1983, with President Reagan adamantly opposing any expansion of the federal government's role in health care, spending hit a whopping $358.6

billion. By 1993, with a new President elected at least in part on his promise of comprehensive health reform, the U.S. appears poised to act on a problem that has grown so immense it threatens American economic viability and international competitiveness. Government actuaries estimate that, absent reform, the U.S. will spend $880 billion on health care in 1993.[3]

Clearly, steadily rising costs as well as the plight of those Americans who cannot afford care are nothing new. So why, if it has eluded so many for so long, is health reform on such a fast track? How well have lawmakers and policy makers learned from the mistakes of the past, and will they manage to avoid repeating them?

WOFFORD RIDES THE WAVE

The current wave of reform began not with Clinton's successful presidential campaign of 1992 but with a special election held in 1991 in Pennsylvania to fill the seat of Senator John Heinz III, a moderate Republican who died in a plane crash. Heinz's death created an opportunity for Democratic Governor Robert Casey to appoint a member of his party to the seat. Several high-profile recruits, including Chrysler Corp. Chairman Lee Iacocca, turned the job down. Finally, Casey turned to his Secretary of Labor and Industry, Harris Wofford, who consented. The 65-year-old Wofford, a former president of Bryn Mawr College and the original deputy director of the Peace Corps, was seen as a caretaker for the Senate seat, and an underdog in November's special election.

Republicans had no trouble recruiting their candidate, U.S. Attorney General Richard Thornburgh, who resigned his Cabinet post to run for the Senate. Thornburgh had served a surprisingly controversial stint as attorney general under Presidents Reagan and Bush — his overly secretive nature had alienated much of the Washington press corps and Democrats on Capitol Hill. Still, Thornburgh had been a very popular former two-term governor of the state and had retained his political network even after six years away from the State House.

Thornburgh jumped to an early lead in the polls, aided by his larger war chest and his high name recognition. In fact, to many Pennsylvanians, it almost seemed like Thornburgh was the incumbent and Wofford the little-known challenger. Ironically, that perception helped Wofford begin the long climb up in the polls (at one point during the summer, Thornburgh was 47 points ahead). The anti-incumbent fever that was to sweep through the country in 1992 was raging in Pennsylvania in 1991.

Thornburgh played right into Wofford's hands by running as an incumbent, emphasizing his connections in Washington. He was also hurt by his loyalty to Bush, who was beginning his rapid descent in the polls. Having just left Bush's Cabinet, Thornburgh could not easily distance himself from the President.

Meanwhile, Wofford was enjoying what many candidates only dream of doing — campaigning on the issues he cared about without worrying about the polls. One of those issues was health care. Having spent much of his time as Governor Casey's Labor Secretary mediating disputes over health insurance benefits, Wofford saw reform not as a liberal Democratic issue but as a middle-class "bread-and-butter" issue that would play to voters' fears. With little to lose, Wofford was able to hone his health reform message without being too specific. By the end of the summer, he had whittled it down to a simple message that he admitted he had borrowed from a Republican physician: "If criminals have a right to a lawyer, I think working Americans should have the right to a doctor." Meanwhile, Thornburgh was pitching a "stay the course" line that rang very hollow in a state being hit hard by the economic recession.

Wofford made steady progress in the polls, cutting Thornburgh's lead in half by Labor Day. In the fall, he continued to hammer on the health reform issue, challenging Thornburgh to come up with a plan of his own. Ironically, Wofford did not have a reform plan, merely a set of principles that could be broadly applied to nearly any reform proposal — Republican or Democratic — then on the table. But Wofford had seized the issue first, making it difficult for Thornburgh to regain ground. Plus, voters' belief that Democrats care more about health care than Republicans gave Wofford the edge. On election day, the incumbent Democrat swamped his opponent, winning by 340,000 votes.

What did Wofford's win mean? Did it, as a poll conducted for the Kaiser Family Foundation of Menlo Park CA suggested, indicate a strong desire for action on national health reform?[4] Or did it, as a poll run for the Health Insurance Association of America found, simply indicate a deep unhappiness with the Pennsylvania economy and with President Bush?[5] Or was it the result of an overconfident candidate taking an election for granted? The answer probably is "all of the above."

Whatever the motivating factor, Wofford's health reform message resonated with voters while Thornburgh's powerful connections did not. Wendy Burnley, communications director for the National Republican Senatorial Committee, said after the election that Wofford was effective because he created a "climate of fear" by tying together the economy, the recession, jobs, and health care costs. Burnley said the mix confused voters, who "never really understood" Wofford's pledge for health reform.[6] But in politics, perception is reality, so the conventional wisdom was that Wofford won because of his calls for health reform.

BUSH ENTERS THE REFORM DEBATE

The proof of that came only a week after Wofford's victory. President Bush, in Rome for an international economic summit meeting, was bombarded with questions from the American press about when he would have a health reform plan. Bush had been playing a delay-and-see game with reform ever since his election in 1988. Forced to address the issue by Democratic presidential candidate Michael Dukakis, Bush had promised a rather nebulous plan involving an expanded Medicaid program. After taking office, Bush shelved that in favor of a series of studies conducted by blue-ribbon panels. The Bush White House had hoped to get through the 1992 election without committing to a specific line of action; Wofford's victory forced his hand. In February of 1992, Bush outlined a $35 billion-a-year program that would make coverage more affordable to uninsured and underinsured Americans through a combination of market reforms, tax credits, and a broader use of managed care.

The Bush plan was perceived as too little, too late. It had no substantive cost containment; it failed to guarantee universal coverage; and it relied heavily on a system of managed care that had not yet fully matured. Most significantly, however, was the belief that the President's heart wasn't really in reform and, if reelected, the issue would drop from his agenda. Bush's critics drew these conclusions from the fact that once he unveiled his plan, Bush rarely mentioned it again. Instead, he spent much of the campaign criticizing Clinton's proposal, charging that it had "the efficiency of the Post Office, the compassion of the IRS, and the cost-effectiveness of the Defense Department." (When his aides pointed out that all three agencies he cited were under his control, Bush changed this sound bite to "the efficiency of the House Post Office and the compassion of the KGB." Either way, the public didn't know what Bush was talking about and concluded that he didn't either.)

THE ROAD TO MANAGED COMPETITION

Bush's plan was not enough to counter the fact that health reform had been the province of a small but powerful group of Democratic legislators, who had struggled to keep the issue alive through the Reagan and Bush years. One of the reformers was Democratic Presidential candidate Nebraska Senator Robert Kerrey, who had a plan that had been introduced as legislation. Former Massachusetts Senator Paul Tsongas also had staked out his position on health care policy early in his bid for the presidential nomination. His plan loosely followed the tenets of "managed competition," a theory under which businesses and individuals would band together in purchasing cooperatives, which would bargain for low-cost, high-quality insurance coverage emphasizing managed care.

At first, Arkansas Governor Bill Clinton issued vague promises of reform but stayed away from details. But he too recognized the political value of health reform. That was no accident. James Carville and Paul Begala, who had advised Wofford on his 1991 campaign, had joined Clinton in early 1992 to help draft a campaign strategy. The two men brought the positive lessons on health care with them to the Clinton camp.

In early January, Clinton threw his support behind the "play-or-pay" model of reform that would offer employers the choice of buying insurance for their workers or paying the government to do that for them. The approach had been adopted in Congress by Senator Edward Kennedy (D) of Massachusetts and Congressman Richard Gephardt (D) of Missouri. It was an attempt to get away from a flat mandate or a broad-based tax on employers. In reality, it achieved neither goal. Opponents of employer mandates argued that play or pay was a mandate in disguise. Foes of a broad tax argued that play or pay was really a new payroll tax.[7]

Clinton was no newcomer to the idea of play or pay. His interest was piqued six months before New Hampshire by an article entitled, "The Pragmatic Road

Toward National Health Insurance,"[8] written by Ronald Pollack and Phyllis Torda, of Families USA, a Washington DC-based advocacy group. In September 1991, Clinton pollster Stanley Greenberg called a meeting in Washington at which Pollack advanced the idea that play or pay offered more possibilities for political compromise than did a single payer approach. Pollack was impressed by Clinton's grasp of policy details and the political terrain. Clinton was able to "synthesize the intersection between good policy and pragmatic politics," Pollack said in an interview in October 1993.

In February, Clinton went public with his reform plan while campaigning in New Hampshire, distinguishing himself from his challengers, especially Kerrey. Adopting a play-or-pay approach "gave Clinton a real working, accepted strategy for dealing with health care," said former campaign adviser Bruce Fried, senior vice president at the Wexler Group, a public relations firm, in an interview.

Tsongas won in New Hampshire; Clinton finished second. The biggest surprise, however, was the miserable showing by Kerrey, who was virtually eliminated from the race. On the surface, this seemed to indicate that while voters wanted the health system reformed, they were wary of massive government intervention envisioned by a single payer approach.

With Kerrey essentially out of the race, the dynamics on health reform changed. Clinton had positioned himself in the center between Kerrey's single payer advocacy on the left and Tsongas' managed competition plan on the right. Most Clinton aides had expected Kerrey to survive longer and Tsongas to drop out. That would have allowed Clinton to move to the right on health reform. With the new results, the Arkansas governor had to stick with play or pay.

In the spring of 1992, the Clinton team summarized his plan in an 11-page policy document, ambitiously titled "National Health Insurance Reform To Cut Costs and Cover Everybody."[9] The white paper claimed Clinton's plan would "cover every American with the money we're now spending on health care by taking bold, specific steps to cut costs." Like others before him, Clinton steered clear of financing specifics. "We don't need to lead with a tax increase that asks hard-working people who already pay too much for health care to pay even more, until every effort has been made to squeeze excess costs out of the system," said Clinton in a speech.

By June, Clinton was ready to issue his "Putting People First" campaign manifesto, complete with financing data, but his aides were struggling to resolve an internal battle over how much money it would take to cover the uninsured.[6] Fried, who coordinated the health policy team in Washington, got an urgent phone call from Clinton adviser Bruce Reed. Reacting to a call from an angry Clinton, Reed demanded to know why health costs couldn't be squeezed fast enough to meet the candidate's goals of covering the uninsured while bringing down health care spending.

Fried contacted Brookings Institution economist Joshua Wiener, who was put in the unenviable position of contradicting Clinton's trusted adviser Ira Magaziner, a Rhode Island business consultant. Magaziner believed Clinton could wring waste out of health spending to such a degree that the candidate could pay for universal access without raising new taxes. A veteran of battles to cut federal health spending, Wiener warned that Magaziner's numbers would not yield the savings he projected. Finding no way to resolve the problem, advisers, with Clinton's approval, finessed the solution. Consequently, no health spending numbers appeared in the document when it went to the presses.

That didn't hurt Clinton, who clinched the nomination early in the summer. At the Democratic convention in New York City's Madison Square Garden, "Health Care For All" banners, posters, and buttons were on carefully-orchestrated and prominent display, highlighting the import the issue had taken on in the race for the White House. In his July 16 acceptance speech, Clinton promised to deliver "jobs, education, and health care." And, borrowing a line from Wofford's successful campaign message, Clinton said he would work toward "an America in which health care is a right, not a privilege. In which we say to all our people: Your government has the courage — finally — to take on the health care profiteers and make health care affordable for every family." While the Democratic Party's platform was mute on the type of reform plan it favored, Clinton continued to plug the play-or-pay model.

Clinton now had to campaign against Bush, who was still fighting the perception that he had only a fleeting interest in health reform, and, at least intermittently, against independent candidate Ross Perot, who favored the testing of several models of health reform.

In August, at the Republican convention in the Houston Astrodome, Bush struggled with his negative image on the issue despite some efforts by his aides to talk up his reform plan. Deciding that going on the offensive might yield better results, Bush blasted Clinton's evolving health reform strategy as a "costly coercive system, imported from abroad." During his acceptance speech, the incumbent said Clinton favored a "massive government takeover of health care, which would ration care and deny Americans the right to choose a doctor." Bush also charged that the Clinton plan would demand massive new taxes.

As the fall campaign began, the dynamics shifted once again. Now that Clinton was his party's standardbearer, the play-or-pay gambit didn't look quite so moderate. It was vulnerable to Bush's attack on Clinton as an old-fashioned "tax and spend Democrat." The Democrat began to look for ways to move to the right without upsetting his liberal supporters in organized labor and in Congress. Senator Jay Rockefeller of West Virginia was a key adviser to Clinton on health reform and he had backed play or pay as chairman of the Bipartisan Commission on Comprehensive Health Care, also known as the Pepper Commission. He cautioned Clinton against going too conservative on reform.

By early September, the Clinton team was in full flight away from play or pay but couldn't figure out where to go. "There is a lot of baggage associated with the play-or-pay term," campaign adviser Judith Feder conceded in an interview.[10]

Worried that those doubts could weaken support, the Clinton campaign staff convened a meeting on September 22 to reshape Clinton's proposal to reflect market-based competition as a mechanism to control costs. Soon thereafter, a team of advisers including Fried, Feder, Magaziner, economist Kenneth Thorpe, health policy adviser Atul Gawande, and Families USA's Pollack met with Clinton in

Lansing, Michigan, to present their views. The aides urged Clinton to drop the play-or-pay approach and instead embrace managed competition. The debate split the staff since Magaziner, Gawande, and others were disciples of the market approach, while Feder, Thorpe, and Pollack preferred a more regulatory tack.

Clinton had also been warmed to the managed competition idea by California Insurance Commissioner John Garamendi, who ran the Clinton campaign in that key state. By combining the employer mandate borrowed from the play-or-pay approach with a restructured delivery system under managed competition, Clinton could achieve his goals of a public-private partnership leading to universal access to health care, the aides said. Recalling that meeting later, Fried said Clinton took to the idea immediately and realized it provided him with a "coordinated strategy that was defensible, politically viable, and served his candidacy."

On September 24, in a speech at the Rahway, New Jersey, headquarters of Merck & Co., Clinton formally shed his support for play or pay. The Democratic candidate's endorsement of the market-based approach of managed competition "pulled the rug out" from the Bush campaign, said Fried in an interview. And it was in that speech that Clinton first made his ill-fated promise to deliver his reform plan to the Congress "within 100 days" of his inauguration.

The Clinton camp got a big boost from a report released by Pollack's Families USA that concluded Clinton-style managed competition would reduce U.S. health spending by nearly $746 billion over seven years compared to only $157 billion under the Bush strategy. From that point until the end of the campaign, Clinton rarely missed an opportunity to cite those statistics for the press and the public.

A BILL IS BORN

It is often true that in politics, appearance is more important than reality. In both the Wofford campaign of 1991 and the Clinton campaign of 1992, health care played a small but significant role in the Democrats' victories. It is likely, however, that the faltering economy and a seemingly disengaged President were much more important in the ultimate results.

But political analysts and the media drew a strong parallel between the come-from-behind election of these two men and their emphasis on health care reform. Post-election polls did show that health care ranked high on voters' minds, but it was far behind the issues of the overall economy and job creation. Still, many pundits attributed Clinton's victory, at least in part, to his emphasis on health reform.

Once he was elected, Clinton seemed to believe his own reviews. Health reform became a central element of his first-term strategy. In fact, if it were not for Ross Perot's success in making deficit reduction a top priority for the new President, it is likely that Clinton would have made health reform the number one issue of his first year in office.

Instead, Clinton asked his wife, Hillary Rodham Clinton, to head a task force to examine the reform issue and report back to him with a blueprint by May 3 (approximately 100 days after his inauguration). He also named Magaziner to head his White House health policy staff (a move that greatly disappointed Feder, who had been considered the leading candidate for the job. Instead, she and Thorpe went to work at the Department of Health and Human Services).

The First Lady and Magaziner pulled together an unwieldy task force that numbered more than 500 (mostly made up of government and congressional staff members but its unusual shroud of secrecy made the membership list one of Washington's most-sought items). Magaziner created a complicated system of discrete working groups to make initial decisions that he described as "tollgates." After nearly three months of work, the panels were no closer to deciding the issue than when they started. Much of the final work was done by Magaziner and his staff at the White House and Feder's group at HHS.

Clinton's difficulty with the budget forced the White House to delay the health reform effort until the fall. And, as is often the case in government, the delay allowed Clinton's advisers to reopen nearly every issue that they had closed in the spring.

Finally, on September 22, Clinton spoke to a Joint Session of Congress and delivered the outlines of his plan and his strategy for selling it. (See appendix, page 231, for a summary of the legislation.) Basing his proposal on a set of six principles (security, savings, simplicity, choice, quality, and responsibility), Clinton said reform must guarantee every American "health care that can never be taken away." Hoping to capitalize the same insecurity that had helped elect Wofford in 1991, the President was gambling that American's nervousness about the future of health care would rally support for his plan.

In mid-October, Clinton and his wife delivered the plan to Congress in the form of a 1,342-page bill. After tinkering with some of the details and deciding key jurisdictional issues, the bill was introduced November 20 by Senate Majority Leader George Mitchell and House Speaker Thomas Foley.

The battle for health reform is on. It is expected to be an intense campaign that will bring out the best and the worst of the American legislative process. But more likely than not, by the end of 1994, a final plan will be back in Clinton's hands and ready for his signature.

THE NO-REFORM SCENARIO

We began this chapter by discussing various scenarios being presented for the post-reform era. There is, however, another distinct set of possibilities raised by the prospect of defeat of the reform movement. After all, there are more examples of defeat than victory in the U.S.' history of health reform debate.

Some believe that there will be reform of the American health care system whether or not Congress enacts a reform bill. Under this scenario, Congress spends many months flailing at reform but is ultimately unable to agree on a final package. Rather than accept incremental reform, the President pulls his plan off of Capitol Hill.

One side of the "no reform" camp believes that reform still would occur even absent legislation. That belief is predicated on the conviction that the current system has become too unmanageable for any of its players. Such a scenario would play out as follows. Health care providers, anxious to preserve their "victory" over reform, voluntarily hold down their prices and effect efficiencies in their profession. Large insurance companies that had favored reform press for industry standards to rid their field of most of the small insurance companies. Hospitals continue to consolidate, with many of the smaller suburban and rural facilities merging. States continue to enroll their Medicaid recipients in managed care plans. And such plans, which grew rapidly in the 1980s and less briskly in the 1990s, get a new head of steam and become the dominant delivery system by the beginning of the next century.

Of course such a scenario would be helped along by some targeted legislation. Members of Congress from both parties agree on certain elements of reform that could be enacted if a broad reform measure fails. For example, passage of insurance reforms that regulate underwriting by small insurance companies would help to reduce the size of the insurance industry and improve access to care. Creation of small, voluntary insurance cooperatives could give some assistance to small employers. And changes in antitrust rules could speed the consolidation of the hospital sector.

However, there is much greater reason to assume that the scenario cited above is the product of wishful thinking on the part of the entrenched lobbies. It is based on the shaky assumption that after decades of profit-driven behavior, the health care industry suddenly is going to right itself. While that may hold true for a short time after defeat of health reform legislation, it is unlikely to remain true for long. After the 1979 defeat of President Carter's hospital cost containment legislation, hospitals did indeed hold down their price increases for a two-year period. After that, however, prices took off and soon surpassed the pattern of earlier years. In addition, the belief that Congress could pass a scaled-down version of reform ignores the likelihood that Democrats, angry at the defeat of comprehensive reform, will dig in their heels and oppose enactment of a Band-Aid approach. That was the pattern after the defeat of the Nixon and Carter reform measures.

A more likely outcome of a "no-reform" scenario is a further deterioration of the American health care system. Absent reform, it has been estimated that the proportion of uninsured Americans will rise from 14 percent to 20 percent by the year 2000.[11] A situation in which one in five Americans is without insurance is sure to create greater pressure on hospitals, physicians, and other health care providers to deliver charity care. In turn, those costs will be passed on to employers and their workers in the form of even higher health insurance premiums.

Absent reform, labor-management relations could continue to fray as health insurance becomes the central issue in negotiations. Rising health care costs could begin to exceed wage increases and result in a real decline in take-home pay.

Absent reforms, hospitals are unlikely to eliminate unused beds or enter into creative arrangements with their competition. Instead, pressure from rising charitable care may well result in the closure of many hospitals — and not necessarily the "right" ones.

The biggest winners from a "no-reform" scenario would be those who are profiting most from the current system. Pharmaceutical companies would continue to reap healthy profits with no controls on their prices. For-profit hospitals would remain strong and perhaps grow stronger as they absorb small facilities at bargain-basement prices. Physician specialists might keep their six- or seven-figure incomes, while primary care providers would remain relatively underpaid.

The result of such a scenario could well be greater pressure to completely overhaul the American health care system. A continuing deterioration of coverage and escalation of costs would create the kind of pressure that the advocates of a single payer health care system believe is needed to make their case.

Cathy Tokarski and Janet Firshein contributed to this chapter.

REFERENCES

1. American Hospital Association. *Hospital Statistics, 1992-1993 Edition*. AHA, 1992: 2.
2. Schieber GJ, J-P Poullier, and LM Greenwald. Health Spending, Delivery, and Outcomes in OECD Countries. *Health Affairs* 12 (2), Summer 1993: 122.
3. National Center for Health Statistics. Health, United States, 1992. Public Health Service, 1993: 168.
4. Blendon RJ, US Szalay, DE Altman, and G Chervinsky. The 1991 Pennsylvania Senate Race and National Health Insurance. *Journal of American Health Policy* 2 (1), January/February 1992: 21-24.
5. Schramm CJ. A Second Look at the Pennsylvania Special Election. *Journal of American Health Policy* 2 (1), January/February 1992: 25-29.
6. Tokarski, C. Wofford-Thornburgh: A Turning Point for Health Reform. *Journal of American Health Policy*, January/February 1992: 19.
7. Duffy M and R Thompson. Behind Closed Doors. *Time*, September 20, 1993.
8. Pollack R and P Torda. The Pragmatic Road Toward National Health Insurance. *The American Prospect*, Summer 1991: 92-100.
9. National Health Insurance Reform to Cut Costs and Cover Everybody, Clinton campaign document, 1992.
10. Clinton Walks Away From Play-or-Pay. *Medicine & Health*, September 7, 1992.
11. Shalala D. Testimony to the Senate Finance Committee, October 28, 1993.

CHAPTER 2

President Clinton's Health Security Prescription

Cathy Tokarski and Janet Firshein

At five minutes to nine on a clear September evening in 1993, President Bill Clinton entered the chamber of the U.S. House of Representatives to deliver what many considered to be the most important speech of his first term in office. A buzz of anticipation filled the resplendent room, as swarms of Senators, Representatives, and Cabinet members — some of whom had invested years into trying to solve America's health care problems — awaited Clinton's plan of action.

Once at the podium and just seconds before his speech was scheduled to begin, Clinton noticed that the text of his February budget speech, not his health care address, appeared on the tele-prompter. Undaunted, the rhetorically nimble President ad-libbed the first few minutes of his delivery while Vice President Al Gore Jr. dashed off to fix the problem.

While the rest of the hour-long discourse was relatively smooth and well-received, Clinton's opening glitch could be an omen of the stumbles ahead as he attempts to engineer the most sweeping social change in more than half a century.

His prescription: a bold call for guaranteed, universal health coverage for all Americans, and new strategies to control spiraling health costs. Together, he said, they would "fix" the "badly broken" health system, which has become "too uncertain and too expensive, too bureaucratic and too wasteful" and fraught with "too much fraud and too much greed."[1]

GUIDING PRINCIPLES

Underscoring his willingness to compromise, Clinton outlined six principles that he said should guide the 103rd Congress as it tries to forge a consensus proposal: security, simplicity, savings, choice, quality, and responsibility. Underlying those broad themes is an exhaustive proposal to overhaul one-seventh of the U.S. economy — the fragmented, nearly $900 billion health care system. Clinton's Health Security Act would impose a dizzying array of policies to expand health coverage to 37 million uninsured Americans, guarantee a package of benefits, wring out waste and abuse, improve quality, lower costs, and preserve patients' choice of doctor through a restructured delivery system — all without raising broad-based new taxes.

Clinton's proposed shotgun marriage of free market forces and government regulation appears to have de-fanged at least some of the special interest groups that killed previous efforts — dating back to the 1930s — to expand health coverage to all Americans. After decades of false starts, it seems that the $900 billion health care gorilla has managed to drag even the most strident opponents of reform to the bargaining table.

Clinton's foray into the treacherous world of health reform dates back more than a year before the 1992 presidential election. Along the way, Clinton considered, rejected, and then adopted a mix of traditional and untested approaches to resolving the nation's health care crisis, with politics playing at least as important a role as policy.

TRANSITION TO POWER

At the Little Rock, Arkansas headquarters, campaign workers were reminded on a daily basis that the overarching theme of Clinton's candidacy was, "The economy, stupid." But as Clinton prepared to take office after his November 5 presidential victory, another sign decorating the campaign "war room" implored, "Don't forget about health care."

With an ambitious deadline looming, Clinton quickly named a health transition team to craft a reform plan that would be delivered to Congress within the first 100 days of his Administration. Housed in an office building on Vermont Avenue in downtown Washington, the team began meeting in November to start affixing details to the broad goals and principles. The team was headed by Judith Feder, an energetic Georgetown University health policy analyst who had devoted much of her career to advancing solutions to cover the uninsured. Feder's more regulatory leanings were tempered by Atul Gawande, the team's 27-year-old deputy director and a former congressional aide to managed competition advocate Rep. Jim Cooper (D-TN), who favored more market-oriented solutions. Working with Brandeis University economist Stuart Altman, University of North Carolina economist Kenneth Thorpe, Wexler Group Senior Vice President Bruce Fried, and congressional health staff aide Christopher Jennings, Feder and staff conducted round-the-clock briefings with health groups to solicit ideas, gather opinions, and gauge different options. But by the beginning of 1993, just weeks before the inauguration, some painful realities — predicted months earlier by some of Clinton's policy advisers — were beginning to emerge.

To keep Clinton's promise of universal coverage without new taxes, the transition team concluded that the new Administration would have to impose very tight cost controls on the health care industry. Phasing in universal coverage by 1997 would cost $270 billion over five years, factoring in the cost of a new prescription drug benefit, according to transition documents obtained by the *National Journal*.[2]

Documents prepared by the transition team also said it would be virtually impossible for Clinton to expand health care coverage in his first term without resorting to fairly dramatic cost controls and finding substantial new sources of revenue, the *National Journal* reported. The issue came to a head in a January 11 meeting in Little Rock with Clinton, Altman, Feder, Thorpe, and others. Playing the role of the messenger, Altman presented a series of options, all of which echoed the same conclusion. Clinton was chastened by the exercise but remained convinced that his goals could be reached through savings wrung from the bloated health system. "He still maintains that view," said Altman in an interview in October 1993.

One day before being sworn in as the 42nd President of the U.S., Clinton told the nation's governors that he wanted a health bill enacted by Congress by year's end. To meet that goal, he announced the formation of a health reform task force whose members included Cabinet officials and which would be chaired by First Lady Hillary Rodham Clinton. A Yale-educated lawyer like her husband, Mrs. Clinton had headed an Arkansas task force for then-Governor Clinton that led to sweeping reforms in that state's education system. Putting Mrs. Clinton in charge of such a high-profile campaign pledge sent a strong signal to the health industry, the Congress, and the public about the seriousness attached to this effort.

Rhode Island business consultant Ira Magaziner, a longtime friend of the Clintons, was handed the task of orchestrating the task force's daily operations. Described as an "intense, shy, eccentric genius and harsh task master who works harder than anyone on his staff,"[3] he immediately amassed a 300-member working group of policy experts and congressional staff, which eventually mushroomed to about 500, to pick up where the transition team left off. Housed in the Old Executive Office Building next to the White House, experts drawn from Capitol Hill, federal and state agencies, and the private sector teamed up into dozens of working groups studying virtually every aspect of the health system.

Putting his consultant skills to work, Magaziner organized the experts into task forces devoted to key topics such as cost containment, health care benefits, and long term care. Crucial decision points were referred to as "tollgates," a process in which task force leaders presented progress reports and participants offered comments and criticism. In a September 20, 1993, *Time* report on the inner workings of the Clinton health reform process, one participant described the tollgate meetings "as a cross between Ph.D. orals and the Spanish Inquisition.[4]

"At each session, task force leaders would present their progress on, for example, the emerging benefits package. Magaziner would listen, ask questions and nudge members in the direction he wanted. Magaziner kept the Clintons abreast of progress, and the President sometimes invited individual members over for briefings in the Roosevelt Room of the White House. Tollgates would go on for 10 or 12 hours, sometimes 16, break for three or four, and then resume, often late at night. The process reached an absurd point when a tollgate continued past 2 o'clock on a Sunday morning."[4]

Despite the intense workings of the task force, Magaziner and his working group soon came under harsh attack for the shroud of secrecy surrounding the process. Critics, ranging from the tradition-bound American Medical Association (AMA) to active health reform proponents, complained that the process was being run by inexperienced "policy wonks" who lacked real-world experience. In response, Mrs. Clinton and the task force began hosting public meetings around the country to demonstrate a willingness to consider different points of view, thereby revealing glimpses of the direction the Administration's proposal was heading.

By and large, Capitol Hill was not pleased with the secrecy surrounding the process either. Recognizing the importance of establishing good working relationships with Democrats and Republicans, the First Lady began paying regular and highly publicized visits to Congress. In a series of meetings with lawmakers, Mrs. Clinton played the role of the able diplomat to the hilt, showing her well-developed grasp of the complex array of issues involved and a willingness to listen to different points of view. But some lawmakers remained uneasy over the degree to which their voices would be heard as the proposal moved ahead.

The 100-day deadline — originally set for May 3 — slipped by one month, then two, then was formally pushed back until mid-September. Between Clinton's inauguration and his September speech, the President and his health advisers floated a series of "trial balloons" intended to gauge political and public support for specific proposals.

Early in 1993, the Clinton team advanced the idea of federal price controls on provider fees and drug prices, eventually dropping that in favor of a voluntary system of short term controls. HHS Secretary Donna Shalala and Office of Management and Budget Deputy Director Alice Rivlin floated the prospect of imposing a value-added tax on goods and services, a proposal that Clinton withdrew after lawmakers denounced it.

In late February, Clinton indicated a willingness to support a tax on cigarettes and alcohol, complaining that the U.S. was "spending a ton of money in private insurance and in government tax payments to deal with the health care problems occasioned by bad health habits."[5] He also tried to test the waters on whether to tax the value of health insurance benefits, a proposal abhorred by labor organizations, which viewed the potential tax as giving back hard-won benefits. But the tax has been favored by Republicans and managed competition proponents as a way to instill cost-consciousness among consumers, who are now shielded from how much health benefits cost. In the end, Clinton bowed to labor's concerns. Finally, a controversial policy for dealing with medical malpractice costs called enterprise liability was advanced by a Clinton aide in late spring but was shot down over opposition by medical groups, especially the powerful AMA.

LAYING THE FOUNDATION

If there had been any doubts about the major direction the upcoming health reform proposal would take, Clinton put many of them to rest at an August 16 speech to the nation's governors one month before the plan was scheduled for formal release.[6]

Clinton defended his widely anticipated decision to rely on an employer mandate to finance universal coverage. Building on the employer-based system is "the fairest way to go," he told the National Governors' Association at the group's annual meeting in Tulsa, Oklahoma. In contrast, single payer would be politically unrealistic, given its requirement for an estimated $500 billion in new taxes now paid via employer-paid premiums. Clinton also vowed to help small businesses cover the cost of health insurance.

As Labor Day neared, much of the details of the Clinton plan had already made their way into the press. But on September 7, a draft copy of the Administration's massive health proposal was leaked en route to Capitol Hill for a viewing by lawmakers, who demanded to read it in the privacy of their own offices instead of viewing it during allotted times set up by the Administration. Copies of the 239-page draft plan quickly became a best-seller on the streets of Washington, putting the Administration on the defensive before the Clintons had the chance to resolve some key issues, including how to design and finance the federal subsidies it had promised to small businesses.

By the time Clinton delivered his long-awaited September 22 health reform speech to a joint session of Congress, it had an anti-climatic quality since most major media outlets had published details of the draft plan. Over the course of the next month, Clinton continued to wrestle with major financing questions. Meanwhile, Mrs. Clinton served as a health reform ambassador to Capitol Hill, where she wowed lawmakers with her political savvy and policy smarts in three days of back-to-back hearings before the key health committees. But her skill at artfully evading the tough questions on the plan's structure and financing didn't keep impatient lawmakers at bay for long. One week after Clinton's speech, HHS Secretary Shalala took a political beating before the same congressional health committees Mrs. Clinton appeared in front of when she glossed over details of the proposal. On October 27, nearly 10 months after Clinton took office, the 1,342-page bill was ceremoniously delivered to Congress, who took a temporary break from their queries about the proposal's structure and financing.

Two days before the November 22 Thanksgiving recess, the Clinton health care bill (S.1757, H.R.3600), accompanied by a slew of revisions made since its unveiling one month earlier, was formally introduced into the 103rd Congress by House Majority Leader Richard Gephardt (D-MO) and Senate Majority Leader George Mitchell (D-ME). In the House, the bill had 100 cosponsors; in the Senate, 30. Only one Republican — Vermont Senator James Jeffords — had endorsed the measure.

THE CLINTON BILL

Major portions of the Clinton bill, including some of the revisions added to the final legislation submitted on October 27 to Congress, are summarized here:

□ **Universal Coverage:** All U.S. citizens and legal residents would get health care coverage through state-created regional or corporate insurance purchasing alliances, set up to help individuals and businesses purchase health insurance. Coverage would continue regardless of whether an individual becomes sick, loses his job, switches jobs, or moves to another state. All eligible persons would get a "health security card" as proof of coverage that would entitle them to coverage through a certified health plan offering a federally defined package of benefits. Persons covered by Medicare, the veterans and military health systems, and the Indian Health Service would not have to enroll in a regional alliance, but Medicaid recipients and federal and state employees would be required to do so.

□ **Illegal Aliens:** Undocumented persons are not eligible for guaranteed health benefits. However, employers are required to pay health insurance premiums for all their employees, regardless of immigration status. Alliances would not share information related to health insurance premiums paid by employers with the Immigration and Naturalization Service. Individuals living in the U.S. without proper documentation may continue to use emergency and other health services as provided under current federal law. Institutions that serve a large number of these patients will continue to receive federal funding, estimated at $1 billion, to compensate for the cost of their care.

Individuals who reside in U.S. territories will receive the comprehensive benefit package through their existing health care systems. States with large migrant labor populations are required to address their needs in state plans submitted to the federal government to implement health reform. States may extend coverage to migrant workers through regional alliances or propose alternative programs tailored to their specific needs.

□ **Individual/Employer Mandates:** Individuals would be obligated to enroll in a health plan in the region where they live. Anyone who misses the 30-day deadline for enrollment is automatically enrolled in the first health plan from which they seek medical care. All U.S. employers would be required to pay 80 percent of the weighted average premium for health insurance coverage in the regional alliances that serve their employees or into their corporate alliance. See Figure 2-1.

Figure 2-1

How You Get Coverage: The New System

Health care reform brings people closer to their doctors and the high quality, affordable care they deserve.

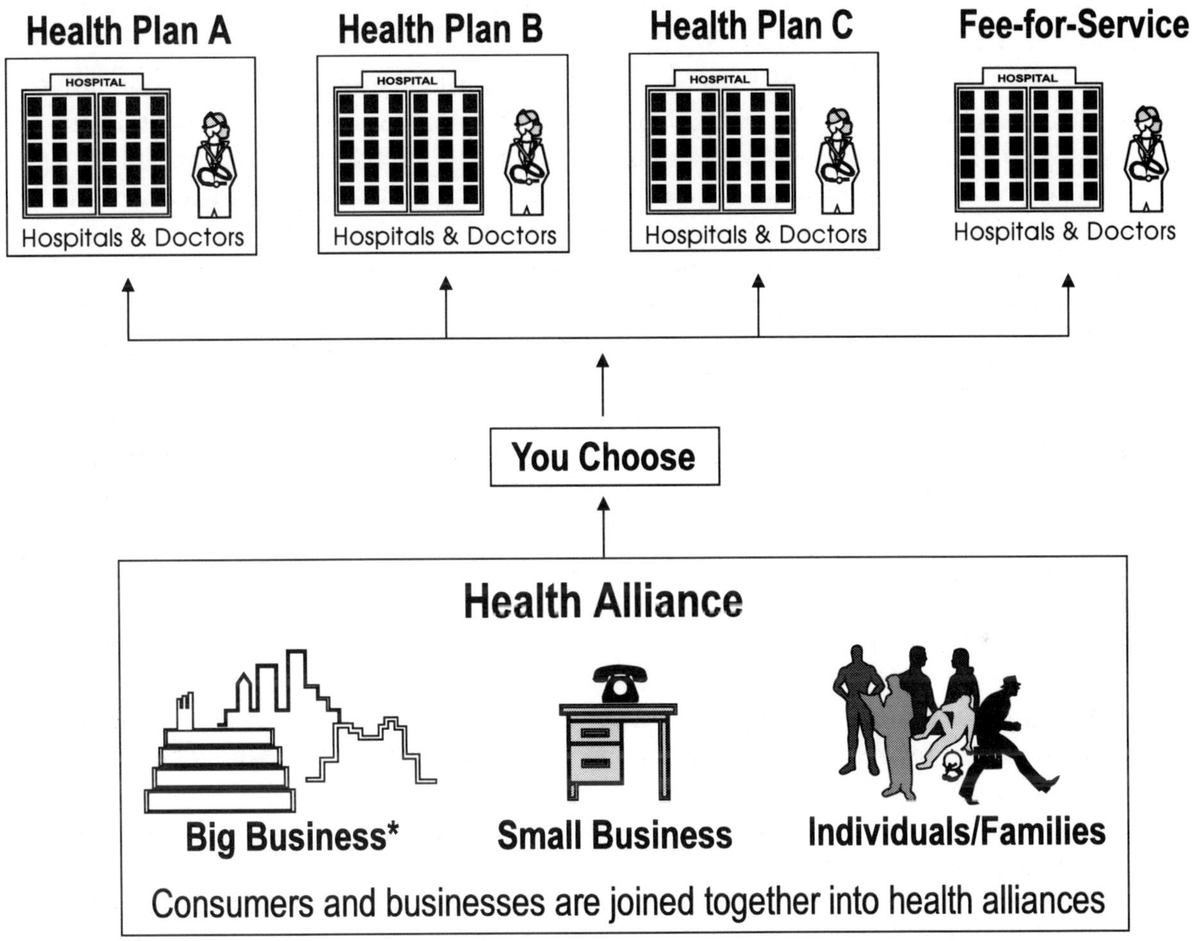

***Large businesses with 5,000 or more employees may form their own corporate alliances.**

Source: Department of Health and Human Services, 1993.

Employers who pay into regional alliances would have contributions capped at 7.9 percent of payroll. Small and low-wage employers with fewer than 75 workers could qualify for discounts off the cost of health insurance that would be subsidized by the federal government; discounts would vary according to the size and average wage of a company. Premium contributions would range from 3.5 percent to 7.9 percent of payroll for small businesses that employ low-wage workers.

Low-income persons who earn up to 150 percent of the federal poverty level would have their premium contributions subsidized so their insurance payments would not exceed 3.9 percent of their income. The majority of workers would be asked to pay 20 percent of the average weighted premium. Employers could opt to contribute all of an employee's share.

□ **Regional Health Alliances:** Each state would set up at least one regional health alliance or large purchasing pool to facilitate the purchase of health insurance for individuals and businesses that employ up to 5,000 workers. A regional alliance could operate as a nonprofit corporation, an independent state agency, or an agency of the state executive branch. The board of each alliance would include an equal number of employer and consumer representatives. Alliances will contract with and pay health plans, guarantee quality standards, provide information to help consumers select plans, and collect premiums. Large corporations have the option of joining the regional health alliance.

Only those state-certified health plans that meet state-determined quality and financial solvency standards can enter into contracts with the appropriate regional alliance to provide the guaranteed benefit package. The alliance would be set up as a mechanism to "promote competition and to protect the consumer." To do this, an alliance may reject a health plan if the plan's premiums are more than 20 percent higher than the average of the other plans in the area. But alliances cannot arbitrarily select or limit the number of fee-for-service plans, or decide that such a plan is not financially viable in an area.

□ **Corporate Alliances:** Companies with more than 5,000 workers could form their own "corporate alliances" but would have to provide the same federally qualified set of benefits and report information about enrollment. Companies that choose this route would have to pay a one percent payroll tax to the regional alliance to help subsidize the cost of its operation. If a company's employee tally drops below 4,800, the company must join the regional alliance.

□ **Benefits:** Benefits covered in the national guaranteed benefits package include hospital and emergency services; services of physicians and "other" licensed health professionals; mental health and substance abuse services; family planning and "pregnancy-related" services, including abortions; hospice; home care; outpatient prescription drugs; outpatient laboratory and rehabilitation services; vision and hearing care; health education classes; and preventive dental services for children.

Each health plan is expected to provide a sufficient mix of providers and specialties and sites to provide adequate access to professional services. The benefit package does not cover services that are not medically necessary or appropriate, private duty nursing, cosmetic orthodontia and other cosmetic surgery, hearing aids, adult eyeglasses and contact lenses, *in vitro* fertilization services, sex-change surgery and related services, private room accommodations, custodial care, personal comfort services, and some investigational treatments.

By the year 2001, a comprehensive, integrated benefit structure for mental health and substance abuse services will replace prescribed limits on individual services. The phase-in period allows states, health alliances, and health plans time to develop quality assurance programs essential to a managed comprehensive benefit. The phase-in also provides incentives for states to implement an integrated system by combining state and local funds that now support separate public systems with health care reform to reduce duplication of services and ensure cost savings.

During the phase-in of the comprehensive mental health and substance abuse benefit, the federal government will support state demonstrations to prove the efficacy of comprehensive, integrated systems of care. By 2001, all states will have to submit to the National Health Board a plan that describes how it would move from the traditional two-tier structure to a comprehensive approach. Limits on outpatient treatment and cost-sharing will then be eliminated, making mental health benefits comparable to other health services.

But until 2001, day and visit limits will be applied, as well as higher cost-sharing for mental health and substance abuse services, such as "intensive residential treatment" and outpatient psychotherapy. Patients would get a maximum of 30 days a year for inpatient or residential treatment; an additional 30 days would be provided for patients if a health professional designated by a health plan in which an individual is enrolled determines that the individual poses a threat to the individual's life or another's or that the individual's medical condition requires hospitalization for drug therapy treatment. Case management services are to be offered by health plans, but plans have the discretion to decide whether certain services should be provided to a patient.

□ **National Health Board:** A National Health Board comprising seven members appointed by the President would be set up to operate like a board of directors. At least one member of the Board must represent state interests. The President will designate one member as chair, who will serve a term concurrent with that of the President. Other board members will be nominated by the President, based on their experience and expertise in such areas as health care finance and delivery, state health systems, consumer protection, business, law, and delivering care to vulnerable populations. Board members may hold no other employment or a pecuniary interest in a health care plan, health care provider, or an insurance, pharmaceutical, or medical equipment company.

□ **Board Responsibilities:** The Board would be given immense powers to set federal standards on quality assurance and would oversee the creation and administration of the new health care system by states. It would also be given authority to interpret and update the benefit package and can recommend any adjustments to Congress and the President. In addition, the Board would: calculate and enforce health insurance premium targets and have broad budgeting powers; establish baseline budgets for health alliances in every state and allocate budgets among alliances; and impose an assessment on each plan whose bid exceeded the target. If the Board determined that a state failed to meet the deadline for establishing health alliances or other federal rules — including cost-containment requirements — it would inform HHS, which could withhold federal health monies. Should a state still fail to meet the deadline, the Treasury Department could tax all employers in the state.

□ **State Responsibilities:** States must ensure that all eligible residents have access to a health plan that complies with federal laws. Each state must establish at least one regional alliance by January 1, 1998; some states that have already launched reform programs, such as Florida, may be ready sooner. The federal government would offer incentives to states to move quickly, including special start-up funds, subsidies, and quick consideration of their plans. Grace periods would be granted to states that make good-faith efforts. States could establish only one regional alliance in each area and must ensure that each alliance enrolls all eligible persons in the geographic area covered by that alliance.

States can establish a single payer health system rather than an alliance system offering multiple plans. A state that wants to adopt a single payer system would get an automatic waiver from the 1974 Employee Retirement Income Security Act (ERISA). States also could integrate Medicare beneficiaries into the single payer systems provided that the benefits are as good as or better than those offered under the Medicare program. Single payer states would have to maintain the 80 percent/20 percent employer-employee split, but they could choose to levy additional taxes.

States cannot regulate premiums charged by health plans except when needed to meet the budget or to ensure plan solvency. States cannot limit enrollment in high-cost plans, set rates for health providers, or institute health planning laws. States cannot rely on a payroll tax or other revenue source tied to corporations or payroll to pay for additional benefits. Each state must operate a guaranty fund to provide financial help to health providers if a health plan becomes insolvent. A state may impose up to a 2 percent tax on other health plans in the alliance to reap revenues to cover outstanding claims from a plan that becomes insolvent. (See Figure 2-2.)

□ **Health Plans:** States would qualify health plans — including HMOs, fee-for-service (FFS) plans, or managed care hybrids — to participate in alliances. Every health plan would have to offer a "point of service" option, under which patients can seek care from a doctor or other provider who does not participate in the plan. This option would cost consumers more. States could waive the FFS requirement if they got approval from the National Health Board. All patients would be guaranteed the chance to seek specialized care at teaching hospitals.

States would have to follow federal rules to determine plan solvency. The minimum capital requirement for health plans is $500,000. Health plans could not exclude participants because of existing medical conditions or impose pre-coverage waiting periods. Plans could not arbitrarily terminate coverage and could not cancel coverage for any person until that person was enrolled in another health plan. Only those plans qualified by the state can participate in the regional alliances,

Figure 2-2

Federal, State, and Alliance Responsibilities

The Federal Government

Sets the basic system framework

- **Federally guaranteed benefits package**
- **Determines premium caps, increases, and enforcement**
- **Insurance reform**

The States

Within federal framework, adopt health reform arrangement of choice

- **Establish alliances**
- **Certify health plans**
- **Monitor quality of and access to care**
- **Implement insurance and malpractice reform**

Alliances

Serve as collective purchasing agents for employers and consumers at the local level

- **Solicit competitive bids from health plans**
- **Disseminate consumer information materials**
- **Enroll all eligible residents**
- **Collect premiums and pay health plans**
- **Administer employer and family discounts**

Source: Department of Health and Human Services, 1993.

and states must ensure that consumers can buy coverage through the alliance at a price equal to or less than the average premium. States can force plans to contract with essential community providers, such as public hospitals and community health centers, as well as academic centers of excellence.

During the transition from enactment of this law to implementation by states, insurers would be prohibited from terminating coverage and benefits. Violations of this rule would be punished by a minimum fine of $25,000. Group health and individual health insurers could not terminate or fail to renew coverage except in the case of nonpayment of required premiums, fraud, or misrepresentation.

HHS would have to establish a National Transitional Health Insurance Risk Pool to ensure access to health insurance during the transition to a national system. This pool would be available to individuals who cannot get insurance coverage from private plans because of their health status. Payments under this pool for covered items and services would be made at rates specified by the Secretary of HHS based on payment rates for comparable programs under Medicare. Providers would have to accept federal payment as payment in full.

☐ **New Benefits:** Medicare beneficiaries would get access to a new $66 billion outpatient prescription drug benefit that would be paid for by limiting Medicare spending growth and imposing more cost sharing on high-income elderly (couples with more than $125,000 in yearly income). Drug makers would have to sign agreements with HHS and pay a 17 percent rebate for brand-name drugs as a condition of Medicare payments. HHS could negotiate a "special rebate" for breakthrough drugs that are deemed to be "inappropriately priced." If a manufacturer refuses to change the price, HHS can blacklist the drug from Medicare.

A new $65 billion long term care program for elderly, disabled, and chronically ill people would be established, which would offer home- and community-based care services funded by the federal government with some help from the states. Individuals would have to pay no more than 25 percent of the cost of premiums and the benefit would be phased in by 2002. The personal needs allowance provided to nursing home residents covered by Medicaid would be increased from the current $30 to $50.

☐ **Quality Improvement:** A new, 15-member advisory council will oversee a sweeping national quality management program, which aims to gauge the performance of the health system and inform consumers of the quality of health plans they select. Specifically, the program would: develop a set of quality and performance measures and consumer survey questions; conduct consumer surveys that measure access to care, use of health services, outcomes, and satisfaction; set national performance goals; establish minimum standards of access and quality that individual plans must meet; evaluate the impact of health reform on quality of care; and use a national network of regional centers to obtain quality management data.

The program also will develop a standard set of performance measures that apply to all health plans, institutions, and practitioners. It will publish annual performance reports that outline the results of those measures for each health plan. Annual reports to the states will compare health plans and state quality programs.

States, health alliances, and health plans each would play a role in the quality management program. States would develop plans to meet enrollment, access, and quality standards; ensure that plans and providers meet national standards through licensure and certification procedures; and prepare comparative reports on the performance of alliances, plans, providers, and practitioners. Health alliances would resolve consumer complaints, grievances, and requests to leave a plan; disseminate information about quality and access to help consumers select a plan; prepare comparative reports on the quality of health plans, providers, and practitioners and ensure that performance and quality standards are met. Health plans would measure and disclose performance on quality measures; report on, maintain, and improve the quality of care delivered by providers and practitioners; and meet national conditions of participation established for plans by the National Health Board.

□ **Malpractice Reform:** The plan calls for changes in tort law and alternatives to costly and time-consuming litigation. Reforms include: alternative dispute resolution mechanisms, such as settlement offers, mediation, and non-binding arbitration; a limit on attorneys' contingency fees to one-third of the award; new rules requiring that awards be reduced by the amount collected from other sources, such as disability or health insurance; and periodic award payment schedules. The plan also requires that lawsuits claiming medical malpractice be accompanied by an affidavit signed by a specialist who practices in a relevant field and permits public access to the National Practitioner Data Bank, which tracks providers who incur repeated malpractice claims and settlements.

□ **Antitrust:** The plan directs the Department of Justice (DOJ) and the Federal Trade Commission (FTC) to publish guidelines that create "safety zones" for hospital mergers and an expedited business review or advisory opinion procedure through which the parties can obtain timely (90 days) assurance that their merger will not be challenged. The plan also calls on DOJ and FTC to publish guidelines for joint ventures and arrangements involving high technology or expensive equipment and services. The federal agencies also would provide guidance for physician joint ventures that do not possess market power (below 20 percent) and that share financial risk.

□ **Long Term Care:** A new long term care program created through Title 15 of the Social Security Act would: expand home- and community-based services (see New Benefits); improve Medicaid coverage for institutional care; provide standards to improve the quality of private long term care insurance; create tax incentives to help disabled individuals to work; and create a demonstration program to study ways of integrating long term and acute care.

□ **Medical Education:** The plan sets a goal of having medical schools on track to train 55 percent of new physicians in primary care as of 1998, including family medicine, general internal medicine and general pediatrics, and obstetrics and gynecology. HHS would determine how many training positions there should be for each specialty based on recommendations from the National Council on Graduate Medical Education, and those programs that failed to comply would be denied federal medical education funds.

Funds to support graduate medical education are pooled from all insurers and the Medicare medical education budget. Payments reflect a mix of residency salaries, costs of faculty supervision, and related teaching supervision. Funds go directly to training programs approved for residency positions, with a preference for non-hospital-based training sites, such as HMOs and community clinics. Transition payments would be provided to teaching hospitals as they readjust their work force.

A national loan forgiveness program would be established to encourage more primary care practice, and programs would be established to retrain mid-career specialists in primary care. Incentives also would be used to encourage more minorities to enter the health professions, and funding would be increased for programs that train nurse practitioners, physician assistants, and nurse-midwives.

□ **Underserved Areas:** To ensure that underserved areas have an adequate supply of physicians, doctors located in underserved areas would receive a personal tax credit of $1,000 a month that could be claimed during the first five years of practice. Physician assistants and nurse practitioners would get credits of $500 a month.

□ **Public Health Initiative:** A total of $29 billion will support improvements in the public health infrastructure. The federal, state, and local public health roles will be strengthened in three ways: improving the core public health functions; authorizing a pool of funds to address high-priority health problems; and expanding federal support for unified data systems and information networks.

Public health activities will shift away from the direct delivery of health services to defending against preventable diseases and conditions, such as AIDS, tuberculosis, and chronic and environmentally related diseases.

□ **Medicaid:** Aid to Families with Dependent Children (AFDC) and Supplemental Security Income (SSI) recipients would be able to choose from any plans participating in a regional alliance, but their payment would come from Medicaid. Non-cash assistance recipients would no longer receive insurance through Medicaid but would be covered by their employer. They would continue to receive supplemental benefits now paid for under Medicaid, including rehabilitation and transportation services. Federal and state shares of Medicaid would continue as they are now. Disproportionate-share payments to hospitals that treat a heavy volume of uninsured patients would be phased out, but some funds would be retained to pay for treating illegal aliens.

□ **Retiree Health:** Employers now obligated to provide health benefits to employees will be required beginning in 1998, to pay individuals 20 percent share of the cost of the comprehensive benefit package for those employees that retire early. The federal government would pick up the remaining 80 percent, at a cost of nearly $12 billion.

□ **Workers' Compensation:** Health plans would provide treatment for individuals who suffer work-related injuries covered under workers' compensation insurance. Workers' compensation insurers, including self-funded employers, would continue to bear the responsibility for the costs of treatment and reimburse plans for services provided. Reimbursement would be based on a fee schedule or would be negotiated between workers' compensation insurers and health plans.

Individuals enrolled in health plans within the alliance would receive treatment for work-related injuries or illnesses from their plans, although emergency treatment may be obtained from any health provider. State laws governing choice of provider for workers' compensation cases would be overridden for individuals covered through health alliances.

□ **Outreach:** States may determine that financial incentives are needed to ensure that health plans enroll disadvantaged groups and provide extra services, such as outreach, transportation, and interpreting services to ensure access to care. Alliances may use financial incentives to encourage health plans to expand into areas that have inadequate health services. Alliances may also organize health providers to create a new health plan targeted to such an area, providing assistance with setting up and administering the plan. An alliance may not assume risk on behalf of a new health plan but may arrange favorable financing to encourage a health plan to operate in an area with inadequate services.

□ **New Spending Initiatives:** The savings and revenues would be funneled to pay for improvements in public health programs, including enhancement in the women, infants, and children nutrition program, new public health initiatives, and new spending on academic health centers ($31.1 billion); a long term care benefit that includes a new home- and community-based care program for disabled persons, tax incentives to encourage the purchase of long term care insurance, and liberalized rules for Medicaid eligibility ($65 billion); a new Medicare prescription drug benefit ($66 billion); a 100 percent tax deduction for self-employed individuals who purchase health insurance ($9.7 billion); and capped premium subsidies for small businesses that need assistance complying with an employer mandate ($161.1 billion).

HOW THE PLAN IS PAID FOR

While employers and employees are expected to shoulder the lion's share of the plan's cost, the Administration estimates the federal government's share to be $331 billion between 1995 and the year 2000. It would raise those funds by: imposing a 75-cent increase on tobacco and tobacco products ($65.3 billion); assessing a one percent tax on corporations that form their own alliances ($24.1 billion); reducing the rate of growth in Medicare through a series of 28 policy changes, including lowered payments to providers ($124.4 billion); trimming Medicaid spending growth, and reducing payments for uncompensated hospital care ($65.3 billion); reaping savings from federal programs such as the Federal Employees Health Benefits Program and health programs covered by the Veterans Affairs Department and the Department of Defense ($40 billion); and capturing expected revenue gains from higher taxes paid by corporations and individuals due to lower health care costs ($71 billion). This would raise $390.1 billion, according to Office of Management and Budget Director Leon Panetta, leaving $58 billion for deficit reduction.

The Administration has a three-pronged approach to cost containment as it approaches the universal coverage deadline of 1998. First, the plan restructures the health care delivery market to encourage wider use of managed care plans that would compete on the basis of price and quality within regional health alliances. Second, Clinton has established a back-up strategy of insurance premium caps or global budgets that would limit the rate of growth in health premiums. Third, the Administration predicts that substantial savings would be wrung from curtailing Medicare and Medicaid spending growth. The Administration also is proposing to impose a cap on the tax deductibility of health insurance benefits as of 2004. The cap would be imposed on all employer spending, including cost-sharing, for the comprehensive benefit package. (See Figure 2-3.)

How the Administration plans to control costs is by far the most contentious issue. Lawmakers are wary of the magnitude of the Medicare and Medicaid reductions and the pace and level of the premium cap proposal, which critics say would, in effect, establish tighter spending controls on health care outlays than any other

Figure 2-3

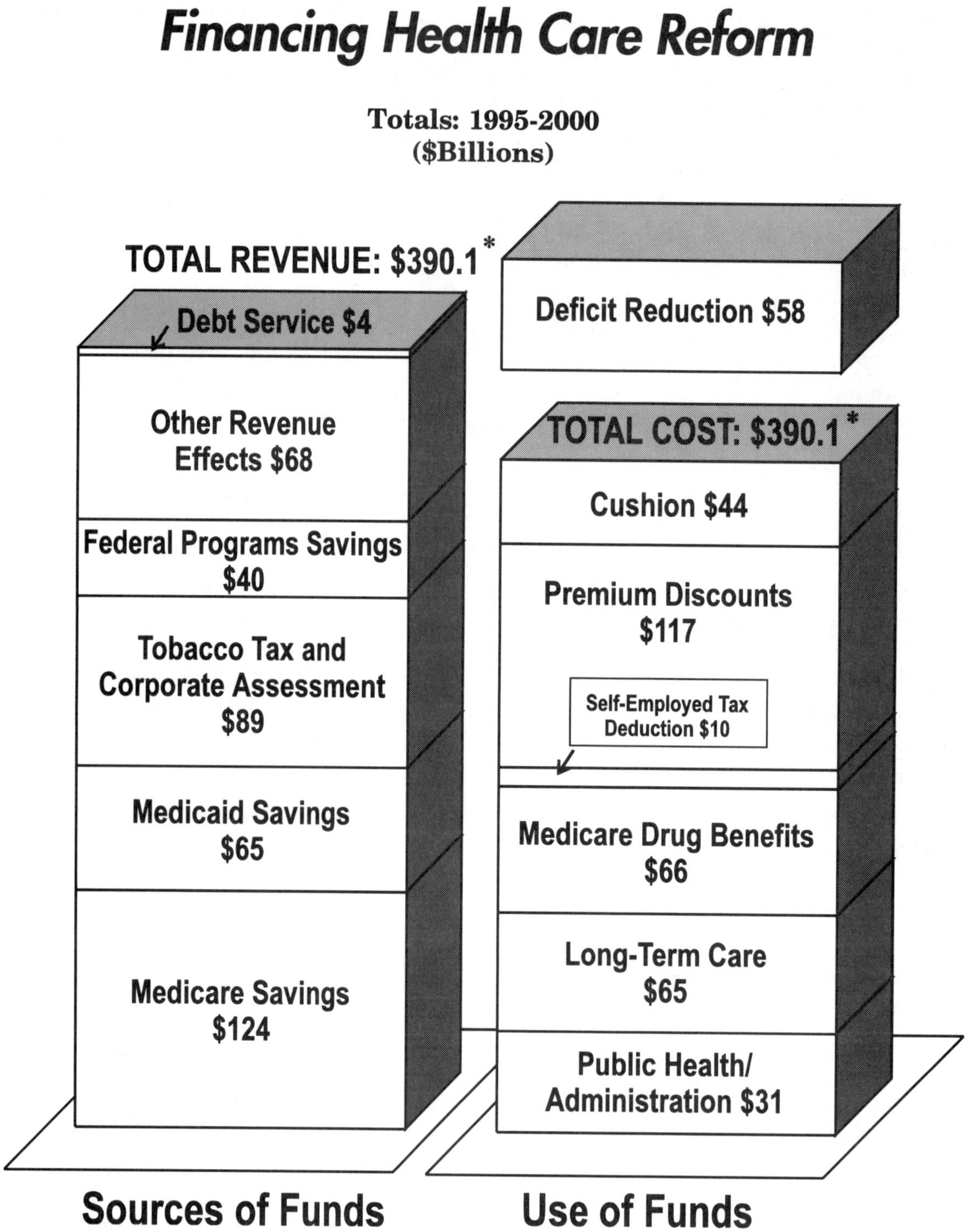

***Numbers do not total due to rounding.**

Source: Department of Health and Human Services, Nov. 4, 1993.

nation — including Canada and Great Britain — by 1999. Insurance premium caps would be enforced through an automatic mechanism that would be written into the final law. If premiums charged by a health plan in an alliance exceed the cap, the alliance operators could negotiate with the health plan to lower its costs. If premiums are not reduced this way, automatic premium reductions would be triggered, and payment to providers would be similarly lowered.

Starting in 1996, the Administration would allow private insurance premiums to rise according to the increase in the Consumer Price Index (CPI) plus 1.5 percent; in 1997, they would rise at CPI plus one percent; in 1998, they would be held to CPI plus 0.5 percent; and in 1999, premiums would be held to the CPI. Population growth would be taken into account in the formula as well.

In 1998, the National Health Board would submit to Congress recommendations on the appropriate level of general private sector health inflation beginning in the year 2000. By January 1, 1995, the Health Board would have to determine a national per capita baseline premium target for the guaranteed benefits package. By January 1, 1996, the Board would also decide a per capita spending target for each regional alliance.

As of late November, the Administration was still compiling its estimates for projected private sector spending growth under its health plan. Currently, private sector insurance premiums are expected to grow at about 8 percent a year. The Administration's goal is to about halve that rate by the year 2000. Medicare payment rates, now growing at about 11 percent year, would grow at less than 8 percent a year if the White House's proposal prevails. National health spending will still rise significantly under reform, an Administration official argues, because more people will have health insurance coverage. But by holding down the rate of increase in premiums, "we're putting some control on the overall system" over the long term.

REFERENCES

1. Clinton B. Address to Congress on National Health Care Reform, Washington DC, September 22, 1993.
2. Kosterlitz J. O.K. Bill, It's Time To Pick Your Remedy. *National Journal*, January 23, 1993: 200-201.
3. Pear R. Washington at Work; An Idealist's Task: To Revamp Healthcare. *The New York Times*, February 26, 1993: 14.
4. Duffy M and R Thompson. Behind Closed Doors. *Time*, September 20, 1993: 62.
5. Clinton Hints at Sin Taxes To Pay for Health Reform. *Medicine & Health*, March 1, 1993.
6. Clinton B. Speech to National Governors' Association, Tulsa, Oklahoma, August 16, 1993.

CHAPTER 3

Access to Care and Health Care Reform

Diane Rowland and Lois Simon

One of the most important measures of a health care delivery system is the extent to which all members of society are brought up to acceptable standards of health. The medical system in the United States is preeminent in the world, but the fruits of the system are not uniformly available to all Americans. An estimated 35.6 million Americans are uninsured, and millions more are underinsured and at risk of financial hardship when serious illness strikes. Limited availability of providers of care in many inner-city and rural areas of the country and the gaps in insurance coverage limit many Americans' access to care.

These gaps in fundamental access for millions of Americans have spurred the call for reform of the American health care system. Improved insurance protection, greater availability of care in underserved areas, and better access to primary and preventive care for all Americans are central to the debate. The success or failure of any health reform proposal will ultimately be judged by whether it reduces financial burdens and improves access to care for the American population.

HEALTH STATUS AND ACCESS TO CARE IN AMERICA

The ultimate goal of any health system is to maintain and improve the health of its population. Health expenditures are intended to advance the health of the population by reducing infant mortality, extending life expectancy, and reducing the incidence of disease and disability by promoting more effective treatment. The United States has been a world leader in medical advances and has pioneered much of the research that has improved medical outcomes worldwide. Yet, despite its cutting-edge research, incredible investment in health care delivery, and substantial expenditures on medical care, the United States often falls behind other nations in securing the health of its population.

Rates of infant mortality, low birth weight, and childhood mortality in Australia, Canada, France, Germany, Japan, and the United Kingdom are similar, and often superior, to those of the United States, but each of these countries devotes a smaller share of its economy to health spending[1]. The United States has higher infant and child mortality rates than these six countries and a low birth weight rate that's among the highest of the six. Within the U.S. itself, there are significant differentials in health status and access to care for subgroups of the American population, especially the poor and minorities.

Health Status in America

Most Americans enjoy relatively good health and have few problems in obtaining access to medical services. Nearly nine out of ten Americans (87 percent) report their health status as either good or excellent[2]. However, nearly a quarter (23 percent) of non-elderly poor Americans rate their health as fair or poor, while only 10 percent of Americans with incomes above 200 percent of poverty (poverty level is roughly $11,000 for a family of three) report fair or poor health (see Figure 3-1).

The association between poverty and poor health is also demonstrated by higher rates of chronic conditions, mental illness, infectious diseases, low birth weight, and childhood conditions for the poor. Chronic conditions, including hypertension (high blood pressure), arthritis, heart disease, and diabetes, often require expensive medications as part of ongoing medical treatment and management and can result in severe disability and even death without appropriate and timely care. Rates of heart disease and diabetes for the poor are twice the levels as among the non-poor[2]. The poor are more than twice as likely to suffer from serious mental illness as the non-poor[3]. Moreover, infectious diseases such as AIDS and tuberculosis hit low-income families disproportionately.

Poor children, especially those in inner cities and underserved areas, are particularly at risk for health problems. Inadequate prenatal care and environmental factors combine to leave many children impaired throughout life by conditions that are preventable during youth. Poor women are at high risk of having babies of low birth weight, a leading cause of infant mortality and disability. In New York

Figure 3-1

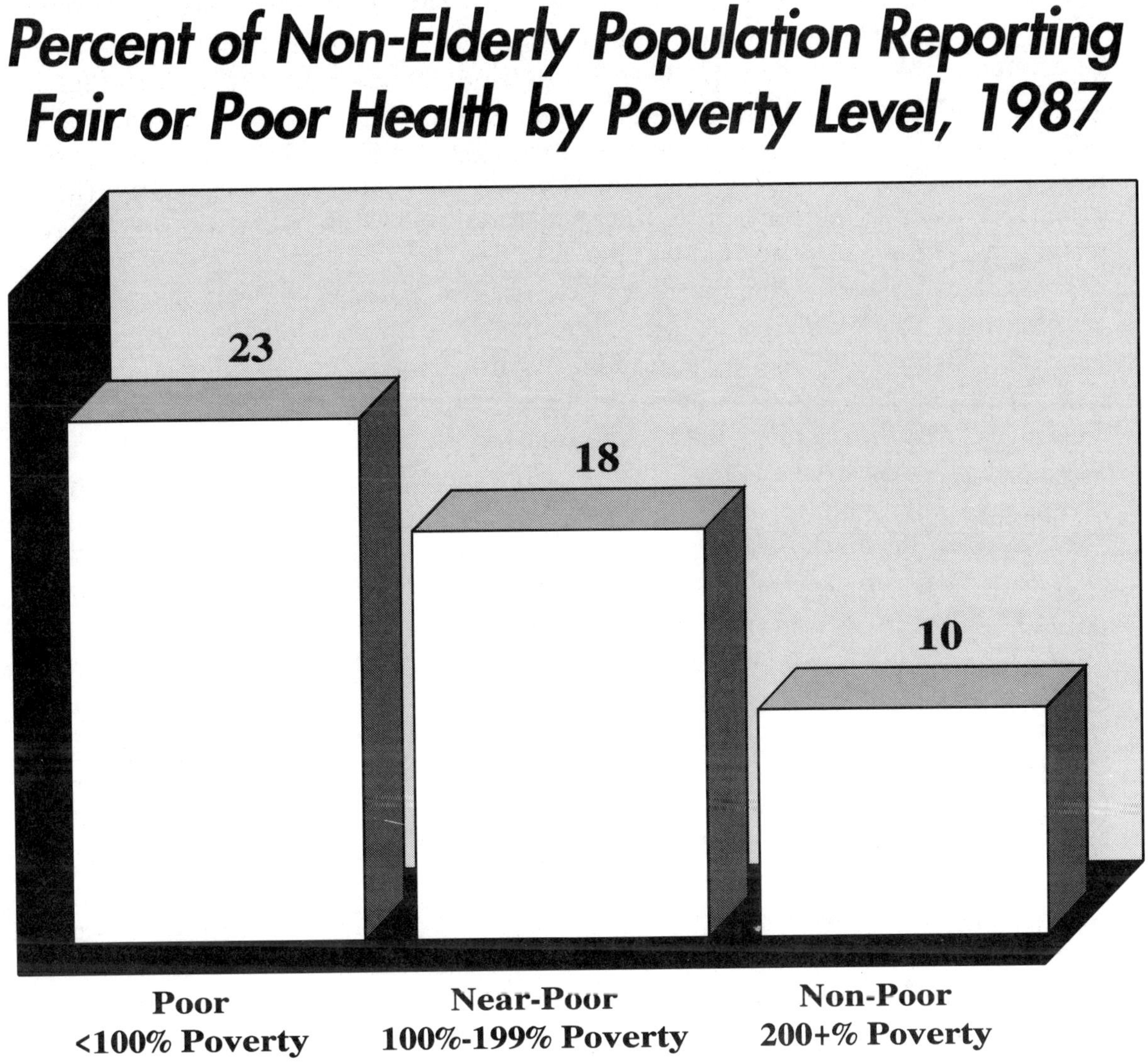

Source: Kaiser Commission on the Future of Medicaid, NMES, 1987.

City, a recent study found that twice as many low birth-weight births occur in the poorest neighborhoods as in the wealthiest neighborhoods[4]. Once children are born into poverty-stricken households, they are less likely to receive health services, which could prevent diseases. Only 38 percent of two-year-old children living below poverty were fully up to date on their immunizations, compared with 61 percent of children living above the poverty line[5].

Many poor children are at risk of greater health problems because of the conditions of their housing and environment. Lead paint in the home is a serious problem in most inner-city neighborhoods and can cause mental deterioration if undetected and untreated. A 1986 study concluded that 41 percent of children living in households with an income of less than $6,000 had lead poisoning, compared with 17 percent of children in families with incomes of more than $15,000[6]. Contamination from lead paint is a prevalent condition among poor children. It could be eliminated with adequate resources and strengthened public health activities but has not received the funding or support to correct the problem in most areas.

Within the United States, there is also a substantial disparity between the health of minority populations and the health of the nation as a whole. Minority groups have higher mortality rates than whites as well as higher rates of low birth weight, heart disease, cancer, and diabetes.

On almost every health indicator, black Americans fare worse than their white counterparts. Black Americans were more likely to express health concerns than white Americans, with 13.4 percent of blacks and 8.5 percent of whites assessing their health as fair or poor[7]. Infant mortality rates for blacks (17.0 deaths per 1,000 live births) were more than twice that for whites (7.7 per 1,000) in 1990[8]. The low birth-weight rate is higher for blacks than whites for both the poor and non-poor — 12 percent for blacks compared to 10 percent for whites for the poor and 8 percent for blacks and 4 percent for whites for the non-poor[9]. In 1990 life expectancy for white males was 8.2 years longer than for black males (72.7 compared with 64.5 years); similarly, life expectancy for white females was 5.8 years longer than for black females (79.4 compared with 73.6 years)[8].

Research also shows that health status tends to be lower for Americans living in rural areas, the South, and other areas with high concentrations of disadvantaged populations. Death rates are 12 percent higher in rural counties and 19 percent higher in counties that include large cities than in suburban areas[10]. Persons living in the South were more likely to report being in fair or poor health than persons in other regions[7]. In 1987, rural populations were 23 percent more likely to have activity limitations due to chronic conditions[11].

Differentials in Use of Health Care Services

The lower health status of the poor, minority populations, and residents of many rural and urban areas would generally be expected to result in higher medical care utilization rates for these populations. In fact, the opposite is true. Within America, too often the benefits of the health system are not uniformly available to all residents. Some lack the financial resources to access routine health care services because of low incomes and lack of insurance. Others live in areas with an inadequate supply of providers, limiting access to health services. Many Americans also face cultural and other non-financial obstacles to use of health care services such as lack of transportation and language barriers.

As a result, Americans experience divergent health care utilization patterns that cannot be explained by health status variations alone. Comparisons of medical care utilization between the poor and the non-poor under age 65 using a comprehensive national survey of health use and expenditures in 1987 reveal striking differentials. Physician utilization is used as an indicator of access to care because it not only measures both direct contact with a medical provider but also captures the physician's role as a gatekeeper for other services. Despite their lower health status, the poor are less likely to have had a physician contact over the past year for either preventive care or medical treatment. More than a third of the poor (34.8 percent) had no physician visits in the previous year compared to 27.4 percent of the non-poor[2] (see Figure 3-2). This indicates the poor are not gaining initial access to the health system.

Given the lower health status of the poor, one would expect higher visit levels for those who access the medical care system. However, among the population with physician contacts over the past year, the poor continue to lag slightly behind the non-poor in terms of average number of visits during the year. The average

Figure 3-2

Percent of Non-Elderly Population With No Physician Visit in Past Year, by Income and Health Status, 1987

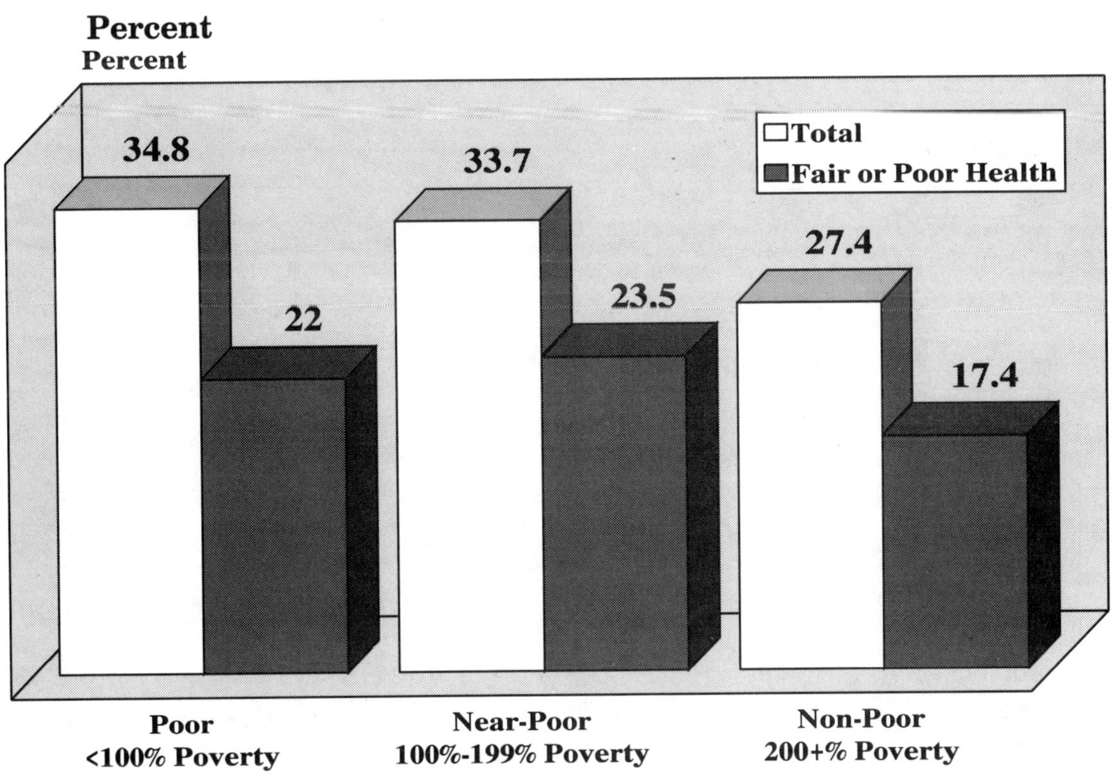

Source: Kaiser Commission on the Future of Medicaid, NMES, 1987.

annual number of physician visits for the poor and non-poor with at least one visit were nearly the same; 6.0 visits and 6.3 visits, respectively. When utilization among those in fair or poor health is adjusted for health status, the poor actually lag behind with 9.6 visits per year compared to 10.7 visits for the non-poor[2] (see Figure 3-3).

Not only do the poor use fewer health services, but when they do seek medical care, their site of care is often different from that of the non-poor. The poor are less likely than their non-poor counterparts to report that the site of care for the majority of their visits is a physician's office. The poor see physicians in their offices 62.9 percent of the time compared with 81.2 percent of the time for the non-poor[2]. Access to care for the uninsured poor often depends on the availability of a community health center, a hospital emergency room, a public health department clinic,

Figure 3-3

Mean Annual Physician Visits Among the Non-Elderly Population With at Least One Visit by Income and Health Status, 1987

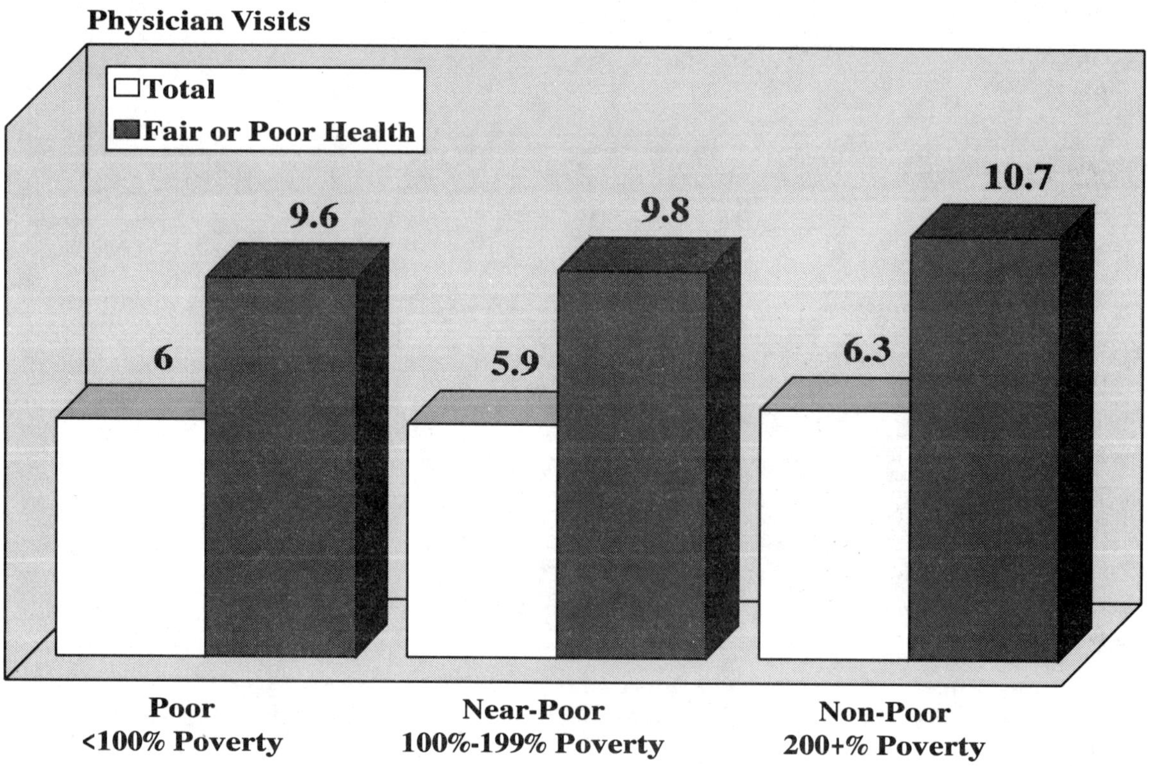

Source: Kaiser Commission on the Future of Medicaid, NMES, 1987.

or charity care from a public or nonprofit hospital. Clinics and hospital outpatient clinics account for more than a quarter (25.9 percent) of the physician contacts by the poor, compared with 12.4 percent of visits by the non-poor. The poor are more than twice as likely as the non-poor to receive care in emergency rooms; 10.6 percent of all physician visits by the poor are to emergency rooms, compared with 5.4 percent of physician visits by the non-poor[2].

Having a regular source of medical care is viewed as a measure of access to care because a stable medical provider relationship helps to foster use of preventive care and early intervention for treatment of disease. In addition to having fewer visits per year, the poor are less likely than the non-poor to have a regular source of care. A quarter of the non-elderly poor, compared with 18.6 percent of the non-poor, do not have a regular source of care[2].

Similar results are found in analyses of access to care among minority populations. Despite their worse health status, minorities use fewer health care services than whites. This inequity persists across income levels and is present even for patients with chronic illness[12]. Even after adjusting for income and health status, blacks have a lower mean number of annual ambulatory visits and are less likely to have seen a physician in the past year than whites[13]. Ongoing medical management of conditions such as hypertension is important to prevent deterioration and the onset of more serious disease. However, 30 percent of blacks with hypertension had not had a blood pressure check in the last year compared to 19 percent of whites[13].

These variations in use of services by income and race reflect gaps in access to care for millions of Americans. Some of these differences stem from these people's inability to pay for insurance coverage. Often such financial barriers are further complicated by physical barriers to care arising from an inadequate provider supply in inner-city and rural areas.

FINANCIAL BARRIERS TO ACCESS TO CARE

Clearly health insurance coverage to help provide the financial means to pay for medical care is an important component of ensuring access to care for all Americans. Without financial access through insurance coverage or sufficient income to purchase care, it is difficult to obtain timely and appropriate treatment and preventive and primary care. Yet, in the United States, more than 35 million people are without insurance coverage, and millions more are at risk of losing their coverage. Most Americans who do have insurance are covered either by their or a family member's employer or else they are aged or poor enough to qualify for public assistance for health coverage.

Sources of Insurance Coverage

Insurance coverage in America is derived from a variety of sources rather than from a single national program. Most Americans (63 percent of the population) receive coverage from private insurance policies that are offered through the workplace or are privately purchased (see Figure 3-4). Another 13 percent of Americans receive coverage through the federal Medicare program because they are aged or disabled. Eight percent are covered by the joint federal and state Medicaid program that provides assistance to low-income individuals. An additional 2 percent are eligible for both Medicare and Medicaid. This leaves 14 percent of the American population — almost 36 million people — without coverage because they do not qualify for public coverage and cannot afford or obtain private coverage.

The only group of Americans uniformly covered by health insurance are those over age 65, who by virtue of their Social Security coverage are also covered by the Medicare program for health insurance. Medicare provides health coverage to more than 34 million people who are either 65 years of age and older, permanently disabled, or have end-stage renal disease. Medicare covers virtually all elderly Americans and provides financial protection to assist with the costs of hospital, physician, and other health care services. It is publicly funded and federally ad-

Figure 3-4

Health Insurance Coverage of Non-Institutionalized Population, 1991

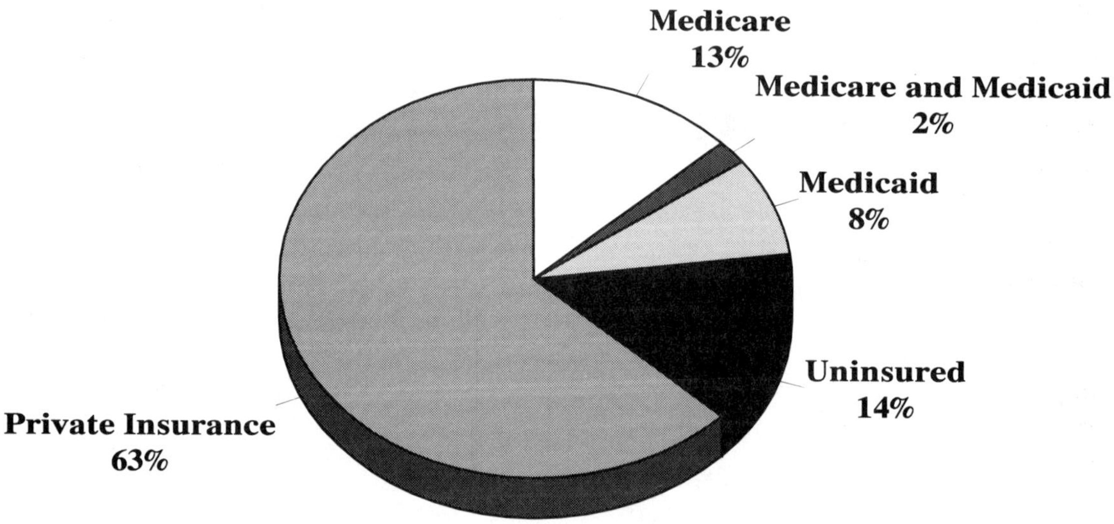

Total = 251 Million

Source: Kaiser Commission on the Future of Medicaid. *Analysis of the Current Population Survey*, 1992; Kaiser Foundation Health Reform Project, 1993.

ministered and thus offers the same benefit package and coverage regardless of the income or residence of the Medicare beneficiary.

For non-elderly Americans, employment-sponsored health insurance finances most medical care. Almost 84 percent of working Americans and their dependents have coverage obtained through employment. Most employers that offer insurance also provide some assistance with the premiums to pay for coverage, but employer contributions are not required and vary by region and by type of employment. Since providing insurance benefits is voluntary for employers, firms may opt out of offering insurance coverage to their employees. Many businesses cannot afford or are unwilling to pay the high cost of insurance for their employees. Private insurers often refuse to cover firms deemed as high risk or individuals with preexisting conditions.

The government-sponsored Medicaid program offers health coverage to some vulnerable populations, most notably families and individuals receiving welfare cash assistance, low-income pregnant women and children, and individuals with severe disabilities. In 1992, the federal and state governments financed care for 29.8 million low-income Americans through Medicaid. Most Medicaid recipients (72 percent) are low-income children and their parents, but the bulk of Medicaid spending is for the aged and disabled. Medicaid spending for the aged and disabled is high because it provides supplementary insurance for Medicare premiums and cost-sharing and pays for expensive long term care services for the elderly and disabled.

Medicaid is the nation's primary assistance program for low-income Americans, but, unlike Medicare for the elderly, it is not a uniform national program. The federal government requires states to provide specific population groups with certain benefits and gives states the option to cover others. States receive federal matching grants for Medicaid spending. Each state determines who will be covered, how much providers will be paid, and how its own program will be administered within federal guidelines. Consequently, Medicaid's scope and role are quite different across the states, and coverage of the poor varies widely across the nation. On average, Medicaid covers less than one-half of one percent of the population living in poverty[14].

While government programs like Medicare and Medicaid have had a positive impact on the financing of care for many Americans, the current system leaves approximately 14 percent of the population without health insurance. In addition, more than one in four Americans had a lapse in their health insurance for at least one month between 1987 and 1989[15]. As shown in Figure 3-5, the likelihood of being uninsured is higher for minorities and the low-income population. At any point in time, millions of Americans are without insurance, and millions more are at risk of losing it.

Gaps in Insurance Coverage

The current system of financing health care in America that splits responsibility between the public and private sectors and relies heavily on employers and

Figure 3-5

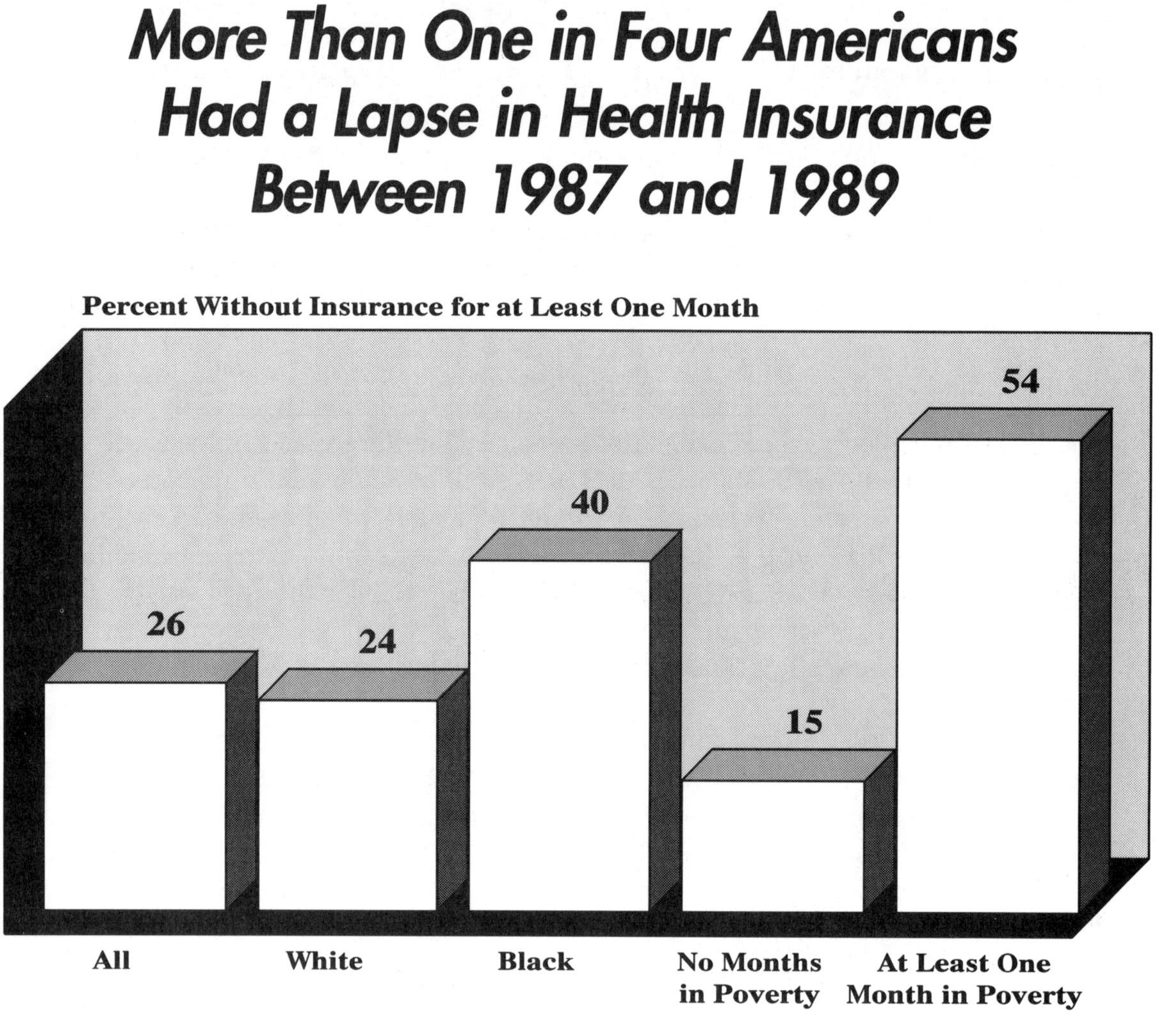

Source: Bureau of the Census, 1992.

individuals to purchase insurance leaves many cracks in coverage. The uninsured population is almost entirely composed of individuals under the age of 65 because Medicare provides universal coverage to virtually all elderly Americans. The composition of the uninsured demonstrates the limits of both employer-based insurance and the public programs for the poor.

Though the U.S. health care system is employer-based, having a job does not guarantee health insurance. Eight in ten uninsured Americans have an attachment to the work force and could potentially receive employer-sponsored coverage but do not because either the employer does not offer coverage or because the cost of purchasing such coverage is too high[16]. Over half (52 percent) of the uninsured are full-time workers or dependents of full-time workers, and nearly a third (30 percent) are from families with part-time workers. Only 18 percent of the uninsured are outside the working population (see Figure 3-6).

The rate of employment-based coverage increases as firm size increases. In 1991, 93 percent of individuals attached to firms with 1,000 or more employees (as either workers or dependents of workers) were insured, compared with 69 percent of individuals attached to firms with fewer than 10 employees[17]. The uninsured tend to be overrepresented in certain employment categories: Agriculture, personal services, and the construction industries have the highest proportion of uninsured workers and dependents.

The particularly high cost of insurance coverage makes it difficult for many employers to offer this voluntary benefit to their employees. Experience rating and lack of administrative economies of scale are obstacles for many small businesses. In addition, insurance companies protect themselves from large claims by practicing medical underwriting and then denying or overpricing coverage for individuals

Figure 3-6

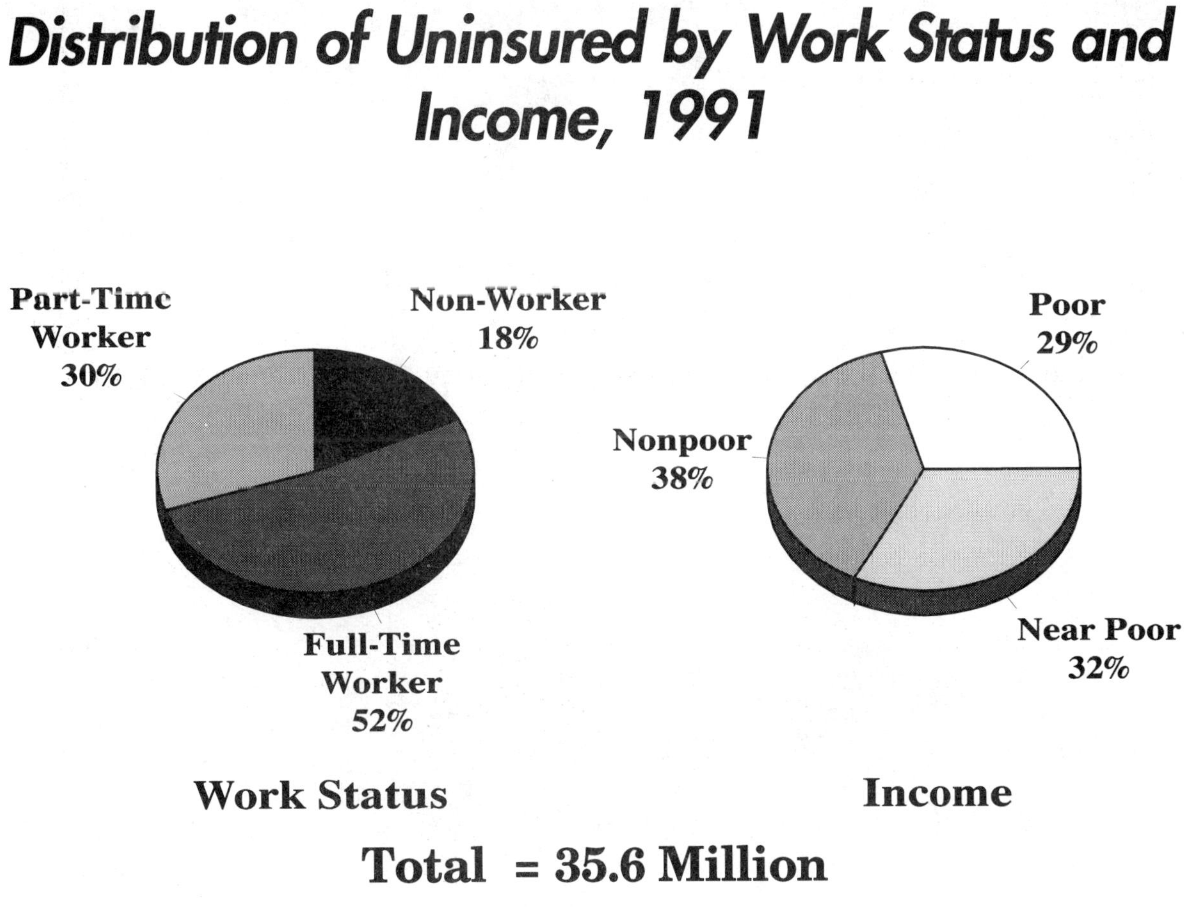

Source: Kaiser Commission on the Future of Medicaid. ***Analysis of the Current Population Survey***, **1992; Kaiser Foundation Health Reform Project, 1993.**

or small groups deemed high-risk. Between one and two million Americans are medically uninsurable because of preexisting conditions[18].

Though most uninsured Americans are in families with incomes above the poverty level, 29 percent of the uninsured are poor. Today, nearly a third of the 32 million non-elderly people in households with incomes below the federal poverty level are without insurance, compared with 9 percent of those with incomes of 200 percent of poverty or greater (Figure 3-7).

Even the poor who work all year at a full-time job are not guaranteed employer-based coverage. Only a quarter of full-year, full-time workers and their families with incomes below the poverty level received employer coverage, compared with 84 percent of the working population with incomes above 200 percent of poverty in 1991[16]. This disparity reflects the fact that poor individuals are more likely

Figure 3-7

Distribution of the Non-Elderly Population, by Health Insurance, 1991

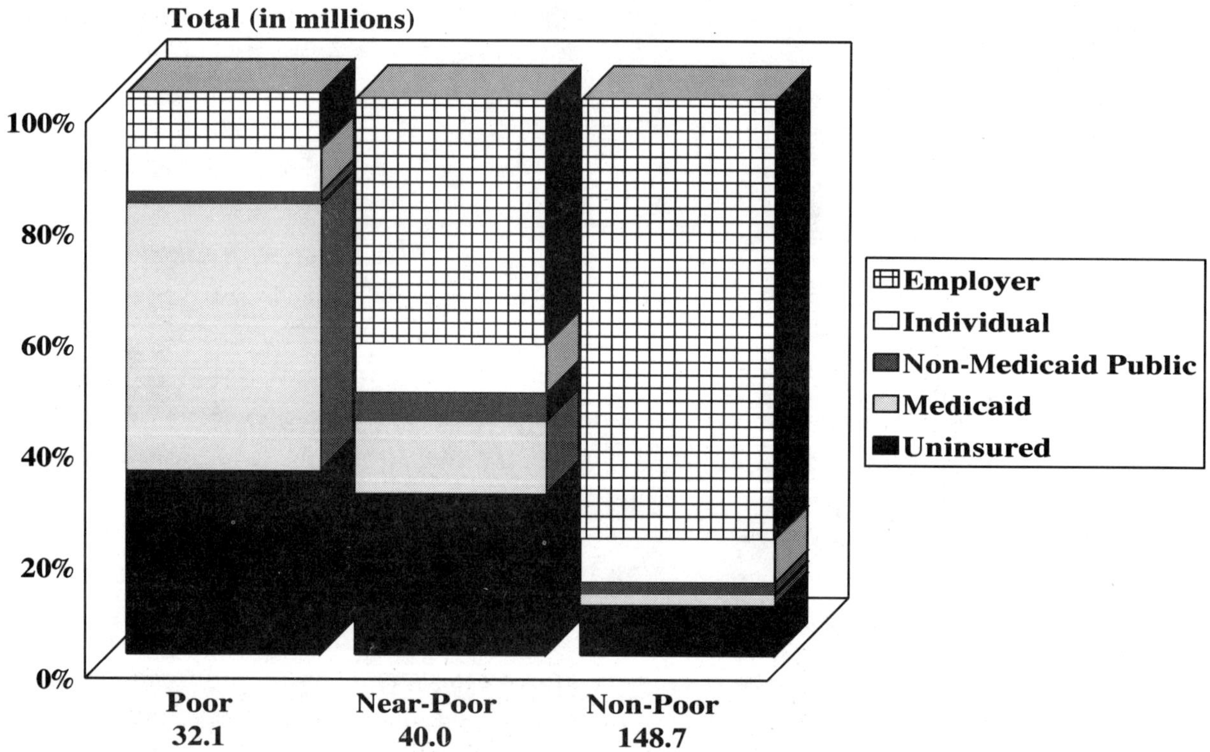

Source: Kaiser Commission on the Future of Medicaid. *Analysis of the Current Population Survey*, 1992; Kaiser Foundation Health Reform Project, 1993.

than the non-poor to work in low-wage and small firms that do not supply health insurance.

Medicaid does not provide full coverage for the population in poverty. Though one in ten Americans receives Medicaid benefits, the program still covers less than half (47 percent) of the poor non-elderly population. Congressionally mandated expansions have broadened Medicaid coverage to two-thirds of all poor children and to pregnant women with incomes below 133 percent of poverty, but most poor single individuals and childless couples are categorically ineligible for Medicaid unless they qualify as disabled under the Supplemental Security Income (SSI) welfare program. Moreover, state variations in income and resource levels for eligibility for Medicaid coverage result in residential differentials in the percentage of the poor covered by Medicaid.

Underlying these differences in coverage by income and employment are regional and racial differences. Minorities are more likely to be uninsured than whites, regardless of their income. In 1991, 33 percent of Hispanics and 22 percent of blacks were uninsured, compared with 12 percent of whites. The southern states also account for a disproportionate share of the uninsured; one-third of the American population lives in the southern states, but residents of these states account for 42 percent of the uninsured population[17].

Lack of insurance coverage has serious consequences for access to care for the uninsured population. Without health insurance coverage or ready cash, many of the uninsured do not obtain preventive care and have to turn to the hospital emergency room when a medical emergency arises. Often care is not received until conditions have worsened, resulting in more serious illness and expensive treatment when care is ultimately rendered. As shown in Figure 3-8, lack of insurance can mean going without needed care. A third (34 percent) of the uninsured report that they did not obtain needed medical care, in contrast to 8 percent of the privately insured population and 10 percent of the poor on Medicaid[19].

NON-FINANCIAL BARRIERS TO ACCESS

While many of the differentials in utilization of services reflect financial barriers, others relate to the uneven supply of providers across communities in the United States. Access to care is frequently limited in inner cities, rural areas, and the South by an inadequate supply of primary care providers. It is estimated that nearly 11,000 primary care physicians would be needed to help underserved areas reach the government's target rate of one physician for every 2,000 residents[20]. In 1993, 70 percent of all U.S. counties were considered medically underserved. This classification is based on high rates of low birth weight, infant death, reported cases of immunizable diseases, hepatitis, tuberculosis, and reported deaths from pneumonia and heart disease, which indicate depressed health status, along with a shortage of primary care physicians, or both. Some 43 million Americans of the 51 million considered at risk for underservice because of their low income and lack of adequate health insurance live in these counties. There are 11 states, mostly in

Figure 3-8

The Uninsured Are More Likely To Go Without Needed Medical Care

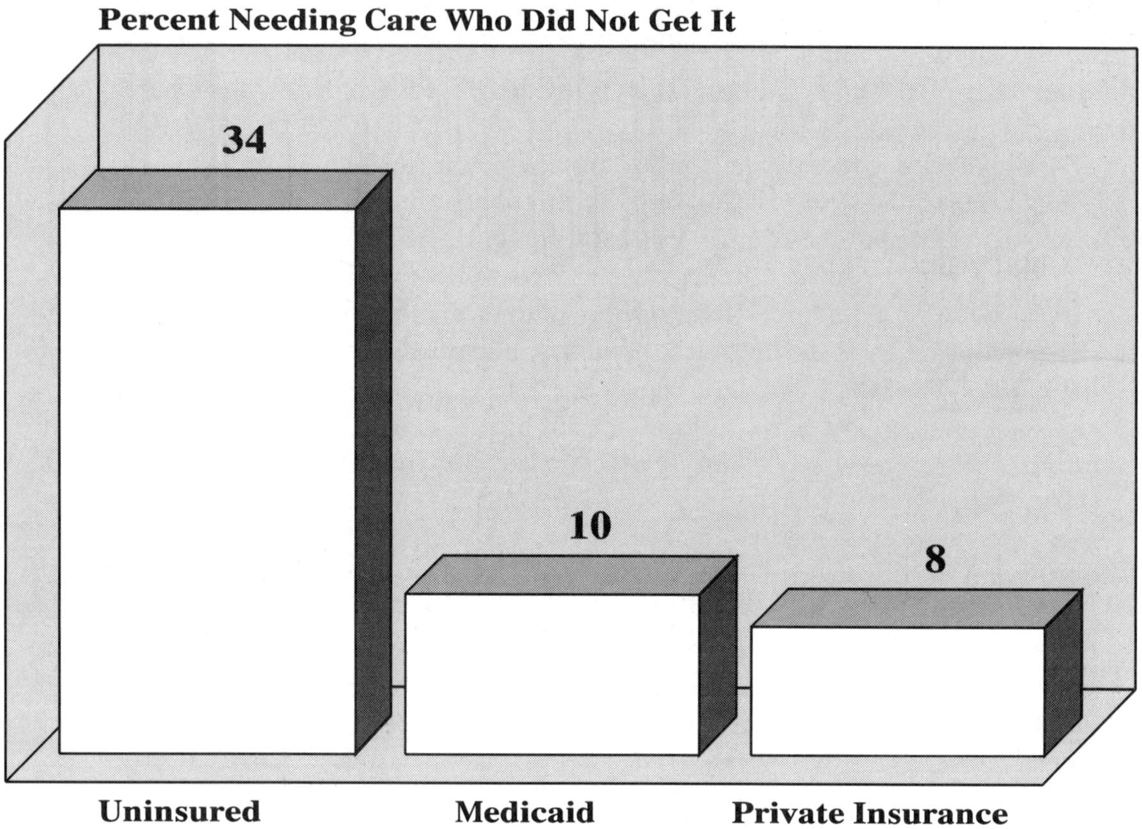

Source: Kaiser Foundation Health Reform Project. Kaiser/Commonwealth/Harris Poll, 1993.

the southern region of the United States, where at least 20 percent of the state's total population are medically underserved[21] (See Figure 3-9).

The lack of providers in medically underserved areas stems from inadequate financial means within the community to attract and maintain physicians and other health professionals. In inner-city areas, an inadequate supply of primary care providers often results in increased reliance on institutional providers, most notably the clinics and outpatient departments of public and teaching hospitals in the city. In rural areas, the inadequate provider base often means long travel times to obtain care and postponed care that contributes to more serious illness.

Many rural areas are faced with a shortage of health care providers, a declining population, eroding economies, and hospital closures. The combination of high poverty rates and a shortage of health care providers contributes to rural residents receiving fewer physician and hospital services than urban residents[22]. Problems related to persistent poverty, unemployment, violence, and drug use in urban communities accentuate the access difficulties in the inner cities. Other non-financial barriers in both areas include language/cultural barriers and a lack of adequate transportation. These problems combined with the lack of insurance coverage for millions of Americans focuses a significant share of the responsibility of providing care on facilities where insurance cards are not required for entry.

Many of the uninsured rely on public hospitals, community health centers, and local health departments as their sole source of available care. Federally supported health care delivery programs supplement insurance coverage by developing health care resources in inner-city and rural areas where poverty rates are high and the supply of providers of care is inadequate. These programs put resources into underserved areas and provide a source of care for many of the uninsured. In 1991, more than 600 community and migrant health centers provided preventive and primary care to six million medically underserved children and adults, regardless of their insurance status or ability to pay[23].

Figure 3-9

Percentage of Population Living in Medically Underserved Areas, 1990

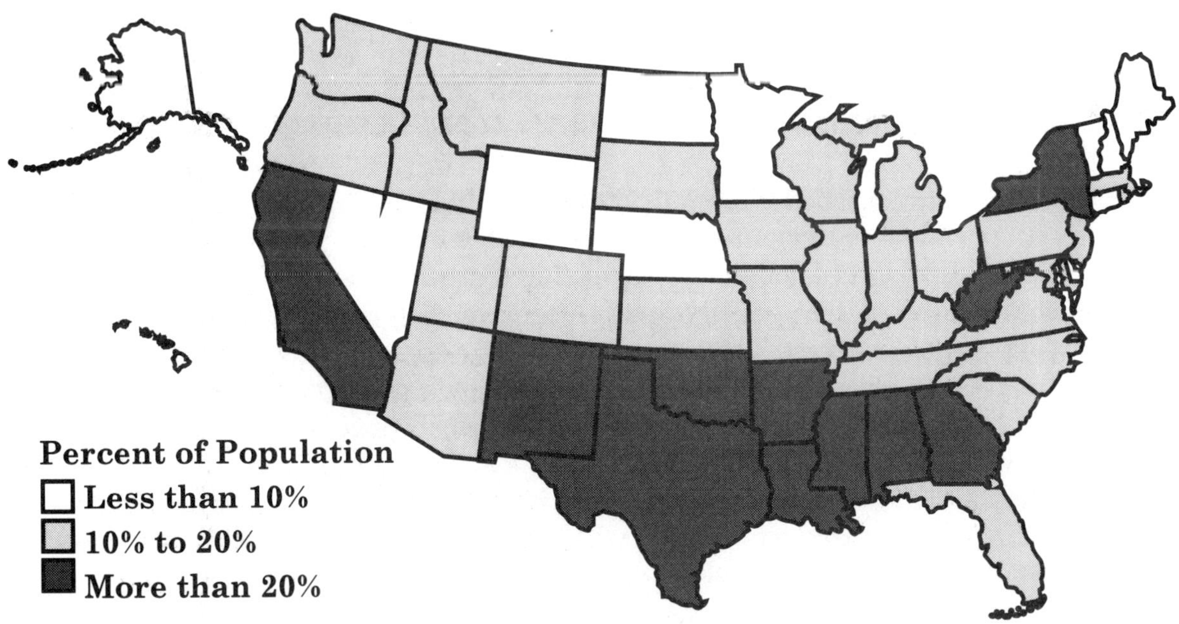

Note: Alaska is treated as a single area in this study.

Source: National Association of Community Health Centers, March 1993

Other public providers, including more than 1,200 public hospitals and 2,932 local health departments, also provide preventive and acute care to medically indigent individuals with no other resources. More than 400 school-based clinics provide a range of care and health education to teenagers in predominantly low-income neighborhoods. Other safety net programs serving disadvantaged populations include the federal Maternal and Child Health Block Grant given to states to provide medical care to low-income children, pregnant women, and mothers; 2,310 community mental health centers; and family planning centers that provide gynecological exams and reproductive counseling to people of any income level.

The National Health Services Corps (NHSC) is the federal government's primary means of recruiting physicians to rural and inner city areas suffering from health personnel shortages. Through loan repayment agreements and NHSC scholarships, the NHSC plays an essential role in moving primary care physicians into the most severely underserved areas.

These safety net providers are faced with a growing demand, and highly constrained resources. The local governments in communities with a large share of uninsured persons are also feeling the strain. Locally funded public hospitals and health centers inevitably incur major financial deficits. The health system is in stress, and millions of Americans still lack access to care.

IMPROVING ACCESS TO CARE UNDER HEALTH CARE REFORM

When Americans use the health care system, they are generally pleased with the care they receive. In 1993, 81 percent of Americans polled about their attitudes on health care reported that they were satisfied with their personal care[18]. Yet, when asked their opinions on the overall health system, only 13 percent report that they are satisfied. This gap between satisfaction with personal care and satisfaction with the system presents the true challenge for health care reform — to preserve what is liked about our system and fix the problems.

What Americans are upset about and what is leading the call for reform of the health system is the way in which care is financed and the cost of paying for that care. Americans fear the loss of health insurance coverage when they switch jobs, lose their jobs, or get sick. They worry that health insurance will not be there when they need it the most. They worry about the rising cost of paying their premiums for health insurance coverage and the costs they incur as part of health insurance — the required cost sharing on covered services — as well as the costs for care not covered under insurance, such as long term care. Policymakers have increasingly joined in the call for reform as more and more of our gross domestic product (GDP) and budget goes to health care at the same time the number of uninsured Americans grows.

The goal of health reform is, thus, to improve access to care and insurance protection while providing constraint on overall spending for health care services. Reform can, however, be accomplished by several different routes, including a transition to government-sponsored insurance or an expansion of the current employer-based system.

A government-sponsored national health insurance program that provides public coverage for all Americans and consolidates payment for health services under a single payer to achieve universal coverage and cost control is one option. This approach would ultimately shift the financing responsibilities from the current split between the public and private sectors to a largely government-financed and government-managed system. This would represent a major restructuring of public and private responsibilities for health care financing, but would be the most direct way to fill the most egregious cracks in today's system.

Under a single payer approach, universal coverage with standard benefits and payment policies would remove the financial barriers to care experienced in the current system. The Medicare program, our single payer approach for coverage of the elderly and disabled, has had notable success in reducing differences in access to care within the elderly population. Among America's elderly, differentials persist between urban and rural areas, but the variations by income have been largely overcome[21].

However, moving to a single payer system would require substantial new taxes. Concern over government financing and control of the health care system leads other reformers to seek immediate solutions to correct the notable problems in the health system; solutions that don't require total restructuring.

Building on the existing employer-based insurance system by providing public assistance for low-income people and low-wage industries and requiring employers to fill in the gaps is viewed as a more moderate and less disruptive approach to health care reform. While considerably more complex and less centralized than a single payer national health insurance program, this approach does not require the substantial shift in financing to the public sector of the single payer system, because employers are left responsible for collecting and contributing to the health insurance premiums of their employees. It does, however, require new responsibilities for employers that do not now offer insurance to their employees and requires a public plan to fill in the gaps in coverage for the non-working population and to assist low-wage businesses with the cost of health care coverage.

The Clinton Administration has selected the latter model for providing universal coverage to the American people. The Clinton plan requires all employers to contribute to the cost of insurance premiums for employees and their dependents and provides federal subsidies to offset the costs for low-income individuals and low-wage employers. All Americans would be insured; those lacking an attachment to the work force would be covered by public funds. Since all Americans regardless of employment status would be guaranteed a comprehensive benefit package that emphasizes primary and preventive health care services, the problems of no or inadequate insurance would be eliminated. Cost control would be achieved by introducing more competition into the health system by creating purchasing cooperatives, called health alliances, to negotiate with health plans to purchase the standard benefit package for the lowest cost.

What do these reform plans portend for improving access to health services in America? If health care reform ensuring universal insurance coverage for all Americans is enacted, it will provide the critical first step toward eliminating financial barriers to care for millions of Americans. With an insurance card and coverage under a health plan, all Americans will have the entry ticket to the health system. The fear of being uninsured and unable to afford care will be removed for all Americans, but especially for the Americans most at risk of being uninsured today — low-wage workers, minorities, and the poor.

If health care reform providing a standard comprehensive set of benefits, including preventive and primary care services, is enacted, it will help ensure that the coverage provided will encourage early treatment and preventive care. Comprehensive coverage should help encourage more Americans to seek care or screening that can reduce the later incidence of serious disease. By eliminating financial barriers, a comprehensive benefit plan should make preventive care more readily available for today's low-income and uninsured population and help reduce differentials in use of care by income, race, and residence.

However, even the most sweeping and comprehensive reform of the American health insurance system will not be sufficient to eliminate all the barriers to equitable access to care among some subgroups of the American population. Targeted programs for resource development need to be coupled with improved financing in underserved areas to ensure that providers are available to inner-city and rural residents. Continued funding and expansion of public health programs and the community and migrant health center programs are important adjuncts to health insurance reform, because even with universal coverage, problems of access will persist.

The health care reform agenda of universal coverage, comprehensive benefits, and targeted resource development activities represents a good strategy to reduce major inequities in the American health care system. All Americans ultimately bear the burden for the care of the uninsured under today's system. The choice before the nation now is whether to pay up-front and directly for covering the uninsured or to continue indirectly paying for their care through subsidies to fiscally troubled health facilities, higher insurance premiums, and increased hospital costs to cover the cost of charity care and paying for the ill health caused by neglect and inadequate access to primary and preventive services.

The most pragmatic approach would appear to be to provide health insurance coverage to the uninsured and use targeted approaches to improve resource distribution and address remaining access differentials. Whether the inequities in access to care in today's health care system will deepen or disappear will largely be determined by the outcome of our national health care reform debate.

REFERENCES

1. United Nations Children's Fund. *The State of the World's Children, 1993*. Oxford University Press, 1993.

2. Kaiser Commission on the Future of Medicaid. *Analysis of the National Medical Expenditure Survey, 1987*, 1993.

3. Barker PR, R Manderschield, G Hendershot, S Jack, C Scheonborn, and I Goldstrom. *Serious Mental Illness and Disability in the Adult Household Population: United States, 1989. Advance Data* No. 218. National Center for Health Statistics, 1992.

4. Greater New York March of Dimes. *Infants at Risk, 1990-1991 Statistics*. May 1992 presentation.

5. National Center for Health Statistics. Estimates from the National Health Interview Survey, 1991.

6. Agency for Toxic Substances and Disease Registry. *The Nature and Extent of Lead Poisoning in Children in the United States: A Report to Congress, 1988*

7. Mathematica Policy Research Inc. *Analysis of the 1990 National Health Interview Survey*, 1993.

8. National Center for Health Statistics. *Health, United States, 1992*. Public Health Service, 1993.

9. Starfield B, S Shapiro, J Weiss, K Liang, K Ra, D Paige, X Wang. Race, Family Income and Low Birthweight. *American Journal of Epidemiology* 132(10), 1991: 1167-74.

10. United States Department of Health and Human Services, press release, September 15, 1993.

11. James Bell Associates. *On the Move: Innovations in Rural Health Care Delivery*. Report prepared for the Office of Health Policy, HHS, 1989.

12. Lieu T, P Newacheck, and M McManus. Race, Ethnicity, and Access to Ambulatory Care Among U.S. Adolescents. *American Journal of Public Health* 83(7), 1993: 960-65.

13. Blendon R, L Aiken, H Freeman, and C Corey. Access to Medical Care for Black and White Americans. *Journal of the American Medical Association* 261(2), 1989: 278-80.

14. Kaiser Commission on the Future of Medicaid. *Medicaid at the Crossroads*, November 1992.

15. Bureau of the Census. *Poverty in the United States: 1990*. Current Population Reports. Series P-60, No. 175., U.S. Department of Commerce, 1991.

16. Kaiser Commission on the Future of Medicaid. *Analysis of the Current Population Survey, 1992*, 1993.

17. Smith M and D Nuschler. *Health Insurance Coverage: Characteristics of the Insured and Uninsured Populations in 1991*. Congressional Research Service, U.S. Congress, April 1993.

18. Bodenheimer T. Private Insurance Reform in the 1990s: Can It Solve The Health Care Crisis? *International Journal of Health Services* 22(2), 1992: 197-215.

19. Kaiser Foundation Health Reform Project, The Commonwealth Fund, and Louis Harris and Associates. *The Americans and Their Health Insurance II Survey*. Administered September 10, 1993.

20. Collins S. Desperate for Doctors, America's Poor Need More Health Care, Not Just More Health Insurance. *U.S. News and World Report*, September 20, 1993.

21. National Association of Community Health Centers. *Lives in the Balance: The Health Status of America's Medically Underserved Populations*, March 1993.

22. Rowland D, B Lyons, and J Edwards. Medicaid: Health Care for the Poor in the Reagan Era. *Annual Review of Public Health* 9, 1988: 427-50.

23. National Association of Community Health Centers. *Community and Migrant Health Centers, Critical Components of Health Reform*, 1993.

CHAPTER 4

Curbing Health Costs: Many Tried, None Succeeded

Cathy Tokarski and Janet Firshein

For decades, solutions to the nation's spiraling health care costs have eluded the nation's top policymakers and economists. Despite efforts to control spending through regulatory and market-oriented strategies, by 1993, health care spending reached nearly $900 billion and accounted for 14 percent of the nation's gross domestic product (GDP).

By the early 1990s, it was clear that health costs were sapping the nation's economic strength, preventing the U.S. from rebounding from a persistent recession and hampering businesses' ability to compete at home and abroad. Despite the $3,358 per person spent on health care in the U.S. — the highest in the world — 37.4 million Americans remained without insurance, while millions of others remained in jobs primarily because of their fear of losing health insurance.[1]

In making the case for comprehensive health care reform, President Bill Clinton has identified the link between exploding health costs and the nation's lackluster economy and warned that unbridled health spending would render all efforts to reduce the bloated federal budget deficit in vain.

Clinton first publicly referred to health spending's drag on the economy just weeks after he won the Presidential election against incumbent George Bush. At a two-day economic summit in Little Rock, Arkansas on December 15 and 16, 1992, the new President-elect grew visibly exasperated when speaker after speaker pointed out the corrosive effect of health care costs on current and future federal spending.

Clinton, who had promised as a candidate to "focus like a laser beam" on the economy, concluded that unless he and Congress dealt aggressively with heath costs, the nation's economic vitality could never be fully restored. "We are just kidding each other," Clinton said, pounding his fist on the table. "We are all just sitting here making this up if we think we can fiddle around with the entitlements and all this other stuff and get control of this budget, if you don't do something on health care. It is a joke. It's going to bankrupt the country."

Nearly 11 months later, Clinton reiterated that message when delivering his 1,342-page health reform bill to Congress. "Rising health care costs are threatening our standard of living," he said in his October 27 letter to the leadership of the 103rd Congress. "The average American worker would be making $1,000 a year more today if health care accounted for the same proportion of wages and benefits as in 1975. Unless we act, health care costs will lower real wages by almost $600 per year by the end of the decade, and nearly one in every five dollars Americans spend will go to health care."

Clinton was not the first President to worry about health care's bottomless appetite for federal dollars. The galloping health inflation that followed the 1965 enactment of Medicare and Medicaid led federal policymakers to experiment with a variety of regulatory and competition-based approaches to cost containment, none of which had more than a limited effect.

REGULATORY RITUALS

Between 1965 and 1971, the six years following the enactment of Medicare and Medicaid, health care spending doubled, rising from nearly $42 billion to $82.3 billion, according to the Health Care Financing Administration (HCFA). In the decade before Medicare and Medicaid, the average rate of growth in health spending was about 8 percent a year; from 1966 to 1971, expenditures grew at 12 percent annually.[2] The cost-reimbursement system used to pay for Medicare and Medicaid was a driving force, along with the practice of most insurance plans to pay full charges.

Alarmed policymakers sought to control the increasing growth rate, and looked exclusively to regulatory solutions. The assumption throughout the 1970s was that "market forces were not capable of keeping costs within an appropriate range," wrote Duke University law professor Clark Havighurst."Providers were seen as autonomous and immune from price competition."[3] Calls for competitive approaches largely fell on deaf ears. Robert Schlenker and Nancy Shanks observed in an article examining the role of the private sector during that period, "The primary governmental response during the 1970s was to impose increasingly rigid regulatory constraints."[4]

The first major effort to clamp down on health costs occurred in 1971 when President Richard Nixon, facing double-digit inflation, singled out medical care for special treatment under a national wage and price control policy called "The Economic Stabilization Program." The Nixon Administration honed in on the health care sector, where prices and expenditures were rising faster than general inflation.[5] Under the Nixon policy, doctors' annual fees were held to a 2.5 percent increase; hospital charges could not rise more than 6 percent a year.

In 1973, controls were lifted for most components of the U.S. economy, but they continued to apply to the health industry for an additional year. That was the only period since 1965 during which health care expenditures grew at a slower rate than the rate of growth in the rest of the economy.

In a 1979 book, David Abernethy characterized the wage and price control program as a "mixed success."[2] The program moderated hospital cost inflation, he wrote, with price increases dropping by half. The stabilization program's policies had "no [lasting] effect" on hospital expenditures, according to a 1993 article in *HCFA Review*.[5]

Once the price controls were lifted in 1974, the short-lived cost-containment gains that had been won evaporated, and hospital and physician expenditures began to climb once again. The Council on Wage and Price Stability reported in 1976 that hospital service charges rose from 4.6 percent when controls were in effect to 14.6 percent immediately after controls were lifted. In 1975, hospital charges rose 13 percent. Physician fees, which had risen 4 percent under wage and price controls, grew nearly 13 percent immediately after they were lifted, and 11.8 percent in 1975 (see Figure 4-1).[6]

Regulatory controls over health spending did not completely thwart development of new forms of health delivery and financing. In a February 1971 message to Congress, Nixon introduced the notion of health maintenance organizations (HMOs) as a cornerstone of his national health insurance plan. Nixon's proposal envisioned a rapid expansion of these new delivery and financing systems as a major way to get control of health costs. The HMO solution had been proposed by Minneapolis pediatric neurologist Paul Ellwood, Jr., MD, then director of the American Rehabilitation Foundation. Ellwood favored a restructured delivery system that would shift away from the inflationary cost-based approach to a capitated payment to compensate providers for maintaining patients' health.

In 1971, 3.6 million Americans were enrolled in some 39 prepaid plans operating in the U.S., mostly in California, where Kaiser-Permanente, the country's first HMO, was based.[7] Nixon's goal was to help create 1,700 HMOs that would enroll 40 million people by 1976. By the end of the decade, he expected almost all Americans to belong to an HMO.[8]

It took Congress two years to pass the HMO Act of 1973. The Act was intended to bolster the formation of HMOs, but some provisions added to the bill during passage may have done more to hamper than spur their growth. While the Act offered federal grants and loans to encourage HMO development, it also stipu-

Figure 4-1

Trends in Annual Increases in Total Hospital Expenses Before, During, and After the Economic Stabilization Program (ESP): 1969-77

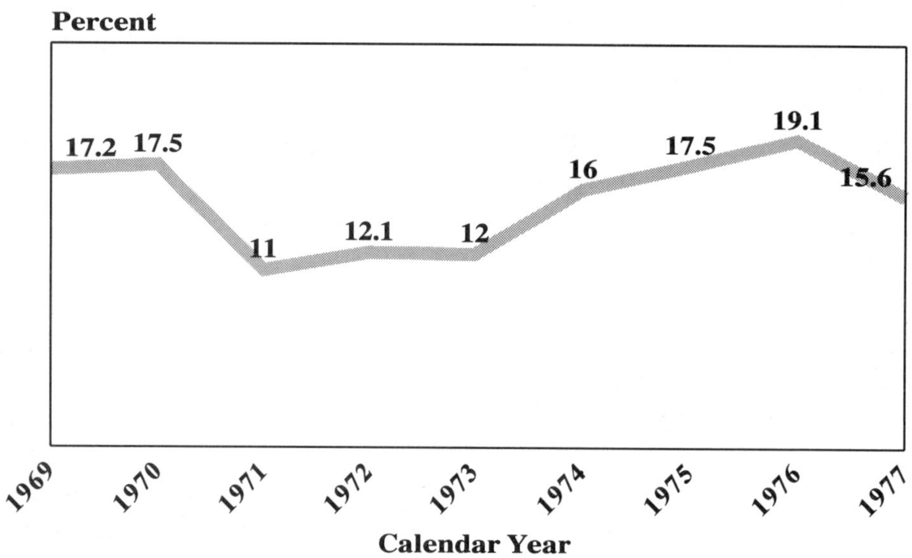

[1]ESP starts in August 1971.
[2]ESP ends in April 1974.
Source: American Hospital Association; National Panel Survey, Chicago, 1969-77.

lated how to organize and operate a plan. To get the federal seal of approval, HMOs had to offer certain types of services, charge community rates, and allow open enrollment for at least 30 days a year, regardless of an individual's health status. Traditional insurers were not subjected to the same standards, however.

The law that emerged from Congress was more limited than what Nixon had hoped for, mostly due to heavy lobbying by the American Medical Association, which feared that a proliferation of HMOs would impede doctors' economic independence. In the end, the Act that Nixon hoped would foster HMO growth "threatened to make HMOs the most heavily regulated part of the entire health care industry and less competitive with conventional health insurance."[8]

Between 1970 and 1974, another 124 HMOs began operating; between 1974 and 1978, the year the Act was improved, only 40 additional HMOs were formed.[7] The Act's restrictions, an economic downturn, and a delay in regulations that would have opened up the HMO market to employers all had a negative effect on HMO penetration.[9]

In 1972, Washington also took steps to staunch rising capital spending incurred by the hospital building craze and to curb unnecessary medical care by doctors. The 1972 Social Security Amendments authorized creation of professional standards review organizations (PSROs), state-wide physician-controlled review groups designed to control costs by reviewing the appropriateness of medical care provided under federal health programs.

But PSROs had a negligible effect on health spending because "by and large [they] lacked the gumption to take on their fellow physicians . . . and did not have the power to deny Medicare reimbursement to profligate providers," wrote former Health Education and Welfare (HEW) Secretary Joseph Califano, Jr.[10] "On the whole [PSROs] did little to check the rise in doctors' fees or to trim the number, intensity, or length of hospital stays."

Critics also noted that the program saved only about as much money as it cost to operate. "It appears unlikely that the influence of PSROs on Medicare outlays, even in the long run, will have more than a slight effect on health care expenditures," wrote Tufts University School of Medicine's William Schwartz, MD, in 1981.[11]

Another amendment to the Social Security law gave Nixon's HEW Department the power to enter into agreements with state health system planning agencies that wanted to review whether proposed major hospital capital expenditures were necessary. Under the Section 1122 review statute, HEW could withhold depreciation and other costs related to Medicare and Medicaid capital expenditures that were deemed superfluous by these agencies. But the certificate-of-need (CON) law had a negligible effect on controlling costs. "The consensus was that health planning had failed because the agencies had no power to enforce their decisions and were dominated by providers, on whom they depended for half their income," wrote Paul Starr.[8]

To strengthen health planning, Congress stepped in and passed a law in 1975 that gave states money to establish mandatory CON programs. The National Health Planning and Resource Development Act established some 205 health systems agencies (HSAs) governed by consumer boards. The HSAs were to collect data, establish health plans in their areas, and make CON recommendations. If a state did not have a program by the end of fiscal 1980, it could be denied federal funding. The 1975 health planning law signified a "more serious effort on the part of the federal government to influence state and local hospital supply decisions while maintaining at least the appearance of a decentralized system sensitive to local concerns."[12]

But intense lobbying by physicians and hospitals watered down the Act, which had originally included provisions to let states set payment rates, decertify health facilities, and regulate physician office equipment.

In the final version of the law, planning boards were not given any decision-making powers over capital spending projects. No effective sanctions or incentives were given to planning agencies to deny CON applications, and no caps were placed on the total volume of projects that could be approved. Boards had an incentive to approve projects because approval meant more services to the community and more jobs. The fiscal consequences of capital expansions were not directly felt by the taxpayers or employers, because costs were diffused broadly through Medicare, Medicaid and private insurance plans, which paid the costs indirectly through patient charges.[13]

Advocates of health planning "put a tremendous amount of expectations on what these agencies could do," said Brandeis University economist Stuart Altman in an October 1993 interview. "But we never gave them the power. . . . We gave them no authority," says Altman, who served in the Nixon Administration.

By the end of the 1970s, it became increasingly clear that CON laws "were ineffective in limiting the overall growth in hospital costs," concluded a 1991 report from HCFA. While CON has shown limited success at reducing costs for specific services, it did nothing to control the rate of growth in total costs, HCFA said.

The soaring inflation of the mid 1970s halted attempts to expand medical care and other social programs. Nixon's health policies had done little to stem the tide of rising health costs. Between 1965 and 1976, real per capita spending on health care grew 79 percent. Medicare outlays were projected to grow a whopping 50 percent in two years, from $17.8 billion in fiscal 1976 to about $26 billion in 1978.[14] In the last eight months of 1977, medical care inflation registered 12.1 percent, compared to 9.5 percent for other services.

CARTER COST CAPS

As a candidate, Georgia Governor Jimmy Carter had promised a national health insurance program. But when the Democrats took over the White House in 1976, budgetary pressures forced President Carter to mothball that pledge. Carter believed that cost containment was the "bedrock prerequisite for national health insurance," wrote Daniel Greenberg in 1978.[15]

At 8 percent of the GDP, U.S. health care spending exceeded that of most other countries that had a national health insurance system. At the start of the 1970s, when Canada introduced a comprehensive health plan, spending comprised about 7.3 percent of GDP in both Canada and the U.S. By the end of the 1970s, however, U.S. spending had climbed to 9 percent, while Canada's had reached 7.5 percent.

From 1975 through 1977, community hospital expenses grew at an annual rate that was 8.7 percent higher than general inflation. In public opinion polls, rising health care costs were among the top three domestic concerns of Americans.[2]

In 1977, Carter introduced legislation that would have imposed an all-payer system on hospital spending and placed limits on capital spending and physicians' fees. By the time Carter proposed his bill, hospital charges were rising 15.6 percent over their 1976 level, compared with a 6.9 percent inflation rate. Under the first version of the bill, Congress would have limited increases in hospital charges to 1.5 times the rate of growth in general inflation. Carter wanted to put a flat 9 percent cap on hospital rate hikes charged to public and private payers.

In an all-out effort to fend off federal price controls, the hospital industry launched a "voluntary effort" to hold down costs while Carter tried to get differing versions of his bill through Congress. By late 1978, the voluntary effort had met and exceeded its goal of cutting the increase in the rate of hospital spending by two percentage points. Industry leaders announced that the rate of increase had dropped 2.8 percentage points from January through August of that year.[8]

By March 1979, Carter reintroduced a watered down bill that would have imposed controls on hospitals only if their costs exceeded a predetermined specific limit; within five years, a commission would develop a permanent prospective payment system for hospitals. The hospital industry, led by the American Hospital Association and the Federation of American Hospitals, pulled out all the stops to kill the Carter measure, claiming the bill was too complex and unnecessary, given their "success" in holding down costs. By November 1979, Carter's bill had died in Congress. Shortly thereafter, hospital costs returned to their inflationary levels recorded before the voluntary efforts began (see Figure 4-2).

By the end of the decade, the evidence was mounting that the regulatory routes taken by Nixon and Carter had done little to hold down the rate of growth

Figure 4-2

Trends in Annual Increases in Total Hospital Expenses Before, During, and After the Voluntary Effort, in Response to Carter Hospital Cost-Containment Legislation: 1974-82

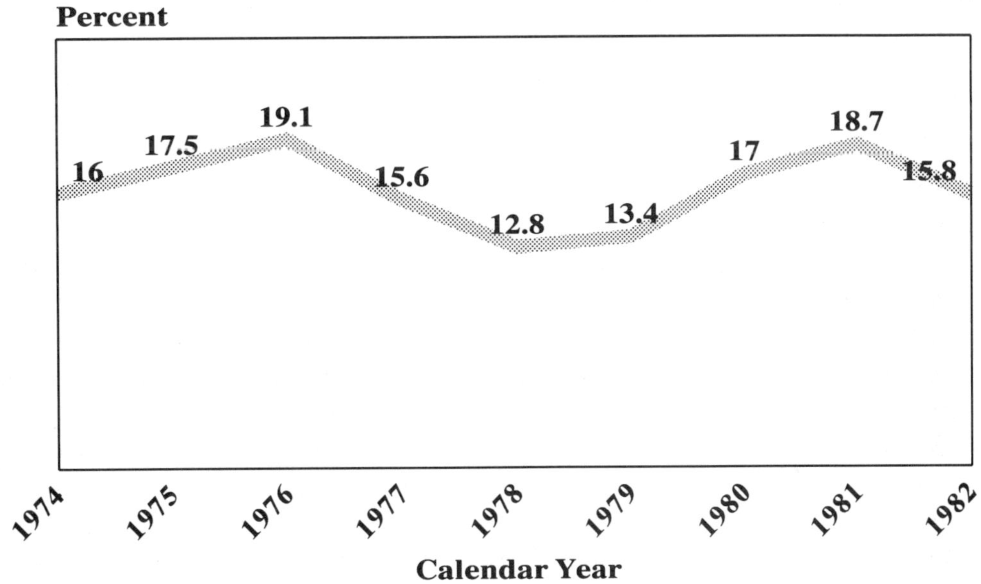

Hospital Cost-Containment Act of 1977 introduced in April 1977.
Hospital Cost-Containment Act of 1979 defeated in November 1979.
Source: American Hospital Association; National Panel Survey, Chicago, 1974-82.

in health spending. Nearly eight million Americans were enrolled in 217 HMOs, far below the 1,700 plans that the Nixon Administration had hoped for. Loopholes in health planning laws thwarted their ability to constrain health costs. HSA recommendations could be and often were overturned by the states. In Massachusetts, nursing homes that had been denied CON for expansions got exemptions for themselves.[8]

On the whole, the cost-containment initiatives of the 1970s were doomed because they were "based on a misconception of the cost problems and an overestimate of government's political ability to contest health care spending decisions taken in the private sector," said Duke's Havighurst. The defeat of the Carter cost caps "put an end at least for the time being, to federal efforts to solve cost problems by regulation."[3]

And, the anti-government rhetoric of California conservative Ronald Reagan, who vowed to voters that he would "get government off our backs," ensured that explicit regulation would not be the preferred route to controlling health costs in the 1980s.

PUTTING FAITH IN THE MARKET

The resounding victory of Republican challenger Ronald Reagan over incumbent Jimmy Carter in the 1980 election held enormous implications for the health care industry and the federal government's approach to controlling health costs. While Carter put his faith in broad regulatory tools to rein in both public and private health spending, the Reagan Administration was intent on containing federal expenditures only and letting the private sector control its destiny.

As Duke's Havighurst observed in 1985, "For the [Reagan] Administration, private health care costs are a private problem, to be solved not by regulation but by competitively inspired innovation in organizing delivery systems and in designing and administering health insurance coverage — all with the object of reintegrating, either contractually or organizationally, the financing and delivery of services. . . . The greatly stepped-up pace of change in the private sector since the defeat of the Carter cost-containment bill indicates, at the very least, that a federal policy of denying regulatory responsibility for private costs is not an irresponsible abdication."[3]

The first target of the Reagan Administration's efforts to control public spending was hospitals. Between 1968 and 1975, the annual growth in Medicare hospital reimbursement per beneficiary stood at 10.3 percent; between 1975 and 1984, it climbed to 15.8 percent a year.[16] Rapid spending growth in Medicare — as much as seven times the growth in the number of Medicare enrollees — prompted the program's trustees in 1981 to predict the Medicare Hospital Insurance Trust Fund would be bankrupt within 10 years if steps weren't taken to restrain the rate of increase or expand the funds flowing to its coffers.[17]

While the Carter Administration opted for all-payer limits on hospital reimbursement, the Reagan team believed a completely different system — one that relied on economic incentives — was needed to make Medicare a "prudent buyer." The interim step toward that goal was the enactment of the 1982 Tax Equity and Fiscal Responsibility Act (TEFRA), which created predetermined limits on hospital-specific Medicare operating costs per patient. The law also required the Secretary of the Department of Health and Human Services (HHS) to develop a legislative proposal for a new Medicare prospective payment system (PPS).

By the end of 1982, HHS Secretary Richard Schweiker delivered the recommendations to control hospital spending that Congress had called for.[18] His plan: the creation of Medicare prospective payment, which would reimburse hospitals based on nearly 500 "diagnosis-related groups," or DRGs, that would reflect the patient's condition as well as the hospital services and resources required to deliver the necessary care.

DRGs were not an untested concept. Ten years earlier, the federal government had signed an agreement with researchers at Yale University to test the idea, and the state of New Jersey had adopted DRGs in 1980 as the payment system used in its cost-containment program that applied to all payers.

Schweiker's plan, submitted to Congress on December 31, 1982, came just two months before the release of two more gloomy predictions about the fate of the Medicare and the Social Security trust funds. But the February 1983 prediction of the imminent bankruptcy of the Medicare Hospital Insurance Trust Fund was different from previous pessimistic reports issued each year by the trustees.

"The trustees said that if Congress didn't act, and act fast, the program would go belly up by 1987, a short five years away," said Richard Sorian in his 1988 book *The Bitter Pill*.[19] Pressure to avert Medicare's looming disaster was intensified by predictions that the Social Security trust fund also would run dry in five years, due to the 1972 law that indexed benefits to the Consumer Price Index, or the so-called "cost of living adjustment."

The twin fortunes of Schweiker's DRG proposal and the Social Security rescue plan were joined in early 1983, which, more than any external pressure to control health costs, ensured prospective payment's rapid adoption in October of that year. But passage didn't occur before Congress altered the proposal significantly, largely delaying the PPS' incentives for efficiency for about two years.

Recalled Sorian: "To smooth out some of the other rough edges in Schweiker's plan, [the House] Ways and Means and [Senate] Finance [Committees] each voted to phase in the system over four years. Separate rates would be set for urban and rural hospitals and for nine regions of the country. . . . A separate fund was created to pay additional amounts for particularly costly cases, known as 'outliers,' and payments for medical education costs and capital projects would continue to be made on a cost basis. The final bill exempted long-term care hospitals, children's hospitals, rehabilitation hospitals and psychiatric hospitals."[19] By using unaudited hospital reports to set payments, hospitals reaped double-digit profits from Medicare in the first few years of the new payment system.

In response, HHS and Congress, acting on recommendations from Congress' Prospective Payment Assessment Commission (ProPAC), tightened the federal spigot. The impact was dramatic: In the five years before PPS, Medicare expenditure for inpatient hospital care increased 93 percent in actual dollars and 45 percent after removing the effects of inflation. By 1989, the fifth year of PPS, Medicare expenditure increases slowed to 24 percent and only 3 percent after adjusting for inflation.[20]

Initial decreases in spending growth were due to a decline in hospital admissions, which fell to 393 per 1,000 patients in 1987, compared to a peak of 431 per 1,000 in 1983. But while the growth in Medicare payments to hospitals has slowed since PPS began, hospital costs have returned to nearly the same rate of growth — between 8 and 10 percent — recorded before the payment system was enacted. "Since costs are increasing substantially faster than payments, many hospitals are now experiencing financial losses from treating Medicare patients."[20] By 1990, hospitals' overall PPS margin fell below zero for the first time; ProPAC estimates that aggregate margins will fall to a negative 8.3 percent in 1992.

What caused the early promise of PPS to control hospital costs to fade? ProPAC Chairman Stuart Altman and Executive Director Donald Young posit several factors. "The PPS incentive to generate a profit by controlling costs was overwhelmed by other, more powerful incentives. Competitive pressures have forced hospitals to provide a full line of the most up-to-date services and technologies, even if they are not economical, to compete with other hospitals on community service, prestige, and perceived quality of care. Hospitals also rely on physicians to admit patients, and administrators do not want to antagonize physicians by cutting the use of resources. In addition, PPS and physician incentives are not aligned, with physicians continuing to be rewarded for providing more, not fewer services."[20]

CHANGING PHYSICIAN BEHAVIOR

Restraining the increases in physician services paid for by Medicare has proven to be an equally daunting task. When Congress launched Medicare in 1965, it set physician payments at either a doctor's actual or customary charge or the prevailing charge in a locality, whichever was lower. Surgeons were more generously compensated than physicians who performed diagnostic work.

But like cost-based reimbursement for hospitals, fee-for-service payments to doctors created cost nightmares. Between 1980 and 1991, costs for physician services in public and private programs jumped from $42 billion to $148 billion, an increase of 252.4 percent.[21] Under Medicare Part B, which pays for physician services, costs increased from $10.7 billion in 1980 to $46.4 billion in 1991. Because physician services have a strong influence on trends in overall health costs, the rising Medicare costs — which more than tripled on a per-enrollee basis in the 1980s — sent policymakers scrambling for solutions.

In 1984, the federal government froze fees for physician services for 15 months; the policy was extended an additional seven months for physicians who did not accept assignment (or Medicare's limits on charges) for patients. The dramatic step had little effect on curbing physician spending, however: the number of Medicare Part B services provided increased by 11.6 percent between 1984 and 1985 and by a whopping 15.3 percent and 17.6 percent in the subsequent two years.[22] Equally disturbing, physician charges per beneficiary skyrocketed by 30 percent between 1983 and 1986.[23]

Many who analyzed this troublesome result concluded that it was due primarily to a trend by physicians to perform more services or to increase the intensity of services provided to patients. Charges by physicians varied according to specialty, with surgeons accounting for 9 percent of the increase, while gastroenterologists contributed 73 percent.[23] Other factors that could have played a role, albeit a less significant one, in the acceleration of physician services included the rapid advances in outpatient surgery and reduced out-of-pocket prices for beneficiaries.

To counteract these trends, in 1989 Congress enacted a fee schedule based on the relative costs of services performed by physicians that took effect on January 1, 1992. A two-year study headed by the Harvard School of Public Health's William Hsiao produced a resource-based relative value scale (RBRVS) for physician payments.

RBRVS formed the basis of the new physician fee schedule. It factors in differences in physicians' time required to render services, practice costs, and malpractice premiums. In addition, Congress required the issuance of volume performance standards for physicians to discourage them from offsetting the effects of any cuts in fees by increasing patient visits or the intensity of services performed.[24]

Doctors' groups agreed to go along with payment reform partly because policymakers promised that RBRVS wouldn't decrease total Medicare payments to physicians in 1992. Congress also sought to soften the blow of the transition by stretching it over the five years between 1992 and 1996.

In its 1993 report to Congress, the Physician Payment Review Commission (PPRC) noted that RBRVS was having some of its intended effect. General and family practitioners, who typically earned the lowest salary among physicians, saw a 10 percent increase in payment rates, while surgical specialties had an 8 percent overall reduction.[25] PPRC Executive Director Paul Ginsburg said the system has "been successful in containing costs." Physicians did not increase the volume or intensity of services as much as Congress had predicted they would, which resulted in savings that were plowed back into the annual increase in physician payments for 1994.

Commonwealth Fund Executive Vice-President Karen Davis, a PPRC member, told the Senate Finance Committee in October 1993 that in the first 10 months of 1993, Medicare Part B outlays increased at about 5.6 percent, compared with 9.5 percent during the same period in 1992.

TIPPING THE SCALES

Two other factors had an enormous impact on the explosion of health costs in the late 1980s and early 1990s. Medicaid, largely untouched by cost-containment policies, consumed federal and state dollars at an ever-increasing rate; while cost shifting, an inadvertent result of federal cost containment, began to hit the private sector.

With policymakers focusing their energy on controlling Medicare costs, Medicaid spending was growing at nearly 15 percent a year by the mid 1980s. Between 1965 and 1980, states had been generous in offering optional eligibility and benefit expansions under the health care program for poor Americans. By the late 1970s, Medicaid covered three-quarters of poor Americans. But a deep recession coupled with the conservative backlash that swept Ronald Reagan into office kicked off a decade-long battle involving the White House, Congress, and the nation's governors over what Medicaid should cover and how its costs should be paid.

In 1981, Reagan pushed Congress to pass cuts in welfare and Medicaid programs, trimming nearly $1 billion in spending and one million beneficiaries from Medicaid rolls. In response, Congress, led by Representative Henry Waxman (D-CA), passed a series of laws starting in 1985 requiring states to cover more pregnant women and children, reforming nursing home regulations, and expanding screening and diagnostic services for children.

Congressional mandates, coupled with rapid medical inflation and growing Medicaid enrollment, caused total federal and state Medicaid spending to hit $71 billion by fiscal 1990, nearly three times 1980's level of $26 billion, according to the National Governors' Association (NGA). In 1990, Medicaid expenditures grew by 18 percent from 1989's level; by 1991, expenditures grew 27 percent from 1990's level. At its annual meeting in August 1989, the NGA asked Congress for a two-year moratorium on Medicaid expansions. The state leaders suggested that federal policymakers focus their energies on comprehensive health care reform and covering the nation's uninsured.[26]

In the meantime, states began using some creative accounting ploys to gain access to millions of new federal Medicaid dollars. Derided by Bush Administration Budget Director Richard Darman as "scams," Medicaid voluntary donation programs and provider tax plans inflated the amount of the state's contribution, which was then matched by federal dollars by as much as a three-to-one ratio.

Richard Kusserow, then HHS Inspector General, issued a report July 25, 1991, on the use of Medicaid provider tax and donation programs, calling them "an uncontrollable virus spreading from state to state" that could "bankrupt" Medicaid. Kusserow noted that these programs would cost the federal government $3.8 billion in fiscal 1991. By fiscal 1993, he predicted, 39 such programs would cost the U.S. $12.1 billion.[27] Donation plans were especially popular in southern states like Alabama and Georgia, where federal matching rates reach 80 percent. In fiscal 1991, 11 states used a voluntary donation program to increase their Medicaid match, reaping a total of $1.7 billion.[28]

A September 1993 report from the Henry J. Kaiser Family Foundation's Commission on the Future of Medicaid noted that increased state use of provider taxes and donations along with disproportionate share payments to hospitals were the "major factors driving the rate of Medicaid spending growth to an all-time high between 1991 and 1992."[29] But a law passed in 1991, strongly backed by the Bush Administration, curtailed state use of these strategies and is expected to slow the growth rate significantly. "Early reports of 1993 Medicaid spending suggest that the legislation may have effectively reduced state use of these strategies," according to the Kaiser report.

In August 1993, when HCFA issued final regulations implementing the 1991 tax and donation law, the agency claimed that forcing states to meet new standards for tax and donation activities will limit the federal portion of Medicaid to $14.4 billion in FY94, $18 billion in FY95, and $22 billion in FY96. New rules for state spending for disproportionate share programs will limit the federal government's contribution to $10.7 billion in FY94, $11.7 billion in FY95, and $13.1 billion in FY96.

THE COST-SHIFTING EXERCISE

As margins flattened, then dipped into the red, hospitals looked for ways to recoup the revenue they lost as a result of federal efforts to restrain payments and from the mounting costs of uncompensated and unsponsored hospital care. A 1993 study by the Employee Benefits Research Institute estimated that cost shifting — hospitals' practice of charging private payers more in order to recoup their Medicare and Medicaid losses — had reached $21.5 billion in 1991.[30]

A 1992 study by ProPAC outlined the pervasiveness of the problem. According to the analysis, Medicare covered about 90 percent of patients' hospital costs, while Medicaid covered 80 percent. Most, but not all of the hospitals that needed to recoup additional revenues to sustain their operations were able to shift their costs onto other payers, ProPAC found.

But this phenomenon, denounced by corporate America, whose profits were being drained by the cost of health benefits, is now more difficult for hospitals to sustain. The ability to cost-shift depends on the extent of managed care in a hospital market, the EBRI report said. "In areas with relatively few hospital competitors and little PPO or HMO activity, Medicaid and Medicare price reductions and uncompensated care burdens will be partially absorbed by higher prices paid by private payers. In more price-sensitive markets and in markets in which prices to private payers have risen to those commensurate with the market power of local hospitals, such cost shifting will not occur," the report said.

THE CLINTON PHILOSOPHY

With more than two decades of cost-containment schemes and their mixed results to guide them, Clinton health advisers didn't seem eager to push either a purely regulatory or a purely competitive scheme. In a 1993 book *Mandate for Change,* which has influenced major policy initiatives of the Clinton Administration, a chapter by Jeremy Rosner warned of the pitfalls of an either-or approach to health care policy.

"Many on the political right . . . suggest 'the market' without fundamental reform, can cure the health care system's ills. Some on the left suggest 'the market' does not apply to health care, and so government must step in to set limits on health care prices, and perhaps to become the sole health insurer as well," Rosner wrote.

"This is a false choice. The proper role for government, on health care and elsewhere, is neither to let broken markets run amok, nor to replace the market with bureaucratic mechanisms that set prices and allocate resources. . . . The new Administration's goal should be to achieve comprehensive health care reform and universal coverage without imposing public price controls and bureaucratic budgeting mechanisms on the U.S. health care system."[31]

While President Clinton's health reform team was guided by those goals of balancing regulation with market forces, critics contend the legislation that Clinton submitted to Congress in October 1993 contains plenty of the "bureaucratic budgeting mechanisms" Rosner warned against.

The Health Security Act sets the ambitious goals of lowering the rate of medical inflation to match the increase in the CPI after the year 2000 while providing health insurance to all Americans. To bring down health costs, the bill targets both public and private health spending through a series of regulatory and quasi-competitive mechanisms and incentives to bring about changes in consumer and provider behavior.

The insurance purchasing clout of large and small employers, individuals, and Medicaid recipients would be tapped through the formation of new regional health alliances, which would encourage a greatly expanded use of managed care and discourage inflationary fee-for-service medicine. At least one health alliance would exist in every state. Under the bill, regional alliances are "designed to encourage competition" but nonetheless have the power to reject a health plan if its premiums are more than 20 percent higher than the average of the other plans in an area.

A seven-person National Health Board, which will have broad powers to oversee the new health care system while remaining accountable to the President, would calculate and enforce the health insurance premium targets. Health plans could not exceed these targets.

The Administration would control soaring Medicare costs by squeezing payments to hospitals, physicians, and other providers; new cost controls would be slapped on drug manufacturers, who stand to prosper from a new prescription drug benefit. Medicare beneficiaries would not be required to enroll in health alliances at first, but the Clinton bill would encourage states to broaden use of managed care among the elderly.

By guaranteeing health insurance to every U.S. citizen, Clinton officials say costs will begin to temper. Instead of turning to high-cost emergency room care, currently uninsured individuals will have a "health security card" that entitles them to health care. Patients would be encouraged to seek less costly, preventive health services through their alliance-sponsored health plans instead of waiting until they need expensive hospital care.

The federal government would make it easier for some hospitals and physicians to form networks and other types of health care arrangements that would prevent costly duplication of hospital buildings, medical equipment, and services.

The Administration says its plan would strike the proper balance between the regulation that marked health policy in the 1970s and the competitive strategies favored in the 1980s.

"Advocates of both purer government intervention and purer competition-based strategies may object to such a hybrid," wrote Clinton adviser Walter Zelman in late 1993.[32] "So too, may cynics who view the hybrid as a political construct aimed at achieving a lowest common denominator political compromise. But as its architects will assert, the Clinton plan's mix of government intervention and market-based reform resulted more from policy than political considerations. That mix may be good politics, but it is also good policy."

Melissa Jee contributed research to this chapter.

REFERENCES

1. Congressional Budget Office. *Projections of National Health Expenditures: 1993 Update*. October 1993.
2. Abernethy DS and DA Pearson. *Regulating Hospital Costs: The Development of Public Policy*. AUPHA Press, 1979: 16, 56.
3. Havighurst CC. The Debate Over Health Care Cost-Containment Regulation: The Issues and the Interests, in *Incentives vs Controls in Health Policy, Broadening the Debate*, Jack Meyer, ed. The American Enterprise Institute for Public Policy Research, 1985: 9, 11, 12.
4. Schlenker RE and NH Shanks. The Private Sector and Competition in Health Care Markets. *Journal of Health Politics, Policy and Law* 8 (3), Fall 1983.
5. Gold M, K Chu, S Felt, M Harrington, and T Lake. Effects of Selected Cost-Containment Efforts: 1971-1993. *Health Care Financing Review* 14 (3), Spring 1993: 183, 186.
6. The Council on Wage and Price Stability. *The Problem of Rising Health Care Costs*. Staff Report, Executive Office of the President, April 1976.
7. Falkson JL. HMOs: A Look Back, A Look Ahead. *Hospitals*, August 16, 1979: 86-94.
8. Starr P. *The Social Transformation of American Medicine*. Basic Books Inc., 1982: 396, 401, 412, 416.
9. Strumpf GB, F Seubold, and M Arrill. Health Maintenance Organizations 1971-1977: Issues and Answers. *Journal of Community Health* 4 (1), Fall 1978.
10. Califano JA. *America's Health Care Revolution, Who Lives? Who Dies? Who Pays?* Random House, 1986: 145.
11. Schwartz W. The Regulation Strategy for Controlling Hospital Costs, Problems, and Prospects. *New England Journal of Medicine* 305 (21), Nov. 19, 1981.

12. Joskow P. *Controlling Hospital Costs: The Role of Government Regulation*. MIT Press, 1981: 80.
13. Davis K, G Anderson, D Rowland, and E Steinberg. *Health Care Cost Containment*. Johns Hopkins University Press, 1990.
14. Enthoven AC. Consumer-Choice Health Plan: Inflation and Inequity in Health Care Today: Alternatives for Cost Control and an Analysis of Proposals for National Health Insurance. *New England Journal of Medicine* 298 (12), March 23, 1978.
15. Greenberg D. Washington Report: Health 'Reform' Massacre on Capitol Hill. *New England Journal of Medicine* 299 (21), November 23, 1978.
16. House Ways and Means Committee, 1985.
17. Hospital Insurance Trust Fund Report, *Trustees Annual Report*, 1981.
18. Schweiker R. *Report to Congress: Hospital Prospective Payment System for Medicare*. Department of Health and Human Services, December 1982.
19. Sorian R. *The Bitter Pill*. McGraw-Hill, 1988: 114-18.
20. Altman SH and DA Young. A Decade of Medicare's Prospective Payment System — Success or Failure? *Journal of American Health Policy* 3 (2), March/April 1993: 11-19.
21. Thorpe KE. *Improving Health Policy and Management: Nine Critical Research Issues for the 1990s*, Foundation for Health Services Research, 1992: 249.
22. Office of the Actuary, HCFA, 1986.
23. Mitchell J, G Wedig, and J Crowell. The Medicare Physician Fee Freeze, *Health Affairs* 8 (1), 1989: 21-33.
24. Wiener JO. Physician Payment Reform: Struggling To Be Born. *Medicine & Health Perspectives*, January 7, 1991.
25. Physician Payment Review Commission, Annual Report to Congress, 1993.
26. Sorian R. Medicaid: Moving Too Fast? *Medicine & Health Perspectives*, September 4, 1989.
27. Pelrine A. The Art of the Deal: Health Policymaking on the Fly. *Journal of American Health Policy* 2 (3), May/June 1992: 23-28.
28. Tokarski C. Medicaid Donations: Scam or Savior? *Medicine & Health Perspectives*, July 22, 1991.
29. Henry J. Kaiser Family Foundation's Commission on the Future of Medicaid. Medicaid Cost Explosion: Causes and Consequences, September 1993.
30. *Hospital Pricing: Cost Shifting and Competition*. The Employee Benefit Research Institute, May 1993.
31. Rosner, J. A Progressive Plan for Affordable, Universal Health Care, *Mandate For Change*, Berkley Books, 1993: 108.
32. Zelman W. The Clinton Plan: With Malice Toward None and Health Security for All. *Journal of American Health Policy* 3 (6), November/December, 1993: 9-13.

CHAPTER 5

Policing the Professions: Malpractice and Antitrust Under Reform

Daniel B. Moskowitz

The relationship between perception and reality is at the heart of the debate over whether the business of medicine should be conducted under the laws that apply to other commerce, or if it needs its own special rules. The question comes up primarily in two areas: antitrust and tort liability. In each case, the advocates of reform insist that society is robbed of chances to get superior medical care by subjecting providers to the general legal rules on what constitutes anticompetitive behavior and professional liability. And in each case, those who insist that the health care industry should live with the same legal rules as other businesses say the medical community is exaggerating the impact of the legal strictures.

Hospital executives, for instance, complain that fears of government prosecution for anticompetitive activity keep them from joining with another institution in a joint venture — to buy expensive new imaging equipment, say — that neither could afford on their own. The reality is that the antitrusters have *never* challenged a hospital joint venture to purchase high-technology equipment — and there is little likelihood that the government will ever oppose a joint undertaking prompted by financial strain and community need. But the perception that there is a threat can prevent two potential partners from ever discussing the venture. Similarly, if a doctor orders unnecessary tests because he perceives that not doing so will make him vulnerable to a malpractice suit, the perception becomes a reality regardless of whether it is founded on the actual probability of being sued.

Because concerns over the threat of antitrust and malpractice actions have become a barrier to doctors' delivering health care in the most efficient and effective manner, any reform proposal has to deal with those issues. What the Clinton Administration's plan tries to do is thread its way carefully between the advocates of reform and those who insist that the present situation is no barrier to effective health care. It is gambling that it can move perception and reality closer together by using modest changes in the legal rules to spotlight how much freedom practitioners really have to practice medicine as they wish. It may be an approach that pleases neither side — a reaction that the White House crew thinks it can sell to the uncommitted as evidence that it has struck a fair balance between the opposing camps.

THE CENTRAL DICHOTOMY

It's not surprising that doctors and lawyers have essentially different views of the import of legal strictures on the delivery of health care services. The dichotomy springs from the difference in world view, inculcated in years of rigorous professional training that begins from radically different premises. As Daniel M. Fox, president of Milbank Medical Fund points out, "Most physicians do not understand the history of the logic of lawyers' claim that formalized conflict between plaintiffs and defendants in a courtroom or around a table resolves disagreements with reasonable equity and preserves social peace. To doctors, the claim that lay jurors can find fact is aberrant nonsense."[1]

While certainly doctors are taught to follow a particular process to arrive at a diagnosis or treat a malady, what really matters to a medical practitioner is the result: the pain alleviated, the illness cured, the patient recovered. The lawyer's enshrinement of process as an end in itself — allowing, say, the overturning of a decision that on its face seems wise because the proper procedures were not used to extract the information on which the decision was based — broadens the intellectual gulf between the two professions.

Moreover, Fox finds, the two professions have profound disagreement over "the purpose and use of politics. For lawyers, politics is a normal and essential aspect of professional life. Most physicians, in contrast, regard politics as intrusive, a distraction from more important matters. Lawyers write or seek to influence laws and regulations as an extension of their other professional roles. Most physicians consider these activities to be so distasteful that, when they are unavoidably caught up in them, they behave petulantly."

When, even a generation ago, doctors were seen as demi-gods with the gift of preserving life, this underlying divergence seldom came to the fore. But, notes Fox, "the conflict between physicians and lawyers, though rooted in the modern history of the two professions, has become more intense in recent years as the authority that most people accord doctors has diminished." Physicians are angry that they must so often now account to lawyers for the way they do their job — the process they use to decide that a particular doctor should not get hospital privileges, the course of treatment selected, or how to use the resources of a medical institution.

THE VELVET SHACKLES

It is perhaps in the area of antitrust that the Clinton Administration has tried hardest to trumpet as an important policy the narrowing of the gap between perception and reality. "You're frustrated because there's no quick or reliable advice from the enforcers of antitrust laws," Hillary Rodham Clinton told an August 1993 meeting of the American Hospital Association. "We've not only heard you, we're going to do something about that."

Antitrust enforcement at the federal level is split between two agencies, the Justice Department in the executive branch and the independent Federal Trade Commission. Just a month after Mrs. Clinton's AHA speech, the two got together to jointly issue policies on how they would exercise that enforcement authority in the health care field. It is the first time there are such public guidelines for a single sector of the economy.

The very fact that the two agencies acted is evidence of how vigorous the objections to antitrust policy have been among the medical community. The government issued the guidelines, explains Anne K. Bingaman, the assistant attorney general in charge of the antitrust division, because "health care is unusual in that it is comprised literally of thousands of local markets. And it is an industry that has faced enormous change and foment."

But the antitrusters argue that most of the criticism it has faced from the medical community is unjust and based on misinformation. For instance, hospital executives fret that trying to solve the problems of a weak institution by merging it with a strong one is likely to bring down the wrath of the antitrusters. The truth is that the government has challenged only eight of the more than 200 hospitals mergers that took place between 1987 and 1992.[2]

Each agency went to some pains to insist that the policy statements were not in fact an easing of the antitrust restrictions but merely an attempt to let medical decision makers know what the rules of the game are. When the policy statements were released, FTC Chair Janet D. Steiger (a Republican holdover in the job, who followed Bingaman's lead on this issue) underscored that the goal was explanation, not liberalization, of the curbs on anticompetitive behavior. In a number of sensitive areas, the agencies have spotlighted "safety zones" and promised that activities that fall within the zones will generally be immune from prosecution. Steiger emphasized that "these safety zones confirm what the agencies' previous enforcement record bears out: that the covered activities normally do not pose a threat to competition or consumers."

The assurances in the guidelines do not go beyond what almost any competent hospital antitrust counsel would have said previously. The safety zones take a most conservative approach. As one major health care law firm, Pittsburgh's Reed Smith Shaw & McClay, put it in a memo to its clients: "In a news conference called to announce the joint enforcement policies, Mrs. Clinton remarked that the statements would 'help lower costs, maintain high quality, and knock down the barriers to collaboration that, unfortunately, are too common in our present system.' In reality, the statements do little more than reduce to writing existing antitrust enforcement policy. The close questions, those that pose the greatest potential risk and are the most difficult to evaluate, are, by and large, left unaddressed in the agencies' pronouncements."

For instance, the pledge is that neither agency will attack a hospital merger if one of partners is more than five years old, has fewer than 100 beds, and has been averaging fewer than 40 patients a day. That is a very sick hospital indeed. The truth is that in very many cases, larger hospitals, and those not running nearly so far under capacity, will be able to merge without antitrust prosecution. But because every market is different, and because some staffer could come up with a scenario in which the disappearance as an independent entity of a 120-bed hospital — or one caring for 60 patients a day — could impede competition, such a deal didn't make it into the safety zone.

The same conservative approach is evident in other safety zones:

- the joint purchase, operation, and marketing of expensive medical equipment is permissible if the deal involves no more hospitals than are necessary to support efficient use of the device.
- hospital participation in surveys about the prices they charge and the compensation they pay staff won't cause trouble as long as at least five hospitals are included, none represents more than 25 percent of the total for any category of data reported, and the figures are at least three months old.
- joint purchasing arrangements among institutions are protected from prosecution if the purchases by the group come to less than 35 percent of the total market for the items involved and as long as each hospital member of the group spends no more than 20 percent of its total revenues through the group.
- physician network joint ventures get the antitrusters' blessing if they are made up of no more than 20 percent of the physicians actively serving in any specialty in the geographic market.

As conservative as those safety zones are, they are not insignificant. In fact, one of the five members of the FTC voted against the policy statement. Commissioner Deborah K. Owen explained that she fears that the government is giving away too much. "The risks of higher prices and reduced output or lower quality of care posed to some health care consumers by the more relaxed enforcement proposed in some of these states far outweigh any benefits generated," she warned in her dissent. For instance, she feels the rule on hospital mergers might allow a big hospital to gobble up an ailing smaller institution when it would be better for consumers to have the small facility ally with another small facility to better compete with the big hospital.

Moreover, says Philip Proger, a Washington DC attorney who specializes in health care antitrust, by publishing the guidelines the antitrusters have given providers an insight into the way the government balances its concerns about the effect of reduced competition in a particular health care market against claims of enhanced efficiency. That will let the individual lawyers advising hospitals and doctor groups speak with more authority.

In addition to the policy statements, the two antitrust agencies issued one more promise: that any time a provider comes to them with a question about the applicability of the guidelines to a particular project under consideration, they will get an answer within 90 days. And if the question is about some antitrust topic not covered by the guidelines, there will be an official reading on the government's view of its legality within 120 days. The first proposal vetted under this quick review policy was for the development of a nationwide preferred provider network of cardiologists, cardiovascular surgeons, and hospitals that would negotiate directly with third party payers to be the provider of choice for treatment of heart conditions in 41 metropolitan areas. The Justice Department assured those putting together the organization that it did not consider the move anticompetitive.

The willingness to provide those advisory opinions coupled with the fact that the antitrusters undertook the guidelines project in the first place should be consoling to those in the health business that the antitrusters are giving them special attention.

Certainly they will continue clamoring for more. Among the issues doctors have been fretting over that were not addressed in the September 1993 document are the power to get together to negotiate with third party payers and the freedom to yank the right to practice medicine from peers who are deemed not to meet medical standards. The antitrusters and the doctors will be battling over those questions in the future.

PLACING BLAME

While the specter of antitrust prosecution hovers over plans of health care institutions, the threat of malpractice litigation directly affects every individual practitioner and so is of tremendous emotional import. Doctors complain that their treatment decisions are being second-guessed by those who could not possibly understand what goes into such a decision, even if the statistics are far less frightening than most doctors believe.

For instance, a study by the General Accounting Office released in the fall of 1993 looked at the malpractice claims made on 374 community and migrant health centers over a six-year period ending in 1991.[3] It found that 64 percent of the centers had no claims at all filed against them during that time, another 18 percent had only one, and only 2 percent had six or more claims filed against them. Moreover, just over half of the cases that had been resolved resulted in no payment whatsoever to the claimant. Yet doctors continue to worry. "There is pretty good evidence that doctors overperceive their likelihood of being sued," notes Herbert Nickens, vice-president of the Association of American Medical Colleges.

Because of that perception, to a lot of practitioners a key element of any health reform scheme is heightened protection against such suits. Doctors are pressing for reforms ranging from caps on the amount of damages a patient can win to a law allowing a physician's having followed established practice protocols to serve as an absolute defense in malpractice suits.

From a practical standpoint, such measures seem to have little to do with health care delivery in this country. "I'm not sure that any of the tort reform items are going to make any difference at all in terms of overall health care," says J. Phillip O'Brien, co-chair of the health care department at the Chicago law firm Katten Mutchin & Zavis. Despite zooming costs of malpractice insurance, total premiums come to just 0.6 percent of the total national health care bill. And the "defensive medicine" that is supposed to be curbed by a lessened fear of malpractice suits is in many cases nothing more than the extra measure of care most patients would want. A report by Lewin-VHI, Inc. on defensive medicine concludes that the concept is difficult to define, that even if there is agreement that a procedure is unwarranted, the decision to order it usually stems from a variety of overlapping motives, and that it is "virtually impossible" to isolate what defensive medicine contributes to overall health care costs.[4]

Moreover, as Sarah Lawhorne, president of the Pennsylvania Medical Society liability insurance company, reports, there is little connection between the professionalism of the practitioner and the likelihood of a suit when the results are less than optimal. The demonstrable fact that there are geographic and demographic differences in both the number and kinds of malpractice suits filed shows that social attitudes are of controlling importance. Urban patients, for instance, are statistically far more likely to sue than those who live in smaller towns. And data released in late 1993 from the extensive Harvard study of 31,000 patients in 51 New York hospitals in 1984 showed that contrary to conventional wisdom the poor — even when they were injured by negligent treatment — are only about 10 percent as likely to bring a malpractice suit as more well-to-do patients. Those over 65 also bring suits at a considerably lower rate than younger people.[5]

It is therefore easy to dismiss the medical malpractice changes included in the Clinton health plan as mere window dressing. But that doesn't make the planks unimportant. Just as window dressing can lure a customer into a store to buy totally unrelated items, the promise of reduced vulnerability to tort litigation can woo doctors into buying other, more profound, reforms.

Georgetown University Medical Center physician-in-chief John M. Eisenberg points out that the Clinton plan "is not very bold in its treatment of malpractice reform." What the Administration wants to do for providers is:

- Shuttle all medical malpractice claims through some sort of alternative dispute resolution scheme.
- Require as a ticket to the courthouse that any plaintiff line up at least one medical specialist willing to attest that the disputed treatment fell short of the established standards of care.

- Hold lawyers who take such cases on a contingency basis — as virtually all do — to a fee of no more than 33.33 percent of the total award, while inviting the states to set lower limits.
- Order courts to slice from any damages awarded by a jury the amount of money the victim gets from other sources, primarily medical insurance.
- Stretch out awards over many years when they are intended to make up for future lost earnings or for treatment costs facing the plaintiff later in life.

Finally, the Clintons suggest some modest testing of two other ideas that might play a bigger role in tort reform down the road: enterprise liability (shifting liability for malpractice from the individual doctor to the health plan with which she is associated), and allowing practice protocols to be a shield against suits as long as practitioners can prove they conformed with the guidelines. Both of those innovations could help plaintiffs or help defendants, depending on exactly how they are implemented.

POLITICAL JUGGLING

The political nature of the proposal is made evident by the number of provisions that sound good but don't really have much potential for changing anything. Start with the cap on lawyer fees. When the Congressional Office of Technology Assessment reviewed six empirical studies of the effect of various moves to reform the medical malpractice system, it found unanimity that limits on attorneys' fees do not reduce malpractice costs and some evidence that they actually significantly increased the amounts paid per claim.[6] Moreover, the 33.33 percent figure is the upper limit of what is generally charged now. Even those who support the lawyers representing malpractice claimants call it unconscionable for any lawyer to take a bigger cut than that. In fact, in many markets, competition in the plaintiff bar has moved the normal fee down to as low as 20 percent of the final award.

Similarly, the requirement for a "certificate of merit" from a specialist before a malpractice suit can go forward looks like little more than a restatement of the current legal reality that a plaintiff can never win a case without testimony from an expert that prevailing professional standards were violated.

The one proposal with the biggest potential for making an impact on malpractice suits, advocates on both sides of the debate agree, is the "collateral source rule," the doctrine that any reimbursement the victim has received or will receive for his injuries should be deducted from the amount the defendant has to pay. That reimbursement might be from workers' compensation, from the patient's own medical insurance, or from settlements by other defendants in the case. "That's a big reform and one I think would make an enormous difference," says Kenneth V. Heland, associate director of the American College of Obstetricians and Gynecologists; "We believe those awards would be significantly reduced."

The OTA study pinpointed a mandatory collateral source rule as one potential change that really has been shown to reduce the cost of malpractice litigation to providers and their insurers. If the rest of the Clinton plan becomes law and almost everyone has health insurance that covers almost all essential treatment, requiring such offsets will be of even more importance, since the cost of care is a big component of most malpractice awards. This is especially true in the most horrifying cases, where a person has been left disabled for life and needs assistance for decades to come. The potential of being liable for medical care far into the future "has been like an albatross, especially in obstetric cases," says Heland. Medical advances are keeping alive seriously deformed infants who previously would have died soon after birth.

In some ways, a reduction in the size of awards is deceptive, since today most insurance payments are made with the proviso that if the patient collects damages the insurance company can recapture its reimbursement, and in fact the insurers are quick to invoke that clause. The rhetoric from some doctors about the collateral source rule being necessary in order to stop victims from collecting twice isn't quite so. A $200,000 award from which the patient then repays an insurance company $100,000 and a $200,000 award from which the court deducts $100,000 is to the patient pretty much the same thing.

But not to society. Those who oppose the provision argue that if a provider's ineptitude harms a patient, the cost of paying for that damage should be placed directly on that person or institution; if a big payout means that that provider's malpractice insurance rates go up, that properly places the blame where it is due. But if the cost of the care necessitated by the mistake is picked up by the patient's own insurance, that means that it will eventually be reflected in the rates paid by a broad segment of policyholders who have played no role in the underlying misdeed. Insurance, this side believes, should cover only the unavoidable loss; the avoidable loss should be paid for by the person whose negligence caused it.

Beneath the policy arguments is a very practical one — the little secret that's seldom mentioned in the debates but one that makes the collateral source rule the most contentious of the Clinton Administration malpractice proposals. It is, simply, that it will cut drastically what lawyers make from such cases. Since lawyers' fees are based on the amount of the award, deducting reimbursed medical costs reduces their slices significantly — by half in the example above, and by even more in many real life situations.

"This could wipe out a large segment of medical malpractice suits," predicts Pamela Gilbert, director of Congress Watch and a leading consumer advocate for tort reform. Because plaintiff lawyers tend to finance most of the litigation costs — not only betting their own time when clients are strapped but also picking up the out-of-pocket costs of investigations and other pre-trial maneuvering — they do a tough, cold assessment of how much a case is going to yield them. Those who calculate incorrectly don't stay in the business long. If lawyers perceive that their likely award is going to be much less, they may turn down cases they previously would have taken.

That collateral source rule is the number one objection plaintiff lawyers have to the Clinton proposals. But it is number one on a long list. In fact, the opening stance of the lawyers who specialize in handling patient claims of provider negligence is an absolutist one: There should be no congressional action at all on the question of medical malpractice litigation — a matter that has always been left up to the individual states. After 12 years of White House hostility to plaintiff lawyers, their professional organization, the Association of Trial Lawyers of America, backed Clinton's 1992 presidential campaign with almost half a million dollars in donations, and they are determined to collect their political chips by battling against congressional interference.

The states' rights position of ATLA is not conducive to the kind of give-and-take compromise at the heart of the Clinton proposals. Both sides see a move to set federal rules for such litigation, no matter how modest the actual impact of those rules may be, as the proverbial camel's nose under the tent. Doctors' groups admit they hope the curbs will move Congress toward setting tougher standards. What they most want are limits on what winning plaintiffs can collect. "Clearly the President has taken a step," notes AMA Executive Vice President James Todd, MD, "This is the first time there has been a national pronouncement on this."

The pioneering Harvard study of New York hospital patients suggests that the overwhelming majority of serious mistakes made by practitioners do not result in malpractice suits, but little of the debate over reforming malpractice law has centered on removing the barriers to those potential claims actually being made.[7] The Clintons have tried to undercut the objection to federal action in the malpractice arena by balancing the pro-doctor proposals with a few changes that would actually make it easier for victims to collect damages. There is the provision to use the National Practitioner Data Bank to finger doctors who repeatedly are found liable for practice mistakes — a proposal the plaintiff bar and its consumerist allies applaud because until now those records have been kept so secret that patients have no easy way of finding out the track record of a doctor they are considering going to. And the Administration has fashioned the ADR proposal so that a patient who isn't happy with the settlement suggested in the procedure still has full rights to take the dispute to court.

But ATLA and its allies fear that once the federal government moves into laying out rules on tort suits, it will push beyond medical malpractice to dictate to states procedures for suits in such heavily lobbied areas as product liability. Warns Jack H. Olender, one of the deans of medical malpractice litigation: "It's a bad precedent. It is a preemption of what had been until now a local right. It's inappropriate, because righting civil wrongs is something the community should deal with rather than Big Brother in Washington."

The odds have to be that the final congressional package will address the malpractice question despite the fierce battle the politically savvy trial lawyers will mount against the idea. That's because the doctors are being asked to accept such radical changes in their way of operating — the AMA's analysis of the Clinton plan calls "fully unacceptable" the caps on medical spending implied in any national health care budget — that the lawmakers are going to be eager to offset those negatives with some goodies physicians want. That includes some action in the malpractice area. Even as she plots the strategy against the provisions, Gilbert acknowledges the importance of the malpractice plank: "They've tried to throw a bone to the doctors because, let's face it, in the long run the doctors are going to be more important in getting this passed than the lawyers."

ACTIONS BY THE STATES

While the debate goes on in Washington, state governments have been addressing the same issues of whether health care providers need special protections from antitrust and malpractice prosecutions. By administrative fiat or legislation, state officials have responded to physicians' complaints with moves meant to assuage their fears. In only some cases have those moves made a substantive difference.

Florida and Ohio are among the states that have passed laws that, in the case of hospitals, override the normal approach to analyzing mergers: looking at how much the combine increases the concentration in the market.[8] Because many communities have only a handful of facilities — often only two — a proposed merger would by the normal arithmetic be unacceptable as putting too much power in the hands of the surviving organization.

Typically, the states are authorizing their health departments to vet such merger plans and decide whether the resulting efficiencies will abate the risk that without meaningful competition the merged institution will be able to gouge the public on rates. If a state gives a deal a go-ahead, it not only immunizes the merging facilities from prosecution under state antitrust laws, but also provides a fair measure of protection from suits brought under the federal Clayton Act.

Similar laws have received serious consideration in more than a dozen other states. The attorney general of Massachusetts in the summer of 1993 acted on his own to try to give hospital managers the same assurances by issuing his own guidelines on hospital mergers, putting in writing that the state acknowledges that "consolidation of unneeded or underutilized hospital facilities is in the interest of consumers."

But as with the federal guidelines, at the same time the Massachusetts officials tried to persuade hospitals that they could go forward with mergers that will benefit their communities, they went to some pains to deny that the institutions were getting a special break. Any industry with excess capacity will be allowed to consolidate for efficiency as long as some forms of competition remain, noted William Brownsberger, the assistant attorney general in charge of the hospital merger guidelines project. "This recognizes at this time the hospital industry is such an industry. We're not changing antitrust law as it applies to hospitals." But even if there is no real change, the guidelines have the potential of changing the perception of how antitrust law applies and thereby encouraging some hospital directors to at least discuss mergers or joint ventures.

In tort law, every state has made some changes since the 1970s, mostly pro-provider amendments to the rules that apply to medical malpractice suits. The trend continues: In 1992 Vermont transformed a voluntary system of arbitrating medical malpractice claims to a mandatory one, and Minnesota decreed that doctors who follow established practice protocols would be completely immune from antitrust prosecution. In 1993 Maryland passed a law allowing doctors to use as a defense evidence that they acted as other practitioners in the same community would have acted.[8]

Probably the most effective protection given practitioners is to cap the amount of damages that can be awarded the victim of malpractice. A total of 22 states now have such a provision on the books, although in only eight of them — including Indiana, Louisiana, and Colorado — is the limit an absolute one, ranging from $500,000 to Nebraska's $1.25 million. More common is to allow a jury unlimited discretion to reimburse a victim for identifiable dollar losses stemming from the injury — lost wages, medical treatment, equipment or assistance to overcome resulting disabilities — but to cap the amount of such non-economic damages as those given for "pain and suffering."

Juries seldom give plaintiffs big money for such losses, but when they do it can be big indeed. A study by the General Accounting Office of malpractice cases closed in 1984 found that just over 2 percent of the cases in which some payment was made accounted for 62 percent of the total money awarded for non-economic damages.[9] Such awards are particularly galling to physicians, because there is no good way to quantify the dollar value of the loss, and they seem to be based on an almost random emotional reaction of the jurors to an unfortunate outcome rather than on a true reimbursement for loss. And for the same reason, they are almost impossible to calculate in advance in trying to decide how large a settlement offer to make to keep a case out of court.

There's little doubt that a cap on damages does reduce the cost to providers of malpractice claims. But, because it may also prevent some seriously injured victims of bad medicine from getting the compensation due them, it is of questionable constitutionality. While courts in many jurisdictions have upheld caps, they have been overturned by the highest court in 15 states, including such major jurisdictions as Ohio, Illinois, and Texas.

The American Tort Reform Association spotlights the 1975 Medical Injury Compensation Reform Act in California as the most effective of all state moves to relieve providers from the threat of ruinous malpractice suits.[8] It includes a relatively low limit on non-economic damages — $250,000 — plus the abolition of the collateral source rule; a requirement that awards based on future costs incurred by the victim be paid in installments; and limits on the portion of the winnings the plaintiff's attorney can claim, which reduce the percentage as the amount of money involved escalates, so the lawyer gets only 15 percent of any amount over $600,000. The statute is now under strong attack from the plaintiff bar and consumer groups that are trying to repeal it or at least water down its key provisions.

Other popular state reforms in medical malpractice law have, according to the OTA survey, not worked at all — at least by empirical measures. For instance, in 16 states no medical malpractice case can get into court until it has been screened by a panel of doctors. A finding by the panel that the case is without merit doesn't prevent the plaintiff from going on with litigation, but the fact that the panel came to that conclusion is likely to strongly influence jurors hearing such a case. The barrier is so significant that mandatory pretrial screening was declared unconstitutional in Florida, Illinois, and Missouri.

Nonetheless, measures of the average size of awards to successful claimants show that it actually goes up once a state adopts a screening procedure. One possible explanation is that the screen procedure is so cumbersome for both sides that they simply get together to settle small claims; only in cases involving major money do they actually work their way through the process and get to court. But regardless of the reason, it seems clear that a technique designed to protect doctors against what was seen as a deluge of unfounded and frivolous claims hasn't achieved that end.

Codifying that doctors are expected to do no more than meet the normal standard of care in the areas where they practice and mandating that payments to victims must be stretched out over time were other "reforms" that the OTA found to have no effect on the overall outcome of malpractice suits.

But in fact the reforms that do not "work" may be politically sound medicine. Opposition, particularly from the plaintiff bar, is weakest to provisions that have little impact on their pocketbooks, but at the same time such provisions at least partially mollify doctors who feel they have become unduly vulnerable to malpractice suits. For political survival always depends as much on perception as on reality, and the policymaker who insists that every decision be based on hard data and ignores the subjective response is likely not to be in a position to make policy for very long.

REFERENCES

1. Fox DM. *Power and Illness.* University of California Press, 1993.
2. Department of Justice and Federal Trade Commission. *Antitrust Enforcement Policy Statements in the Health Care Area.* September 15, 1993.
3. U.S. General Accounting Office. *Medical Malpractice: Estimated Savings and Costs of Federal Insurance at Health Centers.* September 1993.
4. Lewin-VHI. *Estimating the Costs of Defensive Medicine.* January 27, 1993.
5. Burstin HR, WG Johnson, SR Lipsitz, and TA Brennan. Do the Poor Sue More? A Case-Control Study of Malpractice Claims and Socioeconomic Status. *Journal of the American Medical Association* 270 (14), October 13, 1993: 1697-1701.
6. Corrigan JA, study director. *Impact of Legal Reforms on Medical Malpractice Costs.* Office of Technology Assessment, U.S. Congress, September 1993.
7. *Patients, Doctors, and Lawyers: Medical Injury, Malpractice Litigation, and Patient Compensation in New York.* Report of the Harvard Medical Practice Study to the State of New York, 1990.
8. American Tort Reform Association. *Tort Reform Enactments*, annual compilations for 1992, 1993.
9. U.S. General Accounting Office. *Medical Malpractice: Medicare / Medicaid Beneficiaries Account for a Relatively Small Percentage of Malpractice Losses.* August 1993.

CHAPTER 6

Long Term Care: The Looming Crisis

Karen J. Migdail

While the problems of the acute care system are great, they pale in comparison to the outlook for long term care.

The nation's patchwork long term care system is being squeezed by two powerful and competing forces: unremitting demand for services from a rapidly growing elderly and disabled population, and severe financing problems at the state government level, where roughly half of all long term care bills are paid.

There's general agreement the system hasn't yet reached the crisis point; demand has not yet outpaced available services and financing. But demand could easily spiral out of control in the next century as the proportion of persons over age 65 grows larger.[1] The United States is experiencing a demographic revolution: Americans are growing older in record numbers. According to the Senate Special Committee on Aging, by the year 2030, the number of persons over age 65 will be double what it was in 1989 and the 85-plus population will nearly triple (see Figure 6-1).

The aging of the baby boomers will mean that more people will need long term care, either in their homes or in nursing homes. In 1990, approximately seven million persons over age 65 needed some type of long term care. That number is expected to grow to nine million by the year 2005 and to 12 million by 2020.[1] For persons over age 65, the eventual risk of entering a nursing home is 43 percent (some of those people will get other long term care services).[2]

The demographic shift — coupled with the declining size of families and the scattering of family members — will mean that the frail elderly will have fewer informal caregivers on which to rely, and more of them will have to seek professional help. Family members, friends, and other informal caregivers are estimated to provide approximately 60 to 80 percent of long term care services.[3] In some cases, both parents and children will be elderly and in need of care. In others, caregivers will find themselves forced to cope with the needs of their children as well as their parents.

The long term care system also faces a surge in clients drawn from populations that traditionally have not been users of formal services. Increasingly, younger disabled individuals have been seeking access to services as advances in medical technology make it possible for them to move out of acute care settings and back into the community.

Figure 6-1

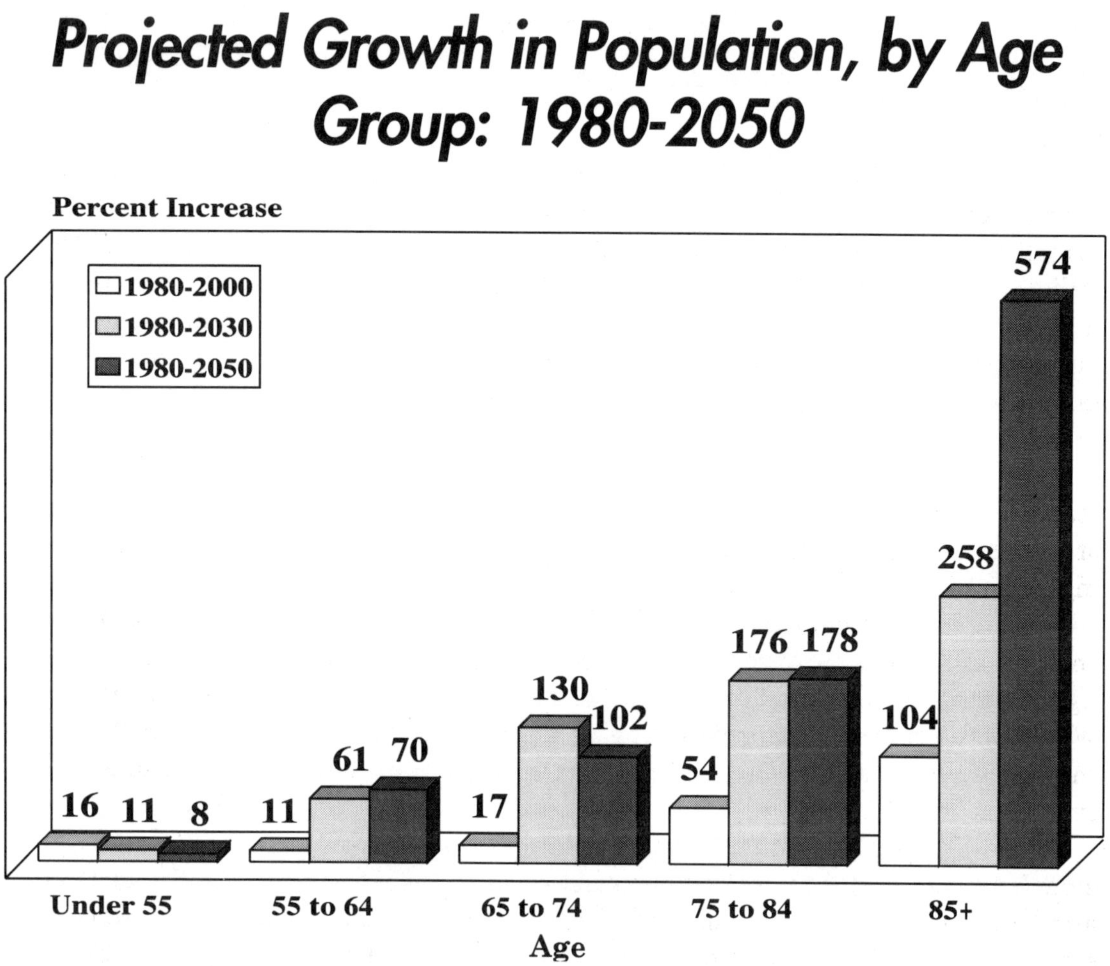

Source: U.S. Bureau of the Census, January 1989; from *Aging America: Trends & Projections.*

Medical advances have extended the lives of infants with birth defects and catastrophic illnesses who otherwise would not have survived childhood. The AIDS epidemic, traumatic brain injuries resulting from accidents, and other conditions are expected to bring younger people into the long term care system in increasing numbers.

Estimates are that more than 30 million persons have some form of disability; between six million and ten million are severely disabled and require special assistance.

Unfortunately, services haven't kept pace even with the most conservative estimates of the potential demand. For example, it's estimated that some five million persons over age 65 will be in nursing homes by the year 2050.

GOVERNMENT HELP

Historically, long term care has been provided primarily by families, mostly by women. Daughters and daughters-in-law care for elderly parents; wives and mothers care for disabled spouses and children. However as women enter the work force in record numbers, the need for more formal caregivers is growing. With the cost of nursing home care approaching an average of $30,000 per year ($50,000 to $75,000 in metropolitan areas like New York City), the need for financial assistance also is increasing.

Over the years and almost by accident, Medicaid — a federal/state program created in 1965 to provide basic services to low-income individuals — became the primary public payer of nursing home care. In 1984, the program spent $10.4 billion on nursing home care (41.5 percent of the $25.1 billion total spent on nursing home care). In 1992, Medicaid accounted for more than 45 percent of the $67 billion spent on nursing homes, covering the bills of nearly 60 percent of the 1.5 million residents living in some 16,000 facilities nationwide.[2]

Although the program was intended as a safety net for the poor, states allow better-off elderly to "spend down" their assets to qualify for Medicaid. In most states, individuals may keep $2,000. Estimates are that approximately 15 percent of residents who enter nursing homes paying the costs themselves end up qualifying for Medicaid within a year.[4]

States have charged that Medicaid costs are rising because wealthy seniors shelter assets to qualify prematurely. In its 1993 budget, Congress estimated that tightened asset transfer rules will save Medicaid $650 million over five years. Whether the modifications will reap this much is debatable: A recent report from the U.S. General Accounting Office suggest that few seniors actually "game" the system in this way.

After complaints from advocates that Medicaid's institutional bias forced poor elderly into nursing homes, Congress created a series of waiver programs in 1981 allowing states to use Medicaid money to cover home- and community-based care services for individuals who would otherwise need institutional care. "Section 2176" waivers can be targeted to a particular population, such as the disabled, AIDS patients, or the elderly, and can cover such services as homemaker/home health aide care, personal care, and adult day care. Medicaid covered $3.3 billion of the $9.7 billion spent nationally on home health care in 1989[5]. Currently, 49 states have Section 2176 waiver programs; Arizona operates under a special arrangement.

Medicare, the $131 billion program covering health care for all Americans over 65, provides limited long term care coverage. The program provides — on paper — a 100-day nursing home benefit per "spell of illness." In reality, the government picks up the tab for the first 20 days, and beneficiaries are responsible for an $87 copayment for days 21 through 100. Beneficiaries also can get a limited home health benefit. Medicare pays less than 5 percent of nursing home bills annually and no more than a third of home health expenses. In 1990, Medicare paid $3.5 billion for home health care and $2.5 billion of the $53.1 billion spent for skilled nursing home care.[5]

The remainder of long term care bills are covered by consumers out-of-pocket — some until they can qualify for Medicaid. A small number of seniors have experimented with the nascent private long term care insurance market. In 1990, only 2 percent of total long term care expenditures were paid by private insurance, according to the Senate Special Committee on Aging. The Committee estimates that the private insurance market will cover only 6.6 percent of long term care bills in 2020.

Consumer advocates criticize the private insurance market, arguing that fine-print policy restrictions — in addition to outright fraud and abuse — render many policies nearly useless. Coverage also is very expensive — annual premiums can run into the thousands of dollars for high-quality policies. As a result, no more than 10-20 percent of elderly may be able to afford coverage.[6]

Proponents of private insurance laud its untapped potential. Arguing that long term care illnesses are insurable events, groups like the Health Insurance Association of America claim private insurance offers a way to plan prudently for future needs. "Consumers must be made aware of the risk of incurring catastrophic expenses, the wide array of long term care services and settings offered, and the numerous types of private insurance products available to finance these services," argues Richard Garner, group vice president and actuary of CNA Insurance Companies.

SPIRALING COSTS

Despite efforts to contain costs, long term care is among the fastest growing sectors of the U.S. economy. Spending for home health care continues to grow at nearly three times the rate of health expenditures as a whole, with nursing home care right behind.[7]

Home health expenditures rose a startling 29.5 percent from 1991 to 1992, from $9.8 billion to an estimated $12.7 billion. In contrast, national health expenditures grew by 11.5 percent to an estimated $838.5 billion. During the same period, spending for nursing home care rose 12.5 percent to $67.3 billion.[7]

Home health expenditures are expected to rise another 30 percent from 1992 to 1993. The hike is attributed to five factors: the availability and use of high technology; higher utilization of health care services; long term treatment for AIDS, cancer, and other diseases; the aging population; and a labor-intensive health care industry.[7]

Spiraling costs, a fragmented delivery system, and burgeoning demand all pose a serious dilemma for state and federal policymakers. The government's safety net is expected to be stretched beyond the breaking point within the next few years as demand outpaces available services and financing. Without substantial reform, long term care is a fiscal time bomb.

OBSTACLES TO REFORM

There is widespread agreement on the goals of long term care reform — providing high quality care in the most efficient, least expensive setting. But experts don't always agree on the best way of getting there.

According to the authors of *The Economics and Ethics of Long-Term Care and Disability*, what has emerged from the debate is "an implicit consensus on some of the basic elements of a system of long term care; for example, greater reliance on community and in-home services, de-emphasis of the medical model, and the desirability of local case management." The essential missing piece, however, has been a viable financing mechanism. Short of that, the long term care system "will continue to have an imbalance between needs and the availability of services for both the elderly and the adult disabled populations."[3]

Lawmakers face seemingly insurmountable obstacles as they undertake the task of reforming the long term care system. First, for reform to be effective, it will carry a high price tag. White House reformers considered four different long term care proposals, with pricing estimates ranging from $5 billion to $126 billion a year. The Clinton Administration settled on a $65 billion-a-year program, which even its staunchest supporters supporters say isn't enough.

Second, no one yet has a precise fix on the extent of long term care services needed, because so many elderly and disabled individuals are cared for at home or through a patchwork of providers that are difficult to track. The fear is that if more formal services are offered, people will take advantage of them. Proponents of the "woodwork effect" theory point to a jump in Medicare payments for skilled nursing facility care after a 1988 expansion of eligibility and benefits. Medicare expenditures dropped after the expansion was repealed a year later. Others dispute the woodwork effect, noting that the majority of disabled elderly continue to live in the community despite the availability of formal services.[4]

Third, policymakers must make tough decisions about paying for systemwide health care reform in the face of mounting pressure from interest groups. For example, the debate could very well pit the needs of elderly and disabled against those of the uninsured. If that happens, it's not at all clear that the elderly wouldn't prevail. Congress is already well aware of the power of the elderly voting bloc.

That power is wielded by, among others, the 35 million-member American Association of Retired Persons (AARP).

AARP's clout was illustrated by a survey of 2,000 adults released in September by the Kaiser Family Foundation, which found that AARP was the most trusted source of information on health reform. The second most trusted: First Lady Hillary Rodham Clinton.

Disability groups demonstrated their mettle as a political force by spearheading passage of the sweeping Americans With Disabilities Act in 1991. Representatives of the Consortium for Citizens With Disabilities, a coalition of more than 100 organizations that fights for the rights of the disabled, testify frequently at congressional hearings.

Taking a more radical approach, Americans Disabled for Attendant Programs Today (ADAPT) has mounted a campaign of disrupting meetings of the American Health Care Association, a national nursing home trade group. In the early 1980s, ADAPT spurred federal and state legislation to make public transportation wheelchair-accessible. ADAPT now demands that 25 percent of Medicaid funding be shifted from institutional care to personal assistance services. Disabled protesters also have taken their cause in person to former HHS Secretary Louis Sullivan, MD, current HHS Secretary Donna Shalala, and President Clinton.

PRIOR REFORM ATTEMPTS

Several years ago the elderly taught Congress a lesson it hasn't forgotten — that senior citizens are loath to pay more out-of-pocket for additional Medicare benefits if they don't include substantial long term care services.

In 1988 Congress passed the Medicare Catastrophic Coverage Act, sweeping legislation that expanded Medicare benefits by adding prescription drug coverage, enhancing the skilled nursing facility benefit, and making other improvements. Beneficiaries, who were asked to pay an additional premium based on a sliding scale, opposed the law with a vigor that shocked lawmakers. The opposition of the elderly forced the repeal of the Act barely a year after it was passed.

Seniors objected to the proposal because they felt they were unfairly bearing the brunt of the financing and because the expansion didn't offer them enough help with the catastrophic costs of long term care — which, according to most public opinion polls, is the expense senior citizens fear most.

As with the acute care system, reforming the long term care delivery system has been discussed for the last several decades. Presidents have convened task forces and conferences, Congress has held hearings, but to no avail.

Long term care reform legislation has been introduced in nearly all the recent congressional sessions. Of the 18 or more long term care bills introduced in the 100th Congress, for example, three bills would have expanded long term care financing options under Medicaid, four would have expanded existing Medicare coverage, and others would have created a Medicare Part C program for long term care.[8] Other bills would have made incremental adjustments and improvements in existing benefits. Another 30 bills were introduced in the same session to spur private financing via individual retirement accounts or by encouraging consumers to buy private long term care insurance coverage.

Congress' only comprehensive attempt at plugging gaps in the nation's health care system began in 1988 when it convened the 15-member U.S. Bipartisan Commission on Comprehensive Health Care, consisting of members from both houses of Congress and White House appointees. Two years later, the panel, renamed the Pepper Commission after the death of its first chair, Rep. Claude Pepper (D-FL), delivered to the full Congress a $66 billion health reform plan.

Of the total, $42.8 billion was earmarked for a national nursing home program that would supplant Medicaid's coverage. The government would cover the first three months of nursing home care for all eligible individuals regardless of income. Individuals would have been required to pay a 20 percent copayment; the federal government would have subsidized payments for persons with incomes below 200 percent of poverty. The Pepper Commission plan also would have increased asset protection levels substantially and created tax incentives to encourage the purchase of private long term care insurance.

The plan also would have expanded home- and community-based care services for all severely disabled individuals needing assistance in three of five activities of daily living (ADLs) — eating, dressing, toileting, bathing, and transferring. Services would have been phased in over a five-year period. The Commission's plan drew fire from critics, particularly because it offered little in the way of explicit financing strategy. In 1992, a coalition of Democratic lawmakers, including panel Chairman Sen. John Rockefeller (D-WV), introduced a bill based on the panel's recommendations.

The legislation didn't go anywhere, but the panel's work provided a strong research base for the Clinton Administration to use in its legislative drafting efforts.

THE CLINTON SOLUTION

To craft its long term care reform proposal, the White House brought together a working group of experts from Capitol Hill, academia, and the federal government. The working group was headed by Robyn Stone, then a policy analyst at Project Hope and now deputy assistant secretary for aging, disability, and long term care policy.

Underlying the group's deliberations was the view that home- and community-based services, not institutional care, should be the basis of a new long term care system and that individuals ought not be required to impoverish themselves in order to qualify for services. A draft of the final plan that was leaked in September outlined the Administration's thinking. Calling the current long term care system "inadequate," the document argued that "many elderly and disabled Americans enter nursing homes and other institutions when they would prefer to remain at home. Families exhaust their resources trying to provide for disabled relatives."

The working group debated four options to present to President Clinton and First Lady Hillary Rodham Clinton: an incremental expansion of Medicaid long term care ($5 billion in fiscal 1994); new federal/state home- and community-based services for low-income, severely disabled people of all ages ($7 billion in FY94); a social insurance program for home- and community-based care that would cover everyone ($15.4 billion in FY94); and, the most expansive and expensive: a social insurance program covering all long term care regardless of income ($6 billion in FY94 and $126 billion at full implementation in 2020).

All but the latter option included a role for private long term care insurance with modification to asset protection rules for individuals seeking nursing home placement. The working group recommended several improvements in the private market, such as consumer education on the benefits and risks of insurance, "minimally acceptable" product and business requirements, monitoring and enforcement of standards, and tax incentives to encourage the purchase of plans. The working group also proposed allowing Medicaid recipients to keep more money — as much as $12,000 — and raising the monthly personal needs allowance from $30 to $100 for nursing home residents.

The leaked draft indicated the group had settled on an $80 billion long term care plan with five components:

- expanded home- and community-based services for the severely disabled and for persons with cognitive impairments;
- improvements in Medicaid coverage of institutional care;
- standards to improve the quality and reliability of private long term care insurance and tax incentives to encourage its purchase;
- tax incentives to help the working disabled;
- a demonstration study to improve integration of acute and long term care services.

Reacting to criticism regarding financing of the entire health reform plan, the White House scaled back the workgroup's long term care proposal when it formally introduced the 1,342-page Health Security Act on October 26.

Generally speaking, the long term care consumer advocacy groups and provider organizations support the Clinton plan's intent and goals. However, they do have some serious questions and concerns. Primarily, they feel that long term care benefits could be vulnerable as Congress seeks to cuts costs.

They are adamant on one point: Health reform without long term care reform makes no sense and is contrary to public opinion. According to surveys conducted by AARP, more Americans would support a health reform program that includes long term care than would support a plan without it (see Figure 6-2).

HOME- AND COMMUNITY-BASED CARE

While the basic structure of the plan remains the same, the White House made a number of changes that dropped the price of the new home- and community-based care program from $80 billion to $65 billion. First and foremost, the Administration proposes delaying implementation of the new benefits for two years. Implementation would begin in 1996 and be completed by 2002.

Figure 6-2

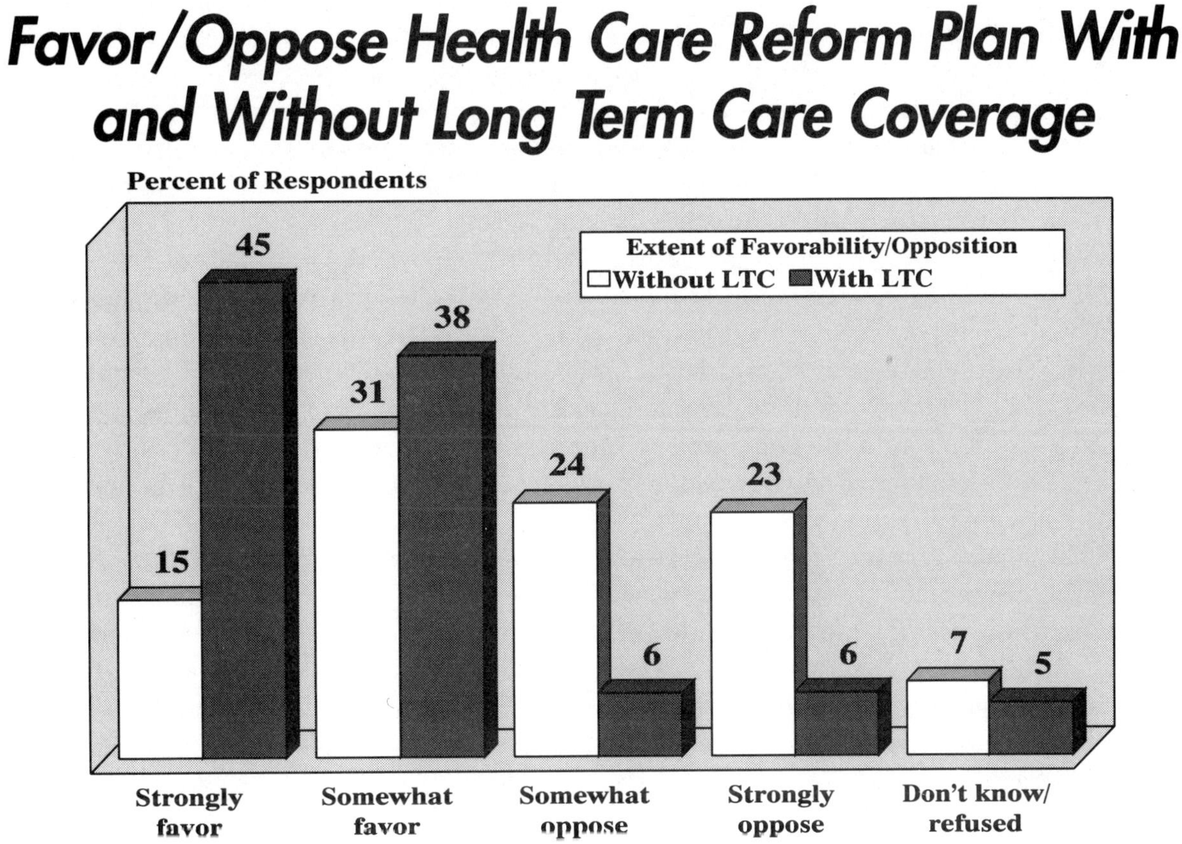

Source: AUS/ICR Survey Research Group, Excel Omnibus Study, April 21-27, 1993. Prepared for the American Association of Retired Persons.

At hearings held by the House Ways and Means Health Subcommittee and the Senate Labor and Human Resources Committee, AARP witnesses argued the five-year delay originally proposed by the White House was longer than the three-year phase-in proposed for other elements of the President's plan. Extending it for an additional two years means that "quite realistically, [AARP's members] will wonder how much of the benefit they will receive."[9]

The final Clinton bill makes the home- and community-based care program optional for states, a disappointment to consumer advocates. Paul McCarty, chair of the Alzheimer's Association's public policy committee, told the Senate Labor and Human Resources Committee that states should be required to participate in the home- and community-based care program, or the plan should provide a "safety valve" to make sure residents get some services in states that don't participate.[10]

Under the bill, states that wish to add services would be required to submit implementation plans to the federal government for approval. Federal match rates are approximately 30 percentage points higher than those currently used in Medicaid. States would get no less than 75 cents on the dollar but no more than 95 cents.

To be eligible, individuals would have to need assistance, supervision, or "cueing" to perform at least three of five ADLs or be classified, based on a gauge specified by the Secretary of HHS, as having either severe cognitive impairment or severe mental impairment or both. Also eligible are persons who display symptoms of one or more serious behavioral problems specified by the Secretary and who need supervision to prevent them from harming themselves or others and profoundly retarded individuals. Benefits also are extended to children under the age of six with a severe disability or chronic medical condition who would otherwise need to be cared for in an institutional setting.

The Consortium for Citizens With Disabilities faults the plan for limiting eligibility for home- and community-based care services to children under the age of six who would otherwise need institutional services. The proposal "would again use institutional need as the yardstick for eligibility, thereby furthering [Medicaid's institutional bias]," Anthony Young, co-chair of the consortium's personal assistance task force, told the Labor and Human Resources Committee. The President's proposal isn't clear about how older children with disabilities could get services, claims Young.[11]

Jenifer Simpson, representing CCD before the Ways and Means Health Subcommittee, argued the criteria proposed for individuals with cognitive and mental impairments is "flawed" and would include only a small percentage of the people who need long term care services. The threshold of an IQ below 36, formerly called "severe or profound mental retardation," covers only about 5 percent of individuals with mental retardation and leaves out many people with severe disabilities, Simpson said. Using IQ as a sole determinant is "outmoded and unacceptable," she maintained.[12]

Under the Clinton plan states would have the flexibility to design their own home- and community-based systems. Services states could provide include case management, homemaker and chore assistance, assistive technology, respite care, home modifications, adult day care, rehabilitation, and home health services not covered by Medicare, private insurance, or the basic benefits package. States would be required to cover personal assistance services. Room and board would not be covered.

All eligible individuals would be assessed and given a plan of care. States would have the option of providing vouchers or providing cash directly to eligible individuals. States could reimburse health plans or providers on a capitated basis and would be required to honor consumer choice whenever possible.

Non-poor recipients would be obliged to contribute to the cost of their care. States could require a "nominal" copayment for persons with incomes below 150 percent of poverty. Persons with incomes between 150 and 249 percent of the federal poverty line would pay 10 percent of the cost of services; for those with incomes above 250 percent, the copayment would be 25 percent. Providers would be required to accept the combined reimbursement and coinsurance as payment in full.

The bill presented to Congress in October included a 40 percent coinsurance payment for persons with incomes of 400 percent of poverty. This was disappointing to advocacy groups because the White House apparently had been considering capping beneficiary contributions at 25 percent. The 40 percent coinsurance payment "is high compared to other copayments proposed in other parts" of the health reform plan, according to the AARP and "could be prohibitively expensive" for some beneficiaries.[9]

The White House has since changed the 40 percent copayment to 25 percent. According to a senior HHS official, the higher figure's inclusion in the final bill was the result of a "drafting error."

Administratively, the program would be managed by states, subject to approval from Washington. Funds would be allocated under a national budget for home- and community-based services that would include administrative costs. States signing on to the plan would be required to cover all individuals now getting Medicaid-covered community-based long term care, and their criteria would have to meet new HHS standards.

Working disabled individuals who need assistance with ADLs and who purchase personal care could get a tax credit for 50 percent of their expenses — up to $15,000 per year. The Internal Revenue Service would be required to issue regulations defining personal care services to include help with completing ADLs, meal preparation and shopping, communication services, work-related support services, assistive technology, and assistance with life skills such as money management.

States would be required to establish "medically needy" programs for all residents of nursing facilities and intermediate care facilities for the mentally retarded. The plan initially raised the Medicaid personal needs allowance (PNA) from $30 to $70 per month — $30 less than what was proposed by the White House in September.

That increase was called "meager" by Max Richtman, executive vice president of the National Committee to Preserve Social Security and Medicare, at a fall hearing in the House of Representatives. He noted that some states and the District of Columbia already have a $70 PNA. Nursing home residents in these areas won't see any increase, he said. The pleas fell on deaf ears; in the final bill, introduced November 20, the White House tried to deflect attacks on the overall plan's expense by raising the PNA to only $50 per month.

"The National Committee frankly is disappointed that the President's plan would not do more for nursing home residents," Richtman told the panel. Unlike the earlier draft of the plan, the Health Security Act legislation would make the increase in Medicaid asset levels optional for states. Pointing out that the Pepper Commission advocated that individuals be allowed to keep $30,000, Richtman maintained that "raising the asset protection to $12,000 is small, and we recommend that it be made mandatory."[13]

LONG TERM CARE INSURANCE

Hoping to encourage wealthier individuals to plan financially for their long term care needs, the Clinton Administration is making a number of changes to spur the private long term care insurance market. These changes are not optional for states.

The plan would require the Secretary of HHS to appoint a five-member Long Term Care Insurance Advisory Council to advise on matters relating to private insurance and to monitor developments in the market. The advisory committee also would advise the Secretary of HHS about whether new insurance regulations would apply to continuing care retirement communities.

The Secretary of HHS would be required to set minimum federal standards for long term care insurance policies, including mandatory nonforfeiture and inflation protection benefits, elimination of preexisting condition limitations, third party notification of lapses, and reinstatements of up to five months if the lapse was due to the policyholder becoming incapacitated. Benefit eligibility would be based on an independent professional assessment.

While they claim to support minimum federal standards, proponents of private long term care insurance are warning that some of the requirements proposed by the Administration would limit the viability of the policies and kill the market's potential. The Health Insurance Association of America argues that mandating that all policies sold offer inflation protection and nonforfeiture — requiring that policies pay out even if the policyholder has missed some premium payments — would cause the price of policies to skyrocket. HIAA has urged Congress to require that insurers offer the benefits as an option.

States would be required to regulate insurance business practices, including establishing an appeals process for beneficiaries, setting standards for agents, limiting agent commissions, and outlawing questionable sales practices. States would be required to submit implementation plans to federal officials within two years of the Clinton plan's enactment. If a state failed to submit a plan or if it wasn't approved, no long term care insurance policies could be sold in the state until a plan was approved. Agents and insurers who failed to comply with business requirements would face civil money penalties, up to the greater of $10,000 or three times the amount involved.

The Administration would establish a grant program for states and private organizations to educate the public about long term care insurance.

The Clinton plan also would amend the tax code to make long term care insurance a more attractive purchase. Under the plan, long term care would be treated similarly to health and accident insurance policies. Among the changes: treating a long term care insurance policy as a guaranteed renewable contract; excluding from taxable income payments for services provided under a qualified long term care insurance policy; making dependency for two ADLs a qualification for favorable tax; and allowing corporate deductions for employer-paid long term care premiums and excluding those premiums from taxable income for employees. The tax code would allow for a maximum $150 per day long term care insurance benefit.

FINANCING WORRIES

The long term care plan's financing is a sticking point for its critics and proponents alike. They argue that the proposed five-year $124 billion in Medicare cuts earmarked to fund the program may be elusive and potentially dangerous. "The proposed new cuts could seriously jeopardize patients' access to care," said Val Halamandaris, president of the National Association for Home Care, who claims that the home health care industry already has been cut to the bone by reductions in Medicare routine cost limits and cutbacks in the five-year budget passed recently by Congress.[14]

American Association of Homes for the Aging Senior Vice President Mike Rodgers told the Ways and Means Health Subcommittee that his organization worries the plan is based on a "prevailing and insidious notion" that home care is less expensive than nursing home care. The opposite is true for individuals who are heavily dependent in multiple activities of daily living, argued Rodgers.[15]

His concerns were echoed by Paul Willging, executive vice president of the American Health Care Association, who expresses serious doubts that the federal and state governments can provide the proposed long term care benefits to such a broad population for the estimated costs. In addition, Willging claims the program may be so ambitious that Americans will believe that they won't need to plan for their old age, further increasing the need for public resources. As evidence, he cites a recent Gallup poll indicating that 45 percent of respondents still believe Medicare will pay for their long term care needs.[16]

Consumer advocates also worry that the financing will fall short. According to AARP, the funding design, which amounts to a capped block grant, raises a number of questions, including what will happen if the program runs out of money before the end of the fiscal year. The organization worries that individuals receiving services would suddenly be cut off. Since the program is capped, it "makes it all the more critical that the data and criteria used to estimate full funding over time are accurate and sufficiently inclusive."[9]

Brookings Institution Senior Fellow Joshua Wiener, who served as a member of the White House working group on long term care, told Ways and Means that the weaknesses of the program are "dictated by fiscal realities." However, the expenditure caps and a limited entitlement don't necessarily reflect potential increases due to inflation and growth in the target population, cautioned Wiener.[17]

ACUTE CARE NURSING HOMES

Ironically, while the Administration is working to provide more social supports in the home and the community, a long term care benefit included in the Clinton plan's basic benefit package could contribute to a "medicalizing" of nursing homes.

Under the basic benefit package, all citizens and legal residents would get 100 days of extended care services after an acute illness or injury as an alternative to continued hospitalization. "We want to provide reimbursement for subacute care at nursing homes rather than in the much more expensive hospital setting," First Lady Hillary Rodham Clinton told the House Labor Committee September 29. "Providing this kind of long term care . . . will help so many families."

Nursing homes are touting their ability to provide more intensive services traditionally provided in acute care settings but at a much lower cost. In recent months, a number of major nursing home chains have indicated that they are shifting to "subacute care." The American Health Care Association, the nursing home trade group, estimates that members can provide services like respiratory therapy and rehabilitation at one-third to one-half the cost of hospital-based care, potentially saving "untold billions per year in reduced federal costs."

The basic benefit package also offers home care services akin to those currently provided under Medicare, with the addition of home infusion therapy and outpatient prescription drug coverage. Services would only be provided as an alternative to care in a hospital, nursing home, or rehabilitation center after an illness or injury. At the end of each 60 days of treatment, patients' needs would be re-evaluated; additional therapy only would be covered if a patient risks institutionalization without it.

The minimum benefit package also includes hospice care — an alternative to hospitalization for terminally ill individuals with a life expectancy of six months or less. Other services covered: nursing and physician care; home health aide and homemaker services; physical, speech, and occupational therapies; and short term inpatient care.

A key question is whether these benefits will be vulnerable to attack by groups claiming the basic benefit package is too generous and thus too costly. In an October 18 letter to President Clinton, National Association of Manufacturers President Jerry Jazinowski argued that the basic benefit package "is too large and ambitious by half." He called for the elimination of long term care coverage, prescription drug coverage, and mental health services, claiming they should be added "only when and if it becomes clear that we can pay for them."

OTHER REFORM PROPOSALS

The Health Security Act is only one of a number of health reform bills pending in Congress. But, at the time of this writing, only two of the competing bills offers a substantial long term care benefit.

A bill introduced by Sen. John Chafee (R-RI) would create a new long term care program under the Social Security Act to replace services currently covered by Medicaid. The new SSA program would not be linked to welfare assistance. Eligibility would be extended to persons with incomes below the federal poverty line with "low" assets who are dependent in a specified number of activities of daily living. Like existing Medicaid "medically needy" programs, the bill would cover persons with greater incomes who have sufficiently high medical expenses.

States would cover nursing home and home- and community-based services, but they would not have to apply for a waiver to pay for noninstitutional care. The bill would allow states, with federal matching funds, to help persons with incomes below 400 percent of poverty purchase long term care insurance, and the tax code would be changed to encourage purchases by more affluent elderly.

The American Health Security Act, introduced by Rep. Jim McDermott (D-WA) and Sen. Paul Wellstone (D-MN), would provide comprehensive long term care services for all who need care. However, the proposal includes a $65 premium for all persons over age 65 with incomes above 120 percent of poverty. Based on the fiasco following the Medicare catastrophic legislation, a seniors-only premium would be very unpopular.

Other reform bills would make smaller, incremental changes. The "Medisave" bill introduced by House Minority Whip Newt Gingrich (R-GA) would provide tax incentives to encourage the purchase of long term care insurance. The bill would permit savings from life insurance, 401(k) plans, and individual retirement accounts to be used to pay for long term care. Funds would be excluded from taxable income. States would be required to offer seniors access to different levels of asset protection programs.

Medicaid would be eliminated and long term care left entirely up to the states under a bipartisan bill introduced October 6 by Reps. Jim Cooper (D-TN) and Fred Grandy (R-IA) in the House. A companion bill is expected to be introduced in the Senate by John Breaux (D-LA) and Dave Durenberger (R-MN).

The Clinton Administration briefly considered — and discarded — a voluntary public nursing home program that would have allowed senior citizens to purchase a public policy on their 65th birthday, with coverage kicking in when they turn 70. Benefits would have been capped at $30,000.

Sen. Edward Kennedy (D-MA) is championing a voluntary public nursing home insurance program. He is planning to introduce a bill that would offer individuals age 45, 55, and 65, who are not in a nursing home or hospital at time of enrollment, a one-time opportunity to purchase coverage with no underwriting or waiting periods. All persons currently over age 45 also would have a one-time opportunity to buy coverage with a three-year waiting period.

Individuals could purchase $30,000, $60,000, or $90,000 of nursing home coverage, and they would be allowed to keep an equivalent amount in assets if they were to qualify for Medicaid. Services would be triggered when an individual became dependent in three of five activities of daily living (bathing, eating, dressing, toileting, and transferring). Premiums would be determined by the Secretary of HHS, and policyholders would be required to pay a 20 percent copayment for the first six months in a nursing home and 35 percent copayment thereafter.

STATE INNOVATION

In the absence of federal reform efforts, states have responded to their swelling long term care/Medicare and Medicaid costs by tinkering with their own systems. A few examples:

California, Connecticut, Indiana, and New York have undertaken a landmark experiment linking the purchase of a long term care insurance policy with Medicaid. Under the Partnership for Long Term Care, funded with seed money from the Robert Wood Johnson Foundation, states are allowing seniors who buy an approved long term care insurance policy to keep higher levels of Medicaid-countable assets. Policyholders in Connecticut, California, and Indiana get dollar-for-dollar coverage. In New York, Medicaid will pick up the entire tab for individuals who exhaust a policy that provides three years of nursing home care, six years of home care, or a combination of both.

Approximately 20 states are pursuing similar efforts. Earlier this summer, HCFA approved a Medicaid state plan amendment submitted by Iowa to develop a long term care partnership between private insurance companies and Medicaid. However, the 1993 federal budget law has put a damper on the expansion of this model. At the behest of Rep. Henry Waxman (D-CA), who has long opposed public-private long term care arrangements, lawmakers required that, in any new states that adopt the model, any money protected be subject to estate recovery programs after the recipient's death.

Under a new universal access program, Florida's rural health purchasing networks are required to provide some level of home health care services and hospice. Networks also must offer adult day care, assistance with ADLs, skilled nursing services, nursing home care, and rehabilitation services available no more than 45 minutes away from the person needing the service.[18]

Vermont's legislature is planning to debate a series of options for reforming its health reform system. Proposals include a social insurance program for long term care. Under this plan, a wide range of services would be covered, including case management, nursing home and home care, homemaker services, and adult day care. Eligible adults would have to require help with two of six ADLs. Benefits would be available after a 90-day deductible period and would be capped at $45 per day in the beginning. For children, the plan only provides for 30 days of respite care. Services would be financed through additional taxes.

LONG TERM CARE IN THE NEXT CENTURY

There's increasing recognition that Congress can't overhaul the nation's health care system without fixing the rickety long term care system. In the future, it's likely that the acute care and long term care systems will be recognized as inextricably intertwined, as large managed care organizations seek to make the most of the resources available and exploit the most efficient path of care.

To that end, Clinton's Health Security Act calls for a demonstration project to test models for integrating the delivery of acute and long term care services to individuals with disabilities and chronic illnesses.

Some say a demonstration is no longer necessary because several unique integration models currently are operating around the country. As the shining and longest-running example, they point to a 21-year-old California program — now replicated elsewhere — as an example of a successfully integrated care network. On Lok Senior Health Services provides a full continuum of unlimited services, including acute, adult day health, home, and long term care to nursing home-eligible elderly in San Francisco. The program first operated on a much smaller scale under a Medicare waiver. In 1983, Congress authorized a special dual Medicare and Medicaid waiver allowing On Lok to operate under a capitated system.

In 1986, Congress extended the waiver to create a national demonstration project based on On Lok, known as Program of All-Inclusive Care for the Elderly (PACE). Currently, nine PACE sites are operating around the country, four sites are in the later stages of development, five are undergoing feasibility studies, and other areas are looking at the model.

The first four PACE sites, which will complete the three-year demonstration phase in 1993, are currently under evaluation by the New York City-based Community Health Accreditation Program. The sites under scrutiny are: Palmetto SeniorCare, Columbia SC; Elder Services Plan, Boston; Providence Elder Place, Portland OR; and Community Care for the Elderly, Milwaukee WI.

The Clinton plan reflects what long term care experts agree is a central principle: that service, not setting, should dictate policy. In other words, the best way to care for elderly and disabled individuals is to provide the services they need in the most efficient, cost-effective way. While this may eventually occur naturally, policy changes such as removing the institutional bias will speed the process along. In the future the traditional lines dividing long term care providers must be blurred in order to best meet the needs of the quickly expanding population of consumers.

REFERENCES

1. Senate Special Committee on Aging, Aging in America, 1991.
2. Health Care Investment Analysts, Inc. and Arthur Andersen & Co, The Guide to the Nursing Home Industry, 1993.
3. Meltzer J. Financing Long Term Care: A Major Obstacle to Reform, in *The Economics and Ethics of Long Term Care and Disability*. S Sullivan and ME Lewin, eds., 1988: 57.
4. Wiener JM and KM Harris. Myths and Realities: Why Most of What Everyone Knows About Long Term Care Is Wrong. *The Brookings Review*, Fall 1990.
5. Senate Special Committee on Aging, Developments in Aging, Vol. 1, February 1991.
6. Rivlin AM and JM Wiener. *Caring for the Disabled Elderly*. The Brookings Institution, 1998.
7. *U.S. Industrial Outlook*. U.S. Department of Commerce, 1993.
8. *Facing the Costs of Long-Term Care*, Employee Benefit Research Institute, 1990.
9. Scarborough R and B Bruan. Testimony for the American Association of Retired Persons to the House Ways and Means Health Subcommittee and the Senate Labor and Human Resources Committee, November 2 and 10, 1993.
10. McCarty P. Testimony for the Alzheimer's Association to the Senate Labor and Human Resources Committee, November 10, 1993.
11. Young A. Testimony for Consortium for Citizens With Disabilities to the Senate Labor and Human Resources Committee, November 10, 1993.
12. Simpson J. Testimony for Consortium for Citizens With Disabilities to the House Ways and Means Health Subcommittee, November 2, 1993.

13. Richtman M. Testimony for the National Committee to Preserve Social Security and Medicare to the House Ways and Means Health Subcommittee and the Senate Labor and Human Resources Committee, November 2 and 10, 1993.

14. Halamandaris V. Testimony for the National Association for Home Care to the House Ways and Means Health Subcommittee and the Senate Labor and Human Resources Committee, November 2 and 10, 1993.

15. Rodgers M. Testimony for the American Association of Homes for the Aging to the House Ways and Means Health Subcommittee, November 2, 1993.

16. Willging P. Testimony for the American Health Care Association to the House Ways and Means Health Subcommittee and the Senate Labor and Human Resources Committee, November 10, 1993.

17. Wiener JM. Testimony to the House Ways and Means Health Subcommittee, November 2, 1993.

18. Economic and Social Research Institute. Health Bulletin, July 1993.

CHAPTER 7

Quality of Care Under Reform: Practice Guidelines and Report Cards

David Strickland

In order to mandate ways to ensure the quality and cost-effectiveness of care, the authors of the quality section of President Clinton's Health Security Act took on the basic tenets of the fledgling outcomes and guidelines movement. In doing so, they inherited not only the movement's principles, jargon, and ambitions, but its uncertainties and detractors as well.

Simply put, an outcome is a result of what happens to a patient on his or her journey through the health care delivery system. Although outcomes are in some sense the consequences of medical interventions, they are also strongly influenced by the patient's overall health before seeking care and such factors as age, habits, genetics, income level, and other demographic elements.

Although health care providers have, over the years, made stabs at measuring the results of their care, the movement to measure these outcomes picked up steam in this country during the 1970s when already-rising costs began to spiral out of control. The movement was spearheaded by those paying for care, who demanded that physicians climb down from their "doctor knows best" pedestals and begin to document performance like any other supplier in a free-market economy. In a sense, payers challenged providers to demonstrate to them that they were actually "getting their money's worth."

Physicians, on the other hand, found themselves tangled in a web created by patient demand for unlimited care, expensive and expanding new technologies, and the constant and growing threat of malpractice litigation, from which "defensive medicine" was born. That web is as sticky as ever and lies at the heart of the reform debate.

The roots of what became a movement can be found in studies conducted in the early 1970s by the Dartmouth Medical School's John Wennberg, MD. Wennberg documented through a system known as "small-area analysis" that variations in levels of health care utilization had more to do with physician beliefs, training, and practice patterns than with the health of similar populations in neighboring communities[1]. Wennberg's seminal research prompted the question, "At what point does more care not equal better outcomes?" Several of medicine's best minds began to grapple with this question in earnest and the outcomes movement, fueled by payer demands, was off and running.

This movement to measure the effects of care, and thereby prove its value, was given a name when Paul Ellwood, MD, coined the phrase "outcomes management" in a May 1988 Shattuck Lecture to the Massachusetts Medical Society. The text of Ellwood's lecture was reprinted in the *New England Journal of Medicine*[2] and was followed soon after by an editorial by then-Editor-in-Chief Arnold Relman, MD, who proclaimed that health care was, at long last, moving into an "era of assessment and accountability."[3]

Although the movement was initially driven by the effort to document the value of care, along the way something synergistic happened. In their attempts to explore cost-effectiveness, researchers across the country found that by closely examining the processes by which care was delivered, the actual quality of care improved in many cases. Thus came the integration of cost-effectiveness and quality, with outcomes as the yardstick for both. An alphabet soup of QI, QA, and QM (quality improvement, assurance, and management) programs bubbled up in hospitals nationwide — many of them staffed by skeleton crews that historically had met infrequently. Pharmaceutical companies, who were traditionally charged with proving the safety and efficacy of their drugs, came under new pressure to demonstrate that their drugs were cost-effective as defined by better patient outcomes.

Throughout this movement are woven practice guidelines. Although they are known by many names and used under different circumstances with differing degrees of force, guidelines are best defined by the Institute of Medicine's Marilyn Field and Kathleen Lohr as "systematically developed statements to assist practitioner and patient decisions about appropriate health care for specific clinical circumstances."[4] The links between outcomes and guidelines run both ways: The best guidelines are based on outcomes research, as opposed to expert consensus, and guidelines are very often used to improve patient outcomes.

The American Medical Association, which prefers the term "parameters" over "guidelines," began cataloging guidelines with its first *Directory of Practice Parameters* in 1989. That first directory identified 700 parameters nationwide. The number has since grown to approximately 1,500. The majority of these guidelines are produced by physician specialty societies, such as the American College of Cardiology and the American College of Physicians. Many payers, utilization reviewers, and local provider groups have also created their own guidelines, which are also known as protocols, standards, algorithms, or decision pathways.

Some physicians scorn guidelines, calling them "cookbook medicine," because they perceive a failure to take into account the "art of medicine" and the multitude of factors that make each patient and encounter unique. These detractors seem to be becoming less vocal, however, as guideline developers take pains to include the very physicians who will be affected by guidelines in the process of creating, reviewing, and updating them. And even skeptics concede that practice guidelines represent a promising means to reduce the unwarranted variation in care first pointed out in Wennberg's research.

While the U.S. Health Care Financing Administration has sought to examine the effectiveness of treatments that it pays for, and agencies such as the Heart, Lung, and Blood Institute have convened expert panels to offer recommendations concerning the best treatment methods, the federal government took a major step toward legitimizing and recognizing the importance of the outcomes and guidelines movement in 1989, when it formed the U.S. Agency for Health Care Policy and Research (AHCPR).

AHCPR has two major responsibilities: sponsoring outcomes research and developing clinical practice guidelines. To date, AHCPR is funding and guiding 14 Patient Outcomes Research Teams, on topics ranging from low back pain to congestive heart failure, and has released six clinical practice guidelines. Those six guidelines are for: acute pain management, urinary incontinence, pressure ulcers (bedsores), cataracts, depression in the primary care setting, and sickle cell disease.

Although the Clintons' Health Security Act calls for creating several new federal advisory bodies, and layers of new bureaucracy, the four-year-old AHCPR figures prominently in the legislation.

THE CLINTON QUALITY PLAN

Quality Measures

The Health Security Act would create a new and powerful National Health Board, that would, among its other duties, oversee the national quality efforts under reform. The bill stipulates that one year after the law's enactment, the National Health Board "shall establish and oversee a performance-based program of quality management and improvement designed to enhance the quality, appropriateness, and effectiveness of health care services and access to such services."

This program, dubbed the National Quality Management Program, is to be administered by a newly created 15-member National Quality Management Council. The Council, which should be "representative of the U.S. population," is to be appointed by the President and composed of individuals representing the interests of government and corporate health care purchasers, health plans, states, providers, and academic health centers. The Council would include individuals distinguished in the fields of public health, health care quality, and related fields of health services research.

Council members are to be appointed for three-year terms, except for those who make up the first Council. The first Council's members will serve staggered terms so that five members will serve for three years, another five members for two years, and a third five members for one year. The President will appoint one of the Council's members as chair. The National Health Board is charged with providing the Council with staff, information, and assistance for carrying out its duties.

The Council is instructed to develop a set of national measures of quality performance to provide information on access to care, appropriateness of care, outcomes of services and procedures, health promotion, disease prevention, and patient satisfaction with care. A draft of the Clintons' legislation called for up to 50 of these measures. The final language in the Health Security Act does not specify how many measures the Council is to select.

The Council is instructed to review and update these measures annually "to reflect changing goals for quality improvement." The National Health Board is charged with establishing and maintaining a five-year priority list of performance measures that the Council should consider adding to its set of measures.

In choosing these quality measures, the Council is instructed to consult with "appropriate interested parties," including states, health plans, employers and other purchasers, providers, a newly created National Quality Consortium, the Director of the National Institutes of Health, the administrators of both the Health Care Financing Administration and AHCPR, and individuals distinguished in the fields of law, medicine, economics, public health, and health services research.

The Health Security Act sets forth the following criteria for the Council's selection of national quality measures:

- ☐ SIGNIFICANCE - The disease, disorder, or condition measured must be significant in terms of prevalence, morbidity (the "state of being diseased," which often includes disease complications), mortality, or costs associated with the prevention, diagnosis, treatment, or clinical management of the disease, disorder, or condition.
- ☐ RANGE OF SERVICES - The set of measures shall be representative of the range of services supplied by health care providers. Many so-called "alternative treatments" not provided by the average hospital could be ruled out under this criterion.
- ☐ RELIABILITY AND VALIDITY - The measures shall be reliable and valid. Reliability is a scientific term that refers to the probability that a measure will be satisfactory according to its rates of failure and accuracy. Validity refers to a measure's ability to be a true indicator of what it is intended to measure.

- ☐ UNDUE BURDEN - The data needed to calculate the measures shall be obtained without undue burden on the entity or individual providing the data. An example of an undue burden would be the Council requiring a data set or data collection system that would cause many providers to become financially bankrupt.
- ☐ VARIATION - Performance under the measure varies widely among individual or institutional providers. For example, if a particular treatment was clearly considered to be the best by almost all physicians, and was in widespread use with very similar outcomes, that treatment and the condition it is used to treat would be unlikely candidates under this criterion. The buzzword "variation" harkens back to Wennberg's research.
- ☐ LINK TO HEALTH OUTCOME - When a measure is of a process of care, the measure shall be linked to a health outcome based on the best available scientific evidence. Process measures often document factors such as immunization rates, screening rates, and hospital length of stay. In these cases, the Council would need to demonstrate that certain immunizations or screenings such as mammography resulted in less incidence of disease, and that patients' length of stay in a hospital affected their health status.
- ☐ PROVIDER CONTROL AND RISK ADJUSTMENT - The outcome measured shall be within the control of the provider and one with respect to which an adequate risk adjustment should be made. There are two important issues addressed here. According to outcomes expert and New York State Health Commissioner Mark Chassin, MD, the rate at which lung cancer patients develop liver metastasis in a six-month period "is a terrible quality measure because we can't do a thing about it."[5] The other issue, risk adjustment, is important because providers must be judged by their outcomes "on a level playing field." If two physicians were compared to one another on the basis of their outcomes, but there was no adjustment made to reflect that one of the physicians treated older, sicker, poorer patients, the comparison would be flawed.
- ☐ PUBLIC HEALTH - The measures may incorporate standards identified by the Secretary of Health and Human Services for meeting public health objectives. It's likely that the framers of this section are referring to the U.S. Public Health Service's national health promotion and disease prevention objectives, known collectively as "Healthy People 2000." This set of measurable targets for the year 2000 include those for cancer, diabetes, heart disease, mental health, oral health, HIV infection, maternal and infant health, and stroke.

Reports on Quality

The Health Security Act makes health alliances responsible for enrolling eligible residents, serving as collective purchasing agents for employers and consumers at the local level, soliciting bids from health plans, and enforcing quality standards, financial solvency, and fair access to health plans.

The Act requires each alliance to annually publish a public report, in a standard format, showing how the plans within that alliance performed with regard to the national quality measures. In introducing their legislation to Congress, both Bill and Hillary Rodham Clinton referred to these reports as "report cards," a new term frequently used to describe published lists of provider quality indicators.

To date, two prominent managed care organizations, United HealthCare and Kaiser Permanente, have used the report card moniker when releasing their own reports that measure levels of care according to a variety of quality indicators. Both organizations showed how they compare with different national, state, and local "benchmarks." These efforts also coincide with the recent efforts of two health care accreditation agencies — the Joint Commission on Accreditation of Healthcare Organizations and the National Committee for Quality Assurance — to develop and test their own quality indicators.

All four groups say the Clintons consulted with them while drawing up reform legislation concerning provider quality reporting. These four have developed lists of quality indicators that vary in the number of indicators and in the ratio between process outcomes, such as mammography rates, and "true" outcomes, such as mortality rates.

The Health Security Act states that in addition to developing quality measures, the National Quality Management Council is to conduct periodic surveys of consumers to gauge health care access, utilization, outcomes, and satisfaction.

These surveys are intended to monitor the reaction of the implementation of the Act and to assess the impact of health reform on the general U.S. population and "potentially vulnerable populations." These surveys are to be administered by AHCPR on a plan-by-plan and state-by-state basis. States may add questions of local interest to the surveys. The Act instructs that survey sampling should take into account "difficult to reach populations" such as those who failed to enroll in a plan, resigned from a plan, or who are members of a "vulnerable population." The results from these surveys are also to be published in the report cards.

The Council is also instructed to do its own assessment of the impact of health reform on quality and access. The Council must annually provide to Congress and each alliance a report that discusses state and national trends relating to quality and access and outlines performance for each alliance and health plan.

Health Care Quality Research

Under the Health Security Act, the Council is to direct AHCPR to support research directly related to the National Health Board's five-year priority list, including research on outcomes of services and procedures, "effective and efficient dissemination of information, standards, and guidelines"; methods of measuring quality and shared decision-making; and the design and components of automated health information systems.

The Council shall also establish priorities for research — and make recommendations for research — taking into account health care quality, appropriateness, and effectiveness. These priorities shall address the highest level of uncertainty concerning treatments; the widest variation of practice patterns; significant costs associated with prevention, diagnosis, and treatment; and high rates of incidence or prevalence for the population as a whole or for particular subpopulations.

The National Health Board is charged with establishing and overseeing "regional professional foundations." Membership for each of these foundations is to include one academic health center, as well as schools of public health, other schools and programs, health plans, regional alliances, corporate alliances, and providers. The foundations are instructed, for their regions, to develop programs of "lifetime learning" for health professionals so that they can keep "abreast of new knowledge, acquire new skills, and adopt new roles as technology and societal demands change."

The foundations are intended to help ensure quality; foster collaboration among plans and providers to improve primary and specialized care; and disseminate information about successful quality improvement programs, guidelines, innovation, and research findings. These foundations will also develop innovative patient education systems that "enhance patient involvement in decisions relating to their health care."

The National Health Board is also charged with creating a National Quality Consortium. This Consortium is supposed to establish continuing education programs for health professionals, advise the Council and AHCPR on research priorities, oversee the development of the regional professional foundations, advise the Council on funding for establishing the regional professional foundations, consult with the Council on choosing the national quality measures, and advise the National Health Board and the Council on other matters.

This Consortium is to be composed of 11 members appointed by the National Health Board and should include five academic health center representatives, and six representatives from schools of public health and other schools, including medical, nursing, and allied health professions schools. These are three-year posts, with the first Consortium to have staggered membership: four members for three years, three members for two years, and four members for one year. The National Health Board will designate the Consortium's chairman. See Figure 7-1.

Practice Guidelines

Under the Health Security Act, the Council is to direct AHCPR to develop and periodically review and update practice guidelines so providers can determine how "diseases, disorders, and other health conditions can most effectively and appropriately be prevented, diagnosed, treated, and managed clinically."

These guidelines shall be "based on the best available research and professional judgment regarding the effectiveness and appropriateness of health care services and procedures." A lack of good, scientific research for forming a guideline is often the Achilles' heel of many such efforts. An AHCPR guideline panel rediscovered this recently while crafting its upcoming guideline for congestive heart failure. The panel's co-chair, Marvin Konstam, MD, of the New England Medical Center, says the panel had a tough time reaching a consensus on revascularization

Figure 7-1

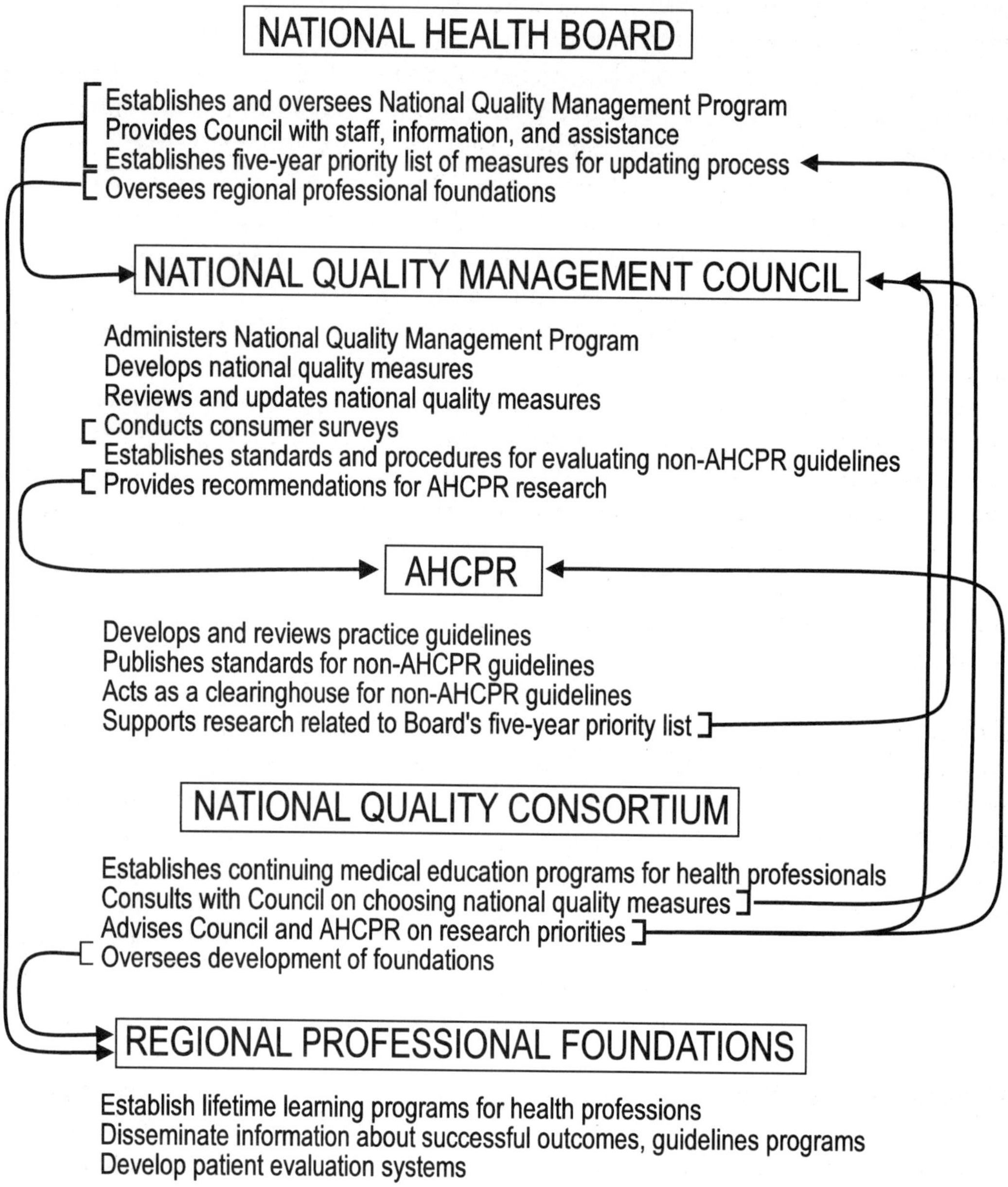

(angioplasty and bypass) because of a lack of good data in the literature they studied. He says the panel was forced to base these recommendations on data from uncontrolled trials because most controlled trials (the "gold standard" for medical research) for revascularization exclude heart failure patients.

The Act stipulates that these guidelines shall be treatment- or condition-specific, and in formats usable by providers, educators, medical review organizations, and consumers. So far, all guidelines released by AHCPR have been accompanied by a reference guide for patients, so that they may better understand the "state of the art" knowledge concerning their condition and available treatments. This is intended to arm patients with the information they need to become active participants in their own treatment plans.

In language similar to that currently guiding AHCPR, the Act states that these new guidelines should "include information on risks and benefits of alternative strategies for prevention, diagnosis, treatment, and management of a given disease, disorder, or other health condition." The guidelines are to include information on the costs of these alternative strategies when cost information is available and reliable. The Council is also charged with establishing standards and procedures for evaluating the clinical appropriateness of guidelines used to manage health service utilization, and with disseminating information documenting clinically ineffective treatments and procedures.

The Health Security Act makes a monumental leap toward influencing how organizations outside the federal government, such as physician specialty societies, shape their own guidelines. This leap comes through instructions to AHCPR to develop and publish standards relating to methodologies for developing guidelines and to develop a procedure so others can submit guidelines to the Council for evaluation and certification. AHCPR is also charged with establishing and overseeing a clearinghouse and dissemination program for guidelines developed or certified according to AHCPR criteria.

It's unlikely that the provision instructing AHCPR to develop standards for guidelines development will create a lot of new work for the Agency: It already employs widely accepted criteria developed by a panel under the auspices of the Institute of Medicine.[6] The IOM drew up these attributes in response to a request from AHCPR shortly after the Agency's creation in 1989. The Agency's own panels and many others outside the Agency adhere to them when developing guidelines. Here is a summary of the IOM's eight attributes:

- VALIDITY - Practice guidelines are considered valid if, when they are followed, they lead to the health and cost outcomes projected for them. Validity assessments should include the strength and quality of the evidence cited, the means used to evaluate this evidence, and the relationship between the evidence and the recommendations. Practice guidelines should be accompanied by a comparison of health and cost outcomes for the recommended interventions and for alternative interventions. Outcomes assessments should consider patient perceptions and preferences.
- RELIABILITY/REPRODUCIBILITY - Given the same evidence and guidelines development methods, another group of experts should be able to produce essentially the same statements. Given the same clinical circumstances, practitioners should be able to apply the guidelines consistently.
- CLINICAL APPLICABILITY - Practice guidelines should define the appropriate patient populations and specify to which populations the statements apply.
- CLINICAL FLEXIBILITY - Practice guidelines should identify exceptions to the recommendations and discuss how to identify and consider patient preferences.

- CLARITY - Practice guidelines must be presented in a logical and easy-to-follow manner using unambiguous language and precisely defined terms.
- MULTIDISCIPLINARY PROCESS - The development process must include participation by "key affected groups" and may include these groups in development panels. Participation by these groups may include providing evidence and viewpoints and reviewing drafts of the guidelines.
- SCHEDULED REVIEW - Practice guidelines must include statements about when they should be reviewed to determine if revisions are needed. Revisions may be warranted in light of new clinical evidence or professional consensus, or in light of a lack of such evidence or consensus.
- DOCUMENTATION - Panels should meticulously document and describe the procedures followed, the participants involved, the evidence used, the assumptions and rationales accepted, and analytical evidence employed while developing the guidelines.

Whether AHCPR determines, under the Health Security Act, that it needs to revise or add to these attributes remains to be seen. If this section of the Act giving AHCPR new power to evaluate and certify others' guidelines is implemented, and the IOM criteria retain their present clout within the Agency, it is highly likely that groups not currently following the IOM criteria as part of their guidelines development process will begin to do so as a means of gaining AHCPR's "seal of approval."

This seal of approval takes on extreme importance because guidelines developed both under the auspices of AHCPR and those developed outside the Agency but certified by AHCPR could be used, under the Clinton plan, in a controversial experiment linking practice guidelines to malpractice liability reform. This experiment is described below.

Practice Guidelines and Malpractice Liability Reform

The Health Security Act calls for reforming our current malpractice liability system in a number of ways. The Act outlines alternative dispute resolution (ADR) systems, under which a final resolution must be reached before any legal actions can be allowed to proceed. The Act puts forth plans to limit attorneys' contingency fees to one-third the total amount of a judgment recovered. The Act also resurrects the idea of "enterprise liability" by calling for a demonstration project, to be established no later than January 1, 1996, that would allow one or more eligible states to explore whether replacing liability for physicians with liability for health plans will bring improvements in quality of care and reductions in defensive medicine.

Guidelines come into play under a demonstration project that would allow physicians, and presumably other professionals providing patient care, to use as a "complete defense" proof that they followed appropriate guidelines as outlined under the National Quality Management Program.

Under the Act, this demonstration project would begin no later than one year after the Secretary of the Department of Health and Human Services determines that appropriate guidelines are available for the pilot project. The HHS Secretary would provide funding for the pilot to one or more states. The HHS Secretary is also required to submit to Congress, three months after the end of each year the pilot is in effect, reports that describe the pilot and contain recommendations that the Secretary considers appropriate, including recommendations relating to revisions to the law governing medical malpractice liability. The Health Security Act does not state for how long this pilot would be conducted.

THE CLINTON QUALITY PLAN: AN ANALYSIS

Guidelines and the Law

The Clinton proposal for a demonstration project linking malpractice defense to adherence to practice guidelines can be traced to similar demonstration projects in Maine and Minnesota. Maine's five-year demonstration project has been under way since January 1992. The Minnesota project could begin as early as spring 1994.

Under the Maine project, which was signed into law in 1990, physicians using 20 state panel-produced guidelines for certain conditions and procedures in the specialties of anesthesiology, emergency medicine, obstetrics/gynecology, and radiology, are allowed to use proof of guidelines adherence as an "affirmative defense" in malpractice cases. Plaintiffs are not permitted to cite failure to use guidelines to bolster their allegations.

The Clinton proposal deviates from the Maine project by signaling a "complete defense" rather that an affirmative defense. In this respect, the Clinton plan more closely resembles Minnesota's project, which is expected to provide physicians an "absolute defense." In cases involving an absolute defense, plaintiffs are barred from further action once guidelines compliance has been established. In cases involving an affirmative defense, plaintiffs may still produce evidence for consideration by the court.

Troyen Brennan, MD, a lawyer and an associate professor of medicine at Harvard Medical School says it's "extremely likely" that the Minnesota law will be found unconstitutional because it offers physicians blanket immunity without permitting plaintiffs a reasonable opportunity to prove otherwise — an opinion expressed by other health law experts as well.

Among these experts is Kathleen Hastings, director of legal medicine for AHCPR and co-chair of a work group that advised the Clintons on malpractice reform. Hastings says her work group told the President that tying guidelines to malpractice reform would be premature at this time because the state-of-the-art for guideline development isn't there yet. Hastings calls AHCPR's guidelines the "most rigorously, methodically developed" guidelines available but points out that the Agency has released only six so far. She says that many guidelines developed by specialty societies and other groups are based merely on consensus panel deliberations and that incorporating those guidelines into federal tort reform would be "irresponsible."

It's likely that the Clintons took this advice to heart when they decided to promote state-by-state demonstrations rather than pushing for immediate use of guidelines in courtrooms nationwide. But the President made his intentions clear as far back as October 1992 when the then-candidate said during a Presidential debate, "I've recommended that our doctors be given a set of national practice guidelines and if they follow these guidelines, it raises the presumption that they didn't do anything wrong."

The American Medical Association supports the demonstration projects, rather than more far-reaching legislation, says John Kelly, MD, director of the AMA's Office of Quality Assurance. He says the projects are "a good way to try out an untested concept" but cautions that it's important that policymakers don't lose sight of the reason why guidelines were developed in the first place. "[Guidelines'] primary goal is to improve the quality of clinical care and the practice of medicine," he says. "They are written for doctors, health care professionals, and the public to provide guidance concerning medical decisions. They are not written for lawyers and the courts."

So far, there have been no cases brought under Maine's pilot project. This does not surprise Gordon Smith, counsel for the Maine Medical Association. "These 20 protocols deal with a very small portion of the medicine practiced in a small state by a small number of physicians," Smith says, adding that "it's going to take a lot more data than we have to examine the liability issue."

Federal demonstration projects could change all that. On the other hand, the use of guidelines in the courtroom is likely to bring challenges to the constitutionality of the effort: Plaintiffs would argue that they've been given an undue burden in proving negligence.

Efforts are already under way to gather data on the Maine pilot's effects on physician practice patterns and defensive medicine. In February 1993 Maine's Senators, George Mitchell (D) and William Cohen (R), ordered the General Accounting Office to launch a study looking into the defensive medicine issue. The GAO study is comparing actual rates of cervical spine x-rays, pre-operative tests for anesthesiology, cesarean sections, and hysterectomies against "expected rates" that may have occurred in the absence of the state pilot's guidelines.

AHCPR is funding a three-year study to examine Maine obstetricians' practice patterns. This study is looking at cesarean section rates and other birth-related outcomes, including fetal distress, fetal pulmonary immaturity, and post-term pregnancy, by examining hospital discharge data and data abstracted from patient medical records for the period between 1987 and 1995. The researchers plan to compare this data with similar data collected for the same period from outside Maine.

Meanwhile, Minnesota officials are planning to adopt for their demonstration project upcoming AHCPR guidelines for treating low back pain and unstable angina. The Agency is expected to release these two guidelines in spring 1994. If the plan goes through, it will be the first time that AHCPR guidelines are permissible for use as a defense in malpractice cases. Minnesota passed its legislation linking guidelines to liability in 1992. Minnesota officials hope the guidelines will also be used to reduce variation, prompt provider internal quality programs, stimulate patient education, and reduce adverse outcomes.

Practicing physicians may not be the only ones landing in court on the basis of decisions involving practice guidelines. Prompted by fears expressed by its panels that they may be held liable for the content of the guidelines they produce, AHCPR has insured its panels and their consultants against any liability award of up to $5 million. The Agency has also distributed to its panels a "guidelines for developing guidelines" manual addressing the dangers of ambiguity, imprecise language, and overstatement.

It's possible that a guidelines panel could find itself in court under a third party suit where a patient sues his or her physician for malpractice and also sues the developers of the guidelines that the physician followed. Some legal experts say it's highly unlikely that a court would grant an award against guideline developers in such a case, because their efforts are perceived by courts to be in the public's best interest. But the Institute of Medicine's Marilyn Field warns, "There's always the chance that you'll get sued." She says that those who are "most potentially vulnerable" are panels that develop a consensus based on opinions of best practices. Field recommends that all guideline developers routinely document every step of their analysis carefully.

AHCPR's Kathleen Hastings says that the Agency's panels' fears "may be overblown," but adds, "We haven't had a lot of experience in this area. It's important to be prudent, cautious, explicit, and clear."

Other Guidelines Issues

The Health Security Act takes another large step into the guidelines arena by granting AHCPR the power to certify guidelines created by other organizations. AHCPR's guidelines panels usually have various physician specialty societies represented in their membership, and drafts of the guidelines are circulated to the appropriate specialty societies for comment prior to their release. But this new provision would go a long way to forcing national standards for guideline development.

The American Medical Association's John Kelly, MD, is afraid that the progress enjoyed through private sector efforts could be undermined by "over-regulation" from the federal government, perhaps even causing a "chilling effect" on the development of guidelines. He says an "inherently arbitrary" system could evolve, in which the government brands conflicting guidelines for the same condition or procedure as "good" or "bad" when, in fact, they might both have merit. Such a system would stifle creativity, he says, and reduce the flexibility that private sector developers currently have to modify and adjust their guidelines as new information becomes available.

One instance of conflicting guidelines is currently being played out in the field of mammography appropriateness. The National Cancer Institute is considering revision of its longstanding guidelines that now call for mammograms yearly or every other year for women in their 40s. The proposed change would suggest that these women consult with their physicians instead to determine the need for mammography. This proposal is based on an examination of several controversial studies that an NCI advisory group says show that mammography screening doesn't lead to lower breast cancer death rates in women under 50.

The American Cancer Society, which also has longstanding mammography guidelines similar to the current NCI guidelines, disagrees with the NCI proposal.

The ACS has no intention of changing its guidelines and says that, to date, there have been no clinical trials yet conducted that answer the mammography appropriateness question with confidence. Other organizations, such as the American College of Radiology and the National Alliance of Breast Cancer Organizations have lined up behind the ACS.

Aside from the issue of conflicting guidelines, there are other problems that a federal certification process could create, says the ACS's Robert Smith. He says he hopes that any federal criteria don't restrict certification to only those guidelines based on findings from controlled clinical trials. "Randomized trials are not always possible for studying certain conditions," Smith says. He cites costs, lengthy study durations, an inability to enroll sufficient numbers of patients, and the ethics of giving sick patients placebos as possible obstacles to controlled trials.

Still others worry about placing AHCPR in charge of certification when the Agency's guidelines have so far generated their own share of controversy. The American Psychological Association refused to endorse AHCPR's 1993 guideline for diagnosing and treating depression in the primary care setting, claiming that the guideline slights psychologists and other mental health professionals and relies too much on medication-based treatment.

A group of ophthalmologists was so irate over certain sections of AHCPR's 1993 cataract guideline that they banded together and released their own cataract guideline. They were upset over statements concerning cataract surgery appropriateness in the AHCPR guideline, and charged the Agency with "trying to frighten seniors away from getting needed care." The AHCPR guideline says that there is not enough scientific evidence to support using specular photographic microscopy and contrast sensitivity, glare, and macular function tests to determine cataract surgery appropriateness. The ophthalmology group disagreed, maintaining that these tests are very useful.

These disputes suggest the need for caution in ceding legislative authority to any one government agency for the purpose of certifying guidelines created in the private sector, especially if those guidelines could take on the force of law in malpractice litigation.

Report Cards

When report cards showed up in the Clinton legislation, few health care leaders engaged in similar efforts were surprised. The surprise, they say, will come when the federal government realizes what an enormous task it is undertaking. Pitfalls along the way include a lack of uniform data, resistance from overburdened providers, different constituencies' conflicting needs, and cumbersome methodologies. These obstacles, however, will be easier to conquer if federal administrators avoid "reinventing the wheel" and seek counsel from outside government.

Those constructing the national report cards "need to seriously consider public/private partnerships at the very beginning of these efforts, so employer groups and providers can bring their experience to the table," says Janet Corrigan, vice-president of planning and development for the National Committee for Quality Assurance, an independent HMO accreditation organization.

One lesson the NCQA learned while crafting its own set of 60 quality indicators is that the majority of health plans it surveyed could only provide outcomes data from administrative data sets, limiting the amount of available clinical data and, in turn, the number of outcomes indicators. "We cast a big net for performance indicators, but the majority fell into the categories of patient satisfaction, health status, and such intermediate outcomes as pediatric immunization and mammography," Corrigan says.

The NCQA plans to release a final version of its indicators soon. But even with a list of indicators for which almost all providers collect some data, the lack of uniformity in reporting is something that both the NCQA and the federal government will be struggling with for a while. Corrigan predicts that it will be several years before either program has truly comparable data to work with.

The Joint Commission on Accreditation of Healthcare Organizations hopes that the federal government doesn't overlook providers' needs in its rush to get comparative data to purchasers and consumers. While mortality rates are of great interest to purchasers and consumers, such rates are of less value to providers because they are "too global" and signal only an "end result," of care, says William Jessee, MD, the JCAHO's vice-president of research and standards. Providers need to know which processes cause bad outcomes so they can move to correct them, he says.

But clinical endpoints are still valuable tools for providers because they signal where to concentrate quality improvement efforts, says Vahe Kazandjian, director of the Maryland Quality Indicator Project, a data-sharing program with 740 member hospitals in 48 states, England, and Japan. He would like to see complication and readmission rates on the list of federal indicators, because these rates are often signs of substandard care.

Consumers find mortality rates helpful for making care decisions, but only if they are for procedures with traditionally high mortality rates, says Arthur Levin, director of the New York-based Center for Medical Consumers. Levin says mortality rates for procedures such as back surgery, which are usually low, "make everybody look good," but tell consumers very little. For such procedures, report cards need to paint a broader picture by including morbidity factors such as pain and disability, he says. And when mortality rates are included, researchers need to "look further down the line" than the 30-, 60-, and 90-day rates that are typically offered, Levin says.

The federal government needs to test a wide variety of data collection, analysis, and dissemination approaches before they finalize their list of indicators, says the AMA's John Kelly, MD. This effort should involve demonstration projects aimed at evaluating the effectiveness — and usefulness — of both old and new systems, he says. "It's possible to collect an enormous amount of data and end up with a lot of information that's not useful to anybody."

JCAHO's Jessee shares those concerns. He warns of "data overload" in which "the state of our ability to handle the available data hasn't caught up with the amount of data that's available." For example, he says, when consumers are told a provider's coronary bypass rates are good, cholecystectomy rates are okay, and cesarean section rates are bad, "most don't know what to make of this." But that shouldn't stop data from being released, he says. "Let's get it out there and say, 'We're just as confused with this as you are. Let's work together to see what it means.'"

Making outcomes information "statistically sound and also manageable for consumers is a fine line," says Joe Martin, spokesman for the Pennsylvania Health Care Cost Containment Council (PHC4). The Council publicly released its third annual Hospital Effectiveness Report for Philadelphia hospitals in late September 1993. The report details outcomes adjusted for patient severity of illness, including mortality rates, for 53 medical and surgical diagnosis-related groups. The PHC4 is best known for its statewide release of surgeon-specific bypass mortality rates, a project that drew fire from many providers who blasted the adjustment methodology and said that the public was not knowledgeable enough to interpret the data properly.

As outcomes data — including the federal government's report cards — become more available, the public will become more adept at using them, says Carol Cronin, executive director of the Managed Health Care Association. "It's primitive to think that people don't have the capacity to understand this type of information," she says. Each public release of outcomes information creates demand for more, and the quality of the information generally improves with each release, she says. "Five to ten years from now we will look back and think it's incredible that there was a time when we didn't have this information."

Cronin says, however, that there hasn't been enough discussion about the cost and labor burden that health plans will have to bear under the federal data collection effort. She calls the kind of infrastructure that the Clinton Administration is proposing "fairly significant," and says the information systems needed to produce the information will require a major investment on the part of providers.

Minnesota-based United HealthCare's (UHC) effort to compile and distribute report cards on its health plans to the thousands of employers it contracts with nationwide is "arduous," says Sheila Leatherman, president of UHC's Center for Health Care Policy and Evaluation. "The final format looks simple but the underlying database, systems, and research are complex and costly," she says.

Leatherman says the data comparison that the report card effort will bring is sorely needed. UHC had an "extremely difficult time" finding up-to-date outside data for comparison with its own plans, she says. A sample UHC report card released in September 1993 on its United Health Plans of New England, which covers members located primarily in Rhode Island and Massachusetts, compares the plan's 1992 cesarean section rate with 1991 National Center for Health Statistics (NCHS) data for the entire northeastern region. The plan's 1992 low birth-weight rate is compared with 1991 NCHS data for the entire country. UHC was unable to locate data for comparison with the plan's hospitalization rate for pediatric asthma. The sample report card compares 1989-1990 liver transplant survival rates for all UHC plans to 1988 national data from United Network Organ Sharing, "the only organization we could find that did a national study on this" says a UHC researcher.

In October 1993, Kaiser Permanente's Northern California Region jumped on the report card bandwagon. Kaiser compared its care on more than 100 indicators with a variety of outside benchmarks, including those furnished by the state of California. Kaiser officials hope that their report card will serve as an precursor for the federal report cards. But in a remark that shows how far the science of creating report cards still has to go, a Kaiser official says, "What we've put together is a Model T Ford of quality measurement. . . . It's incomplete and there are flaws with the comparisons, but we think it's a major step forward in measuring quality and improving patient care."

Once the quality measures called for in the Clinton plan have been selected and the data have been collected and disseminated, the major hurdle of using these reports to actually improve care will still remain. While consumers can use this information to "vote with their feet" by gravitating toward the providers in their area that demonstrate the best outcomes, it will still be up to providers to develop innovative ways to meet the quality improvement mandate.

OTHER LEGISLATION

As expected, lawmakers outside the Clinton camp have risen to the health reform challenge with their own legislation. The quality proposals contained in these various legislative initiatives are, so far, nowhere near as comprehensive as those in the 1,342-page Health Security Act. But many of them are founded on the same principles — and on the outcomes and guidelines movement.

A revamped version of the managed competition proposal introduced in 1992 by the Conservative Democratic Forum was introduced in October 1993 in the House of Representatives by Jim Cooper (D-TN) and Fred Grandy (R-IA). This legislation calls for report cards that would list mortality, complication, and recovery rates. These report cards would also include process outcomes such as the percentage of health plan enrollees who have had immunizations and mammograms. There is no mention of a role for practice guidelines in the bill's section on malpractice reform.

Senator John Chafee (R-RI) hopes to introduce bipartisan-sponsored health reform legislation in late 1993. An outline released by the Senate Republican Task Force on health care reform in September 1993 calls for a Federal Administrative Standards panel to provide consumers with information on health plans' outcomes and quality. The outline also calls for using guidelines approved by AHCPR as a "presumptive defense" in malpractice cases.

Legislation introduced in September 1993 by House Minority Leader Robert Michel (R-IL) steers clear of allowing adherence to practice guidelines as a malpractice defense. Instead, the bill calls for an alternative dispute resolution system, limits of attorneys' contingency fees, and caps on non-economic damages as ways to tackle high liability premiums and defensive medicine. The only area of this bill that addresses outcomes research and quality measurement is contained in a section that would require states to publish data on the "comparative value" of care from providers. Michel's legislative aide says that this language was intentionally vague, but may very well encompass outcomes measurement and reporting.

WARNINGS FROM THE OUTCOMES WATCHERS

In 1988, the *New England Journal of Medicine's* then-Editor-in-Chief Arnold Relman, MD, announced the "era of assessment and accountability."[3] In 1993, the *Journal's* current Editor-in-Chief Jerome Kassirer, MD, issued warnings about the dilemmas that this era has brought.

"From a system that until recently was dominated by reliance on intelligent and thoughtful decision making by individual doctors, we seem to have embarked on a path of codifying the practice of medicine," wrote Kassirer. "In part, we are doing so in the name of quality. To be sure, we are developing the tools to measure and monitor quality, but before we embrace them, we must be sure that they are equal to their intended tasks and that the benefits of standardization are worth the costs."[7]

AHCPR's own leaders urge caution for the road ahead. The Agency's Deputy Administrator Risa Lavisso-Mourey, MD, told a group of providers recently, "The good news is that outcomes and guidelines will play a central role in health care reform. The bad news is that we don't know everything about outcomes and guidelines, and we need to learn more."

REFERENCES

1. Wennberg J and A Gittelsohn. Small Area Variation in Health Care Delivery. *Science* 182, 1973: 1102-8. *See also* Wennberg J et al. Changes in Tonsillectomy Rates Associated With Feedback and Review. *Pediatrics* 59, 1977: 821-26; Wennberg J and A Gittelsohn. Variations in Medical Care Among Small Areas. *Scientific American* 246, 1982: 120-29; and Wennberg J et al. Are Hospital Services Under-Utilized in New Haven or Over-Utilized in Boston? *Lancet* 8543, 1987: 1185-89.

2. Ellwood P. Outcomes Management: A Technology of Patient Experience. *New England Journal of Medicine* 318, 1988: 1549-56.

3. Relman A. Assessment and Accountability: The Third Revolution in Medical Care. *New England Journal of Medicine* 319, 1988: 1221-22.

4. Field M and K Lohr. *Clinical Practice Guidelines: Directions for a New Program*. National Academy Press, 1990: 8.

5. Report From the Field: Interview With New York Health Commissioner Chassin on Appropriate Care. *Medical Outcomes & Guidelines Alert*, April 8, 1993.

6. Field M and K Lohr. *Guidelines for Clinical Practice: From Development to Use*. National Academy Press, 1992: 8.

7. Kassirer J. The Quality of Care and the Quality of Measuring It. *New England Journal of Medicine* 329, 1933: 1263-64.

CHAPTER 8

The States: Laboratory for Reform

Richard M. Sorian with Allan Holmes

While lawmakers in Washington DC were fiddling with stop-gap solutions to health care problems, the states were eager to fix their own systems rather than wait around for federal reform. Several states have instituted major reforms, while dozens of others instituted lesser changes. As 1993 began, there wasn't a state in the union that hadn't at least debated health reform.

Governors and state legislators were driven by several factors, chief among them costs. States, through their government employee health benefit programs, workers' compensation programs, and, most significantly, Medicaid contributions, were devoting increasing sums of money on health care delivery without any material benefits to their residents. In fact, by 1992, the National Conference of State Legislatures (NCSL) reported that spending on Medicaid had outstripped all other items in states' budgets — more than education, job training, and infrastructure maintenance. And the NCSL predicted that the 16 percent gulf between state college and university outlays and Medicaid spending recorded in fiscal 1993 would widen to 24 percent by FY94.[1]

The dramatic increase in state spending on medical costs in the 1980s was a result not only of more poor and elderly persons on the Medicaid rolls, but also the rising cost of hospital and physician care and of prescription drugs. From 1980 to 1991, the average annual cost per person for hospital care, physician services, and prescription drugs rose by between 8 percent (Alaska) and 11.6 percent (New Hampshire).[2] In 1991, that figure for all the states averaged $1,877 per person, more than double the $697 spent in 1980.

The states also were fed up with the gridlock in Washington. The failure of the federal government to address health system reform in the 1980s was frustrating enough for state lawmakers. But to sit by as federal lawmakers imposed new burdens on the states to plug the holes in the leaky national system was adding insult to injury. Beginning in the mid-1980s, Congress mandated state expansion of Medicaid coverage of women, infants, and children. While such voluntary widening of eligibility was popular among the governors — and in fact, had been originally suggested by the Southern Governors' Association — the mandates were irritating and costly to the states. After all, if a state acted in response to federal orders, local lawmakers could get little or no credit for expanding coverage. And if they refused, they risked not only federal penalties but wound up looking like Scrooges. And, to make things worse, those same governors and legislators frequently had to raise taxes to pay for the benefits promised by Washington.

State lawmakers, being closer to their constituents than federal officials in Washington, also were able to pick up on constituent demands for health reform much earlier than those in the national capital. By detecting those early yearnings, state lawmakers signaled their national brethren — people like Harris Wofford and Bill Clinton — that health care would be a potent issue.

With many states well down the road of expanding access and controlling costs, the states' reform models will offer federal policymakers a menu to choose from as they formulate a national plan. And states' head start has given them a bargaining chip with the Clinton Administration. The National Governors' Association, in particular, has worked hard with the White House to ensure that any final health reform package allows for state flexibility so that all the hard-won efforts achieved at the state level are not in vain.

This chapter looks at some of the more sweeping state reform efforts that could influence the course of federal legislation, starting with the trailblazing states of Hawaii, Florida, Minnesota, Vermont, and Washington.

HAWAII

If any state has provided a model for national reform, it is Hawaii. One of the last states to join the union, Hawaii was the first in the nation to adopt a policy of universal coverage.

In 1974, convinced that the federal government was about to enact comprehensive health reform legislation, Hawaii took the reform plunge. Following the lead provided by President Richard Nixon, the state enacted the Prepaid Health Care Act of 1974, which requires all employers in the state to offer health insurance to their workers and to pay at least 50 percent of their premiums. This so-called employer mandate was at the center of a Nixon reform plan introduced in Congress in the same year.

In a bit of fortuitous timing, Hawaii enacted its plan just before Congress passed the Employee Retirement Income Security Act (ERISA) of 1974. That law contains an important provision that has kept other states from following Hawaii's lead. To protect large interstate companies that choose to self-insure, Congress prohibited states from imposing requirements on large firms that do business in more than one state. ERISA provides for no administrative waivers of the rule, so any state that wants to impose an employer mandate must go to Congress for a legislative waiver.

Although Hawaii's law was enacted before ERISA, it was challenged in court and temporarily suspended in 1977. Hawaii went to Congress and, in 1982, got an ERISA waiver to allow the program to continue. The state has been frustrated in further attempts to modify its 1974 law — to broaden mental health benefits, for example — by the need to get further ERISA waivers.

Hawaii hoped that the employer mandate, combined with Medicare coverage of the elderly and Medicaid coverage of the poor, would achieve near-universal coverage of the state's population. To get to full coverage, the state took advantage of changes in federal Medicaid rules to expand its Medicaid program to cover more of the "near-poor." In 1989, Hawaii created a separate program known as the State Health Insurance Program, or SHIP, to cover those remaining uninsured. SHIP targeted about 30,000 to 35,000 poor Hawaiians — about 3 percent of the state's 1.1 million residents — who had little access to primary care doctors. Enrollment now stands at about 22,000.[3]

In addition, in July 1993, the federal government granted Hawaii a Medicaid waiver to set up a five-year project to funnel 88,200 low-income and uninsured people into managed care plans.[4] Today, only 2 percent of Hawaiians are uninsured, compared with nearly 15 percent of all Americans.

Hawaii's near-complete success in covering its residents has had a dramatic impact on its health costs. When it began its reform efforts, Hawaiian health care costs were three times higher than the national average. Today, despite the facts that Hawaii has one of the highest costs of living in the nation and that 80 percent of the state's 4,600 physicians are specialists, Hawaiian health costs are below the national average.[3]

An important factor in that success has been universal coverage. But the biggest contributor is probably the fact that competition among insurers for patients is very low. The vast majority of the insured population gets its coverage from one of two insurers — Blue Cross/Blue Shield or Kaiser Permanente. Both plans use community rating to set their insurance premiums even though no state law requires such action. In fact, attempts to pass such a law have failed in the state legislature.

Hawaii's lead on employer mandates has not led other states to adopt that tack — primarily because of the ERISA quandary and strong opposition from the small business community. Small businesses in Hawaii can hardly pick up and move to the next state and take jobs with them the same way they could on the mainland.

In 1988, Massachusetts adopted a modified version of the mandate by offering its employers the option to either insure their workers or pay the state a per-worker head tax to allow the state to buy the coverage for them. This so-called "play-or-pay" approach was favored by then-Governor Michael Dukakis as he ran for President. After his defeat by President Bush, Dukakis retired from state service and his successor, William Weld (R), has delayed the employer mandate until 1995 while he tries to convince the legislature to repeal it.

FLORIDA

Coming from the opposite direction of Hawaii's regulatory approach, Florida attempts to achieve universal coverage through a voluntary, competitive model of reform.

As in other states, Florida tinkered with installing a Canadian-style single payer model. In 1988, a single payer bill was introduced in the Tallahassee statehouse. Although it had little chance of passage, the bill goaded more moderate lawmakers into action. Rep. Elaine Gordon, the North Miami legislator who introduced the bill, called it "a two-by-four between the eyes of the system."[5]

Indeed, the bill woke up lawmakers to Florida's health care troubles. Because 95 percent of Florida's workers are employed by businesses with 25 or fewer workers, more than 18 percent of the state's 13 million residents are uninsured. That rate is far greater than that of other states leading the nation in health care reform, such as Minnesota, which has an 8 percent uninsured rate, and Vermont, where 10 percent are uninsured. The state's health care costs, pushed up by a higher-than-average number of elderly, have been skyrocketing, growing to $31 billion in the early 1990s and expected to reach $90 billion a year by 2000. As a result, said then newly elected Gov. Lawton Chiles (D), "the salary of working people will seem like a fringe benefit because their main compensation will be in health benefits."[6]

Chiles, who spent much of his 18 years as a U.S. Senator advocating for improved maternal and child health, defeated Republican Gov. Bob Martinez in 1990. Chiles ran on health care reform, and behind his leadership, Florida passed the 1992 Health Reform Act, which guaranteed all Floridians access to health care by December 31, 1994, and created a new state agency, called the Agency for Health Care Administration (AHCA). By using various incentives, Florida hopes to entice employers to cover everyone by January, 1 1995. But if the private market approach to reform fails to achieve universal coverage, a regulatory ax will fall. In that event, the AHCA has the power to enact a play-or-pay system or any other model to guarantee universal coverage.

The 1992 law also reformed the small group insurance market by requiring insurers to make their product available to any group that wants it, limiting the use of experience rating to price insurance products, and improving portability of insurance by eliminating waiting periods for coverage for those with preexisting medical conditions.

The state also set up a health service corps to provide doctors and other health care professionals to medically underserved areas; improved state data gathering; and tightened the state's certificate of need program to restrict the building of new health facilities.

The legislation was a legislative tour-de-force and won the support of business and health care providers. The state legislature, sold on its economic advantages, passed it, with only two senators voting against it. But some managed competition supporters object to the short time allotted for achieving universal coverage before heavier regulation kicks in. State Senator Alberto Gutman (R) from Miami, chairman of the state Senate Health Committee, has said the deadline is unrealistic and a ploy so that AHCA can "scrap the existing system and set up a single payer one."[6].

The 1992 law set the stage for broader action in 1993. The AHCA recommended a managed competition model similar to President Clinton's proposal. With that recommendation in hand, Chiles went back to the legislature to create a structure that would help meet the goal of universal coverage by 1995. In April 1993, the governor signed the Health Care and Insurance Reform Act, which builds on the state's experience with managed care by creating 11 regional community health purchasing alliances (CHPAs) to assist businesses in finding accountable health plans (AHPs).[6]

Chiles was forced to curtail CHPAs' scope, however. Initially he wanted to put all state residents into the CHPAs, but opposition forced him to limit membership to small businesses with up to 50 workers, Medicaid recipients, and state employees. CHPAs cannot directly offer insurance, but serve only as a conduit between business and insurers.

To provide insurance coverage to those outside the full-time working population, Florida created a program known as Med-Access, which offers low-cost coverage to anyone with income below 250 percent of the federal poverty level. Those individuals also will get coverage through the CHPAs.

Each CHPA will offer a variety of AHPs, including health maintenance organizations, preferred provider organizations, and fee-for-service plans. Small firms buying coverage through the alliances will have to offer their workers a choice of at least two of the plans offered. State employees get a choice of at least 10 plans, including five HMOs and five PPOs.

To cut its Medicaid costs, Florida has also embarked on an ambitious campaign to enroll those recipients in managed care. A new law requires all HMOs in the state to participate in Medicaid. Also, Florida has a new program, known as "Healthy Kids," that seeks to cover uninsured children. The design and funding of that program is left to local government.

MINNESOTA

Another of the big leaders on state-based health reform is Minnesota, a state with a long history of health care ingenuity. Beginning in 1992, the state launched a dramatic effort to control health costs and reduce its total uninsured residents. As with Florida, it is too soon to know if the laws enacted in Minnesota will achieve those ends, but policy makers in Washington DC, are paying close attention.

With its deep penetration of HMOs and its tradition of system delivery innovation, Minnesota was ripe for reform. But the process sputtered at first. In 1991, Republican Gov. Arne Carlson vetoed a bill that would have reformed the state's health insurance system and put Minnesota on the path to universal coverage. In less than a year, however, Carlson, reacting in part to the state's 370,000 uninsured, reached out to the Democratic legislature to achieve a bipartisan agreement on reform.

The best-known feature of the Minnesota reform plan — known as MinnesotaCare — is its adoption of a form of global budgeting that attempts to drive the growth rate in health costs down over a five-year period. The plan, which uses growth targets, intends to reduce the growth rate by 10 percent a year.[4]

At the same time, Minnesota moved to reform its small group insurance market by limiting the use of experience rating to set premiums, requiring insurers to offer coverage to any firm that wants it, and eliminating waiting periods due to preexisting medical conditions. It also barred insurers from canceling a policy because of changes in a worker's health status.

As with many reforming states, Minnesota came back a year later to further define and refine its system. Changes made in 1993 helped to create what are called integrated service networks, or ISNs, structures that resemble the health alliances in the Clinton health proposal. An all-payer system will be created for providers who decline to participate.

To deal with the uninsured, Minnesota created a state indigent care program aimed first at families under the Medicaid eligibility level but unqualified for Medicaid coverage. A 1988 initiative called the Children's Health Plan, provides coverage to families with income up to 185 percent of poverty. MinnesotaCare's goal for 1993 was to cover all residents with income under 275 percent of poverty, and to provide their dependents with inpatient and outpatient care for a low copayment.

In 1994, coverage will extend to all Minnesotans who have been uninsured for at least four months and who have not been covered by an employer for 18 months. But even with these programs, Minnesota will fall short of universal coverage. The law will reach only about 40 percent of the uninsured.[7]

To pay for the expanded coverage, the state raised its tax on cigarettes and imposed a 2 percent tax on most providers in the state (one percent on HMOs). The financing of the $265 million-a-year plan was the most controversial part of reform. The provider tax, scheduled to take effect January 1, 1994, is targeted not only at Minnesota doctors and hospitals but also at health providers in neighboring North Dakota, South Dakota, Wisconsin, and Iowa that treat Minnesotans. The state hopes to raise $166 million in 1995, $3 million of which will come from the four neighboring states. But collecting that $3 million will be difficult. The state is already trying to collect a previously enacted 2 percent tax on out-of-state hospitals and surgical centers that treat at least 20 Minnesota patients a year. That tax went into effect February 10, 1993, but no out-of-state provider has paid it. The American Medical Association spearheaded a legal challenge to the second tax, brought by 11 doctors from Wisconsin, Iowa, and South Dakota, which was dismissed for technical reasons in November 1993. Three hospitals have brought a second suit, which is still pending. Both suits claim it is unlawful for the providers to pay a tax to another state.

Minnesota may also be headed for other financial troubles. Enrollment in HMOs in the state is declining as an increasing number of employers take advantage of self-funded plans made possible under the 1992 law.[8] The decline could affect the primary source of funding for insuring 35,000 high-risk uninsured individuals. The drop in enrollment may also conflict with the state's strategy of containing costs by enrolling the majority of Minnesotans in the new integrated service networks.

VERMONT

Despite being one of the smallest states in the union, Vermont took giant steps on health reform beginning in 1992. That movement placed the state ahead of much of the nation and made Vermont a model for other states.

In 1992, the state instituted community rating for setting insurance premiums, limiting insurers to broad rates for family and individual coverage. Waiting periods for those with preexisting medical conditions were banned, and insurers were required to offer insurance to all comers.

Vermont expanded its Medicaid program by liberalizing its income eligibility rules. An existing program, known as "Dr. Dynasaur," was expanded to include children as old as 17 from families with incomes up to 250 percent of the federal poverty line. The state also promised to work to place providers in rural underserved areas and to develop a common claims form to reduce paperwork for health care providers.

A key player in the recent reform effort is Gov. Howard Dean (D), the only sitting governor who is also a physician. Dean became governor in 1991 upon the sudden death of incumbent Richard Snelling. His active leadership on health reform earned him easy reelection in 1992 and a major role in the National Governors' Association deliberations over health reform. He also has been a key health reform adviser to President Clinton and First Lady Hillary Rodham Clinton.

Like Florida, Vermont created a new agency known as the Vermont Health Care Authority (VHCA), a three-member panel appointed by Dean to oversee the reform effort. It was directed to devise two alternatives to achieve universal coverage of Vermont residents by 1994. One was to follow the single payer model used in Canada; the other was to use a multi-payer approach. In 1994, those two plans will go to the legislature, which then must either choose one of them or come up with a compromise plan. Vermont wants to enact legislation by May 1994 to cover all Vermonters by July 1, 1995.

Under either the single payer or the managed competition model, the VHCA estimates it will cost an additional $714 million to cover the state's 563,000 residents, including 60,000 uninsured. Both models would offer a generous standard benefits package that includes a broad array of services, many of which would be available with a $5 copayment.

The $714 million would go a long way toward paying the $1.3 billion the VHCA estimates Vermonters, including Medicaid and Medicare patients, will spend on health care in 1994. To raise that amount under a single payer model, the VHCA proposes instituting a 7.7-to-8.5 percent payroll tax and raising another $28 million by imposing higher taxes on tobacco, beer, and gasoline. Under a managed competition model, the VHCA suggests mandating that employers pay 80 percent of insurance premiums to raise the whole $714 million.

Despite the report's effort at balance, the single payer model has a slim chance of passage in the state legislature in 1994. Even though Democrats hold a majority in the state's House of Representatives, Republicans control the Senate. In 1991, with support from Gov. Dean, a single payer bill never made it out of committee. Yet, demographics and economics are pushing the state toward adopting a single payer model eventually. Vermont, the second least populated state in the nation, remains mostly rural, making it difficult to form competing health plans. And resources are minimal; Burlington (pop. 39,000) is the state's only city with two hospitals. "Managed competition is ludicrous because we simply don't have enough providers," scoffs Veronica Celani, an authority member. "We will become single payer by default."

WASHINGTON

In 1993, Washington state finally achieved what it had been striving for since 1988: broad health care reform. Basing its system on the managed competition model, Washington promised universal coverage by 1999.

Like the model proposed by President Clinton, Washington relies on an employer mandate to cover most of the working population, a uniform standard benefit package, regional health insurance purchasing cooperatives, and premium caps to control spending growth.

The Washington law created a new five-member commission that will develop by January 1995 a uniform benefits package and establish a maximum premium that can be charged for those benefits. Employers will be required to pay at least 50 percent of employees' premiums, with workers picking up the rest. Smaller businesses will be given more time to adjust to the mandate, but by July 1999, all state residents — including the 600,000 uninsured — must have coverage.

The rise in insurance premiums will be limited so that, over time, the rate of growth will come down 2 percentage points a year until it reaches the state's general inflation rate. Premiums will be based on community rating, and insurers will be prohibited from canceling policies because of changes in workers' health status.

Much like the Clinton plan, Washington plans to set up four regional health insurance purchasing cooperatives. Within each cooperative, a minimum of 150,000 members will choose among a number of certified health plans, all of which will offer a standard uniform benefits package. Plans will compete on quality measurements and premium rates, which will be subject to caps.[10]

Washington offers subsidies to the low-income population through the state's Basic Health Plan, which 95 percent of enrollees rated "good" or better, according to a state survey. Previously, the program was offered in only parts of the state, and the benefit package was limited. It now covers the entire state and, beginning in 1995, it will include the standard benefits package. In October 1993, the plan was expanded to 102,000 more residents and began covering prescription drugs.[10]

To raise the money needed to pay for these additional benefits, Washington hopes to raise $231 million in the next two years through increased excise taxes on cigarettes and alcohol and a new 1.5 percent tax on hospitals. Surprisingly, the Washington State Hospital Association abandoned its longstanding principle of opposing any hospital tax and endorsed the plan. "We were seeing increasing numbers of uninsured," explained association President and CEO Leo Greenawalt, "and we had to do something to get the incentives in the system straight — or we might have gone to a government-run system."[10]

Others were not so compliant. An anti-tax group succeeded in getting an initiative to repeal the tobacco and alcohol tax increases passed in 1993 to fund universal coverage onto the state's November ballot. The initiative, however, was rejected by 56 percent of voters. Both large and small businesses complained that the managed competition model would not work and that the mandate would bankrupt them. "There are 4,000 years of experience that show that price controls don't work," declared Steve Hill, senior VP for human resources at the giant Seattle-based logging company Weyerhauser Co.[10] Despite a five-year $150 million fund to help businesses with fewer than 25 employees pay health insurance premiums, a survey conducted by the National Federation of Independent Business, a small business lobbying group that opposes mandates, found that 26 percent of its members would lay off workers or close their doors if they had to pay $50 a month to provide health insurance for each worker.[10]

As a result, passing health reform was anything but easy for Washington lawmakers. Despite a Democratic majority in the state legislature, reform passed the House by a slim 56-42 margin and the Senate by a 28-21 vote. Because Washington's plan closely resembles Clinton's proposal, the state's difficulties in passing reform may foreshadow what Washington DC, lawmakers will encounter in 1994.

REFORM IN OTHER STATES

While the preceding five states are the best examples of comprehensive health reform, many other states have been active on reform as well. Elements of the following plans may also find their way into the national debate.

California. The nation's largest state may be the best testing ground for managed competition. The state groups its 900,000 government employees into a single program known as the California Public Employees Retirement System or

CalPERS. Using the clout gained from its broad purchasing power, CalPERS has recently been able to demand much lower premiums than other payers. Premium rates for 1993 increased only 1.5 percent, compared with about 11 percent nationally, and CalPERS officials announced 10 months ahead of schedule that they planned to demand the 18 managed care groups it does business with roll back rates by 5 percent in 1994. In all, CalPERS estimates it has saved Californians nearly $200 million.[11] Ironically, under the Clinton health plan, cost-saving plans like CalPERS would be banished. State employees would be forced to join regional alliances that would be run by nonprofit organizations, which would negotiate health insurance purchases for employees and individuals.

State officials are trying to bring the same savings to patients in its Medicaid program, Medi-Cal. The state has moved 600,000 recipients into managed care programs and hopes to have half of the 5 million Medi-Cal enrollees in managed care plans by 1996. And California became the first state to test voluntary health insurance purchasing cooperatives in 1993, when 15 insurers began offering a standard benefit package to small businesses. The state claimed that pooling small employers will push down the cost of health insurance by 6-to-23 percent.[4]

Colorado. Unlike other states that have tried to expand on employer-based insurance, Colorado is going in the opposite direction, choosing to sever the job tie to insurance. ColoradoCare, which is now being studied by a state commission, would offer state residents, including 500,000 uninsured, a choice of private health plans via a new health authority. Employers and employees would each contribute to the cost of insurance, but workers would select the plan.

In September 1993, a commission formed by the state legislature and appointed by Gov. Roy Romer (D) concluded that ColoradoCare's goal to provide continuous, universal health coverage for all Coloradans was "feasible." Echoing the financing scheme in the Clinton Administration plan, the commission reported that universal coverage and a standard benefits package could be provided "at a lower average cost than . . . if ColoradoCare were not enacted."[12]

The commission estimated that a "bare-bones" benefits package, which requires a 50 percent copayment with a maximum out-of-pocket expense of $3,000 a year, would cost each Coloradan $77 a month. A more generous package with a $250 deductible and a 10 percent copayment would cost $103 a month. The most generous health plan, which would require only a $5 copayment per visit and cover all services including dental and eye care, would cost each Coloradan an average of $121 a month. Extending benefits to Medicare recipients would require the state to increase spending by between $100 million and $570 millon, depending on the benefits provided. The commission outlined four financing schemes, which included different levels and combinations of payroll and income taxes, and relief to the poor. Like the Social Security wage base, payroll taxes would not be levied on income earned above $59,700.[12]

Kentucky. While advocates like Gov. Brereton Jones (D) had hoped that the Bluegrass State would be an example to the nation of how reform is done, it may actually be best used as an example of how not to achieve progress. Jones, elected in 1991, was an avid advocate of universal coverage. He wanted to institute a

Massachusetts-style play-or-pay system to cover all Kentuckians, including the state's 450,000 uninsured. But Jones could not achieve consensus on how to implement such a system. The Kentucky Chamber of Commerce claimed an employer mandate would force businesses to relocate to one of the seven states bordering the state, and the National Federation of Independent Business warned that the mandate would cost 37,000 jobs.[13] The plan eventually died on the question of how to pay for broader coverage.

Jones offered a revised plan that changes the employer mandate to an individual mandate; lowers premiums by 25 percent; institutes a 3-to-4 percent payroll tax; establishes a purchasing group for state employees, Medicaid recipients, the uninsured, workers' compensation beneficiaries, and prisoners; and forms a five-member health care authority to contain costs. A special legislative session called to debate the proposal ended abruptly May 27, 1993, without any action. Many lawmakers who want to phase in universal coverage blame Jones' insistence on achieving it by 1995 (when he's due to leave office) and for failing to involve them. But Jones says the stubbornness lies with the legislature. "Everything seemed so logical to me, but I couldn't get the legislature to move," Jones admitted.[14] State legislative leaders failed to meet Jones' October 15, 1993, deadline for a written health reform bill, and chances that health reform legislation will be passed in 1994 are growing slimmer as a dozen state lawmakers have pleaded guilty to fraud, extortion, and embezzlement under an FBI investigation.

Maryland. Building on its historic commitment to health care reform, Maryland has recently adopted legislation that seeks to expand access while retaining the state's hammerlock on costs. Since 1974, Maryland has controlled hospital costs through a rate review commission, which has held the rate of growth in costs per hospital admission to half the national rate. Under a law passed in April 1993, the state will expand that effort to physicians. If doctors have not voluntarily held down fees by January 1995, a newly created cost commission will impose a fee schedule. By using modified community rating and insurance reforms, the state hopes to expand coverage of the medically uninsurable. About half of Maryland's 650,00 uninsured work in small businesses, but under reform, HMOs must guarantee issue and renewal to firms employing between 2 and 50 workers. By January 1, 1995, no insurer can deny coverage to persons with preexisting medical conditions. A new state-funded indigent care program will provide coverage to those who are poor but don't qualify for Medicaid. This system most closely resembles the concept known as global budgeting.

New Jersey. The first state to adopt the cost-controlling diagnostic-related groups (DRGs) was the first state to repeal them. DRGs, government-set payment rates for specific hospital procedures and treatments, were designed to hold down rising medical costs. New Jersey had developed them in the late 1970s, then put them into effect in the early 1980s, requiring all payers to reimburse hospitals at the same level. But a New Jersey judge ruled the state's hospital reimbursement system violated ERISA because the system forced self-insured funds to pay a 19 percent tax for uncompensated care.

In two bills introduced and enacted over a seven-day period in November 1992, New Jersey stepped back to a deregulated market when it jettisoned DRGs in favor of allowing hospitals to set their own rates. In return, hospitals now are responsible for their own bad debt. Still, the state legislature thought it was necessary to make $54 million available in 1993 for 43 hospitals that serve large numbers of uninsured and $163 million for hospitals that serve more patients with AIDS, tuberculosis, and other high-cost illnesses.[15] The law also set up community rating for individual and small group insurance. Subsidies for charity care, about $1.8 billion a year, eventually will be replaced by Jersey Shield, a program for the uninsured, unemployed, and part-time workers. Ironically, in May 1993, a federal appellate court reversed the New Jersey judge's decision and ruled that the state's surcharge did not violate ERISA.

New York. Across the river, Governor Mario Cuomo (D) and the New York legislature also are leading the way in health reform — although all is not going well. In July 1992, New York became the first state to institute broad community rating, which requires that rates be based on the demographics of an area and prohibits any insurer or HMO from rejecting an applicant. HMOs are required to pay into a rate-stabilization pool based on the medical condition and demographics of their members. The pool's funds will be used to compensate insurers that cover older and less healthy populations. Like New Jersey, New York's 13 percent surcharge on hospital bills also was challenged in 1993, and the court found it in violation of ERISA. The state hopes the U.S. Supreme Court will hear its appeal of the case. Despite the court battles, Cuomo is forging ahead with more reforms. The governor hopes to extend the rate-setting plan to all outpatient services by 1996 and the certificate of need process to physicians. Increases in reimbursement rates for doctors working in underserved areas and use of health networks to reach those areas are also ideas the governor is pursuing. But none of the ideas found their way into legislative form in 1993.

Oregon. No discussion of state health reform is complete without a discussion of the Oregon plan. The subject of great national debate since the mid-1980s, the state's controversial reform system rationing health care services for its Medicaid population goes into effect in February 1994. Faced with a large number of uninsured residents, the state chose to expand its Medicaid eligibility to include all people under the federal poverty line and the uninsured, a total of 120,000 Oregonians. To finance the expansion, Oregon decided to rank all of the medical procedures provided under Medicaid. The legislature then agreed on a cut-off point below which Medicaid would not provide coverage, choosing to exclude high-cost procedures and treatments that were deemed marginally effective. After nearly two years of consideration, the federal government granted Oregon the federal waivers it needed to implement the $6.5 billion, five-year program.[16] To receive the waiver, Oregon had to agree to 29 terms, including ensuring no bias against persons with disabilities. To raise the $64 million needed to fund the reform program, the state legislature raised cigarette taxes 25 cents a pack. Included in the reform is a requirement that all businesses will cover workers health by January 1, 1998, a deadline that is somewhat later than Gov. Barbara Roberts (D) wanted but a bow to small business opposition.

REFERENCES

1. Eckl C, K Hayes, and A Perez. *State Budget Actions 1993*. National Conference of State Legislatures, November 1993.
2. Health Care Financing Administration. *Personal Health Care Expenditures by State and Region*. May 1993: 11-12.
3. Neubauer D. Hawaii: A Pioneer in Health System Reform. *Health Affairs*, Summer 1993: 34.
4. Firshein J and M Jee. States Take Their Own Reform Steps. *Medicine & Health*, July 19, 1993: 3-6.
5. Brown L. Commissions, Clubs, and Consensus: Florida Reorganizes for Health Reform. *Health Affairs*, Summer 1993: 14.
6. Kent C. Florida Builds on Managed Competition. *Medicine & Health Perspectives*, January 18, 1993.
7. Leichter H. The Trip From Acrimony to Accommodation. *Health Affairs*, Summer 1993: 50.
8. StateLine. *Journal of American Health Policy* 3 (6), November/December 1993: 53.
9. Holmes A. Vermonters Balk at Reform Options. *Journal of American Health Policy* 3 (6), November/December 1993: 51.
10. Kent C and M Jee. 'Other' Washington Launches Major Health Reform. *Medicine & Health Perspectives*, May 24, 1993.
11. Managed Competition It's Not, Says CalPERS Official. *Medicine & Health*, March 15, 1993: 3.
12. Weil A. *ColoradoCare*, report for state legislature, September 1993.
13. Jee M. Small Business Wins Big Exemption in Kentucky Health Reform Battle. *Journal of American Health Policy* 3 (3), May/June 1993: 50.
14. Kentucky Offers Health Reform Lesson. *Medicine & Health*, August 30, 1993: 2.
15. Berliner H and S Delgado. From DRGs to Deregulation: New Jersey Takes the Road Less Traveled. *Journal of American Health Policy* 3 (4), July/August 1993: 44-48.
16. At Long Last, Oregon Gets Medicaid Waiver Approval. *Medicine & Health*, March 22, 1993: 1.

CHAPTER 9

Unlearned Lessons: What Other Nations Might Teach America

Richard A. Knox

"One can count on Americans to do the right thing, once they have exhausted all other alternatives." — attributed to Sir Winston Churchill

In this century, America has considered health care reform once every twenty years or so. The 1993-94 debate differs in many ways, most notably in the high level of public interest and sense of political urgency, which imply that something significant may actually occur this time. Another difference, which also suggests the seriousness and relative maturity of the U.S. debate, is the unprecedented attention Americans are paying to other nations' experience with health care.

AMERICANS' GRADUAL ACCEPTANCE OF "FOREIGN" IDEAS ABOUT HEALTH

For the last few years, international comparisons have crept into U.S. public discourse on America's health care problems. Speeches and articles began to include an almost incantatory reference to the U.S. and South Africa as the only two developed nations to remain outside the circle of "civilized" societies guaranteeing health coverage to their members. As the debate evolved, more detailed allusions to the U.S. health system's dubious distinction as the world's most expensive and most inflationary cropped up in standard diagnoses of the American crisis.

The foreign system most Americans are familiar with is Canada's. References to Canada, as an example to be either emulated or avoided, have become part of U.S. public discourse on health care — although Americans' knowledge of Canadian health care remains shallow and distorted by hyperbolic claims of both proponents and opponents about what has come to be known by the shorthand phrase, "Canadian-style" single payer health care.

THE GERMAN INFLUENCE

Germany's health system, the world's oldest national social insurance scheme for health care and arguably its most successful, garnered an increasing share of attention in the early 1990s. While the average American may read or hear only passing references, the German example has had significant impact on policymakers and opinion leaders as they have become more aware of its exemplary record of cost control and its blend of public goal-setting, off-budget financing based on statutory mandates, private negotiations over reimbursement, and a largely private delivery system.

When Democratic leaders of the U.S. Senate were in the final stages of crafting their health reform proposal in May 1991, they seized upon Germany's federal goal-setting board, called Concerted Action in Health Care, as an answer to intraparty critics who said their draft proposal did not contain sufficient cost control mechanisms.[1] The concept of a National Health Board to set a global spending limit on covered services and oversee private, regional negotiations turned up again as the central structural features of President Clinton's 1,342-page American Health Security Act proposal unveiled in October 1993.

Clinton, a German-speaking student of European social insurance systems, acknowledges his debt. On the day after he outlined his health reform plan to Congress in September 1993, he said the German system "is the most like what I propose." He characterized it on national television as "a private system where large groups of employers and insurers can work with health care providers to provide a wide range of services at low cost, but the administrative cost is much less than we have — although they cover more people and [offer] about the same number of services."

Crossing the Social Insurance Threshold

More important than the particular influence of the German system on the Clinton plan is the fact that this President has given unprecedented prominence to two internationalist ideas:

- governmental mandate and continuing government involvement is essential to achieve universal access to affordable health care; and
- secure health care for individuals in a society is linked to the economic health and competitiveness of the nation at large.

The first idea is embodied in Clinton's argument that citizens are entitled to "health security," which he defined in his October 27 speech unveiling the plan as "a comprehensive package of health care benefits that are always there and that can never be taken away." This is the concept at the heart of the social welfare schemes that first arose in Chancellor Bismarck's late 19th-century Germany, subsequently spread throughout Europe, and now characterize the systems of Japan, Australia and, most recently, Taiwan. It is a highly significant departure from the traditional American view that health care belongs largely in the private realm, as a matter of choice and individuals' ability to pay directly for care or for coverage.

Contrary to the expectations of many social welfare theorists, the enactment of Medicare and Medicaid in the mid-1960s eroded but did not supplant this powerful American commitment to a voluntary approach and the free market. The prevailing idea for most of this century was that employment-based health insurance would achieve near-universal coverage, once the gaps were filled for the elderly and the poor. That belief has foundered on the shoals of risk-based insurance, with its strong incentive to avoid or shed bad risks and shift the costs to some other payer.

Worry among insured Americans that they will lose coverage or that it will become too expensive is a much broader political phenomenon than public concern over the estimated 37.4 million Americans who lack health coverage at any given moment. "We've reached a kind of critical mass where something has to be done, and everyone understands that," Sen. Edward Kennedy (D-MA) said in September 1993. "No one contends, as they did in the past, that the private sector alone can end this festering crisis."[2]

Significantly, many Republicans and conservative Democrats now accept the idea that government must intervene to ensure that Americans have access to health care. Many in the opposition party, such as Senate Republican leader Robert Dole and Sen. John Chafee of Rhode Island, have embraced the goal of universal coverage. This suggests that an important threshold is being crossed; once political consensus jells on universal coverage and the need for government prescription, the debate will have moved into a landscape new to Americans — and quite familiar to the citizens of virtually all other developed nations.

A Matter of National Health

The second large theme in Clinton's argument, that health care and national productivity are linked in an essential way, is also new to the U.S. debate. But it is familiar to Europeans as far back as Bismarck, who understood in the 1870s that a government guarantee of health care and sickness pay was a building block of the German nation he was trying to build (and a trump to the socialists). This idea spans political philosophies abroad. It was evident in post-war Great Britain's decision to create a National Health Service as one of that nation's first steps to economic recovery. It was central in the Communist regimes that emerged from the rubble of eastern Europe. It has been embraced by continental conservatives and Canadian Tories as an indispensable element of national life.

While it was not yet clear in late 1993 whether Clinton's "economic health" argument will strike a resonant chord, it is a prominent theme in his effort to "sell" reform to a reluctant and fragmented Congress. Introducing his Health Security Act, Clinton declared that the legislation "literally holds the key to a new era for our economy, an era in which we can get our health care costs under control, free our businesses to compete better in a global economy and make sure that the men and women who show up for work every day are more productive because they're more secure and they feel that they can do two important jobs at once: be good members of their family, good parents and good children, as well as good workers."

The good news for Clinton and other advocates of universal compulsory health insurance is that the first precondition for such a change — acknowledgement of the failure of the voluntary approach to health insurance — was in place in late 1993. The bad news, from this point of view, is that sufficient agreement on the replacement system still seemed remote and uncertain. As Joseph White of the Brookings Institute put it in October 1993: "All serious U.S. health reform proposals accept that risk-rated insurance, as opposed to international social insurance models, has to go — though they vary on whether they would effectively require community rating. But, aside from President Clinton's and the single payer plans, the other alternatives, such as the Senate Republican Health Care Task Force, Sen. [Phil] Gramm's, and Cooper-Grandy [sponsored by Democratic Rep. Jim Cooper of Tennessee and Republican Rep. Fred Grandy of Iowa], not only ignore but aggressively reject the lessons of international, and I believe our own, experience."[3]

White points out that Clinton's conservative opponents reject government involvement in setting health care providers' fees or system spending limits, or in limiting system capacity — two hallmarks of social insurance systems. To control costs, conservatives prefer instead to rely on either competition among insurers and providers and on making consumers more "price-sensitive" by increasing their out-of-pocket costs — strategies not widely employed in foreign systems, at least to date.

OVERCOMING AMERICAN EXCEPTIONALISM

The very idea that America can learn something useful from other nations' health systems meets resistance from many, in and outside the health care field, who argue that the U.S. is the exception to the developed world's rule. Victor G. Rodwin of New York University calls this "American exceptionalism," and he notes this outlook is not unique to Americans. "Nations throughout the world rely on [an] 'assumption of uniqueness' to reject ideas from abroad," Rodwin says. This attitude "tends to make the U.S. conservative; and, therefore, it supports the status quo in the United States."[4]

In the health care reform debate, exceptionalism takes a number of forms. American individualism and distrust of government, it is often argued, are fundamentally at odds with compulsory health insurance, fairness-based financing, and government constraints on health system pricing and capacity.

This ideology, as suggested above, may be losing some ground as its adherents acknowledge the failings of a voluntary and private health insurance system for most of the population. But antagonism to government is still a major constraint on the Clinton Administration's reform blueprint, and it is certain to exert a major influence in shaping whatever compromise might emerge. Conversely, as will be discussed at greater length later, the American belief in the utility of markets also holds appeal for health care reformers abroad — though always within the context of firmly established principles of universal coverage and government control.

A second manifestation of American exceptionalism is ostensibly based not on ideology but on material fact: the special problems of U.S. society and the unique burdens they place on the U.S. health care system. This position is often advanced to explain the large differences between U.S. per capita health spending and other developed nations', and to suggest that the need for major U.S. health reform to narrow that gap is less justified than often believed. "If Canada, Germany or Sweden had our social problems, a comparably poor population and behavioral risk factors, their sickness and death rates surely would be much worse and their health care costs would be much higher," argue Leroy L. Schwartz, MD, and Mark W. Stanton of Health Policy International, a New Jersey consulting firm.[5]

Health Burdens and Advantages

This argument undoubtedly contains some truth and deserves serious study. However, the picture is complex and difficult to quantify; no firm conclusions are possible at this point. In the U.S. and other developed nations, there are factors that cut both ways. Some factors appear to justify higher U.S. health care spending, while others suggest that some nations have greater burdens of disease and disability — and thus should have higher health costs than they do, relative to the U.S. Sweden, for instance, has the world's highest proportion of residents over age 65, almost 18 percent in 1990 compared to 12 percent in the U.S.[6] Yet Sweden spends only half the amount on health per capita that the U.S. does.[7] A more detailed comparison of the U.S. and Germany illustrates the point. In 1991, the U.S. spent 73 percent more per capita on health care than Germany, on a purchasing power parity basis that corrects for national currency distortions. Between 1985 and 1991, U.S. per capita health spending grew at an annual rate 1.5 times that of Germany's.[7] Poverty may explain part of the difference; about 6 percent of Germany's population received welfare payments in 1990, while 13.5 percent of

U.S. residents had incomes below the federal poverty standard. Teenage pregnancy, a factor associated with poorer pregnancy outcomes, was much higher in the U.S. Only 1 in 166 German mothers is under age 16, versus 1 in 21 American mothers.[8] Though data are unavailable, there are undoubtedly more expensive-to-treat "crack babies" and infants with fetal alcohol syndrome in the U.S.

However, other presumed U.S. disadvantages are more apparent than real. America had 6 times more new AIDS cases than Germany in 1991 but, corrected for population differences, the U.S. incidence of AIDS was only 1.56 times higher. The incidence of active tuberculosis, a disease classically linked to poverty and poor living conditions, is actually twice as high in Germany.[8]

On the other side of the ledger, Germany has important populationwide disadvantages related to behavioral and demographic factors that ought to increase some health costs compared to the U.S. Smoking is still much more prevalent in Germany, especially among men; 45 percent of German men over age 25 were smokers in 1988, compared with 31 percent of comparably aged American men. Since tobacco use is associated in the U.S. with 19 percent of all deaths and a corresponding proportion of disease,[9] Germany's higher smoking rates must be costly to its health system. Similarly, blood cholesterol levels at virtually every age are much higher in Germany, which also has about twice the rate of obesity as the U.S.[8]

Perhaps most important, given the attention paid in the U.S. to the disproportionate medical costs associated with the elderly, the proportion of Germany's population over age 65 is actually 25 percent higher than America's, and the percentage of Germans over age 80 is 37 percent larger. Given these facts, it is hard to say which nation bears the greater health burdens.

Pointing to Others' Troubles

The third and most recent manifestation of "American exceptionalism" is the observation that virtually all other developed nations are having troubles of their own with health care costs, prompting the question: "Why should we look to them for solutions?" Implicit in that attitude is a hopelessness about the possibility of achieving universality, equity, and cost control in health care.

It is true, and important, that most other nations are engaged in some form of health care reform in the 1990s, whether they have high health spending patterns, such as the U.S., Canada, and Sweden, or low expenditures, such as the United Kingdom and New Zealand. The underlying premise is that there has been a sudden worldwide "failure" of health care systems, and an "explosion" of health care costs, notes Robert Evans of the Centre for Health Services and Policy Research at the University of British Columbia. In fact, he says, "the data do not support such rhetorical claims. The general problem has been a decline in overall rates of economic growth."[10] Many nations, beset by recession, are engaged in vigorous attempts to hold health spending costs to a constant share of national economies growing much more slowly than medical costs.

Instead of discouraging reformers and invalidating international comparisons, this reality ought to stimulate more serious interest among Americans in how other nations are doing, and what strategies they are trying in order to cope with remarkably similar problems: stagnating economies; aging populations; expensive medical technologies and expanding indications for their use; provider pressures to do more; and insatiable public demand for medical care.

Up to now, most comparative studies have been descriptive, focusing on the "anatomy" and "taxonomy" of foreign health care systems instead of their "physiology," notes the National Institute of Medicine's Council and Board on Health Care Services.[11] But the time is ripe, given similar health policy struggles across national borders, for deeper examination of what has worked and what has failed. "There are very strong convergences of the health care problems faced by the developed world and to some degree the solutions being tried," notes David Mechanic, director of Rutgers University's Institute for Health, Health Care Policy, and Aging Research. "We can't just pluck other nations' techniques [for health care reform], but we have to use available knowledge of the possible lessons that could be adapted to our particular history and culture."[12]

Despite other nations' better performance on measures of both spending and health outcomes, none has found the secret of keeping costs under control without damaging the health of its citizens. On the contrary, as Evans points out, many developed nations have lived with intrinsic flaws in their health care systems, such as hospital overcapacity, inflationary fee-for-service incentives, wide and inexplicable variations in medical practice, and overcapacity (or undercapacity) of certain medical personnel and physical facilities. In the face of such widely known problems (known, that is, among health services researchers and many policymakers), "The social consensus was more easily maintained by simply adding more funds, while this could be afforded," Evans says. "Now, in all systems, people are trying to address problems which have always been there."[10]

MORE DOES NOT EQUAL BETTER: THE LESSON OF AMERICAN HEALTH EXPENDITURES

When it comes to health care, the main difference between the United States and virtually all other developed nations is that the others are dealing with their health care problems with greater success, in terms of both health outcomes and control of spending. By any measure, the U.S. far outpaces the rest of the world in both the amount it spends on health care and the yearly rate of increase in spending.

This in itself is not necessarily a bad thing. If the high value America apparently places on health care were buying better health, by standard measures of mortality, morbidity, and quality of life, that would be a powerful argument in favor of the world's highest spending levels. If health spending had been increasing rapidly in recent years because the U.S. had been implementing a national commitment to universal access, that would be cause for international congratulation, not disapproval.

Of course, neither is true (see Table 9-1). Eight other developed nations, which spent between 36 percent and 67 percent of the U.S. per-capita level on health care in 1991, all had lower rates of infant mortality. (Among the 24 nations of the Organization for Economic Cooperation and Development, or OECD, only Portugal and Turkey had higher infant mortality rates than the U.S.) The same eight nations had higher life expectancies among newborn males in 1990, and all but one (the United Kingdom) had higher life expectancies among females at birth.

The U.S. does better than almost any nation in expected years of remaining life for 80-year-olds. This may reflect America's more intensive style of care for the most aged; but, interestingly, Canada performs equally well on this index, despite its reputation south of the border for rationing high-tech care.

Table 9-1

Value for Money? Spending Levels vs. Health Outcomes in Eight Nations

Per capita spending levels for 1991, outcome measures for 1990

Nation	Percent by which U.S. health spending exceeds	Infant mortality (deaths per 1,000 live births)	Life expectancy at birth, males (years)	Life expectancy at birth, females (years)	Life expectancy at age 80, males (years)	Life expectancy at age 80, females (years)
Australia	103 %	8.2	73.9	80.0	6.8	8.6
Canada	50	6.8	73.8	80.4	7.1	9.3
France	74	7.2	72.7	80.9	6.8	8.6
Germany	73	7.1	72.6	79.0	6.1	7.6
Japan	119	4.6	75.9	81.9	6.9	8.7
Netherlands	111	7.1	73.8	80.1	6.6	8.6
Sweden	99	6.0	74.8	80.4	6.6	8.3
United Kingdom	175	7.9	73.0	78.5	6.2	8.2
United States	--	**9.1**	**72.0**	**78.8**	**7.1**	**9.0**

Spending calculations are based on purchasing power parity conversions.

Source: Schieber et al., 1993.

These are all crude measures of health, to be sure. Health care is not the only — undoubtedly not even the most important — determinant of a society's health. It would be desirable to have international comparisons on such indices as disability rates, functional rehabilitation following severe illness or trauma, and outcomes for the treatment of common disorders. Nevertheless, the available data clearly do not permit the conclusion that the U.S. is getting proportionate value for the extraordinary sums of money it is spending.

It is more difficult to defend per-capita expenditures 50 percent higher than the next-ranking nation (Canada) in light of the fact that all the other nations guarantee health coverage to all residents, while at any given time 37.4 million Americans are without insurance. The uninsured receive 50 to 70 percent of the medical care provided to those who are fully insured;[13] when they cannot avoid seeking treatment, they must hope for charity. The number of uninsured Americans who do not get medical care when they need it is "particularly alarming," says Karen Davis, executive vice president of the Commonwealth Fund.[14] In 1992-93, 71 percent of Americans postponed needed care, and 34 percent did not get needed care — both more than double the proportion found a year earlier, according to a 1993 survey commissioned by the Commonwealth Fund and the Kaiser Family Foundation.[14] "Although most people enjoy access to the best and latest care in the world, an increasing number of people are shut out," observes Robert D. Reischauer, director of the Congressional Budget Office.[13]

The World Champion of Health Spending

The U.S. record of health spending is recited so often that readers are at risk of becoming inured to it, as if it were a fact of nature. Yet it is worthwhile to consider it once again. The numbers can help us understand what is driving the American health reform debate; but beyond that, they illustrate the large opportunity the U.S. has to curb its ominous rate of health inflation while enjoying a medical standard of living that would still outpace the rest of the world.

When U.S. per-capita health spending is made comparable to other nations' by using purchasing power parities — a medical "market basket" approach considered more stable and meaningful for international comparison than fluctuating currency exchange rates — it stands apart from any other nation's (see Table 9-2). The U.S. rate of spending in 1991, $2,868 per person, was 50 percent higher than Canada's, 74 percent more than Germany's, 119 percent more than Japan's, and 175 percent more than Britain's.

In the seven-year period between 1985 and 1991, U.S. per-capita spending was also growing from this high baseline at a much higher rate (9 percent) than any nation except Japan (8.7 percent). The U.S. annual growth rate during this period was 36 percent higher than the average of Australia, Canada, France, Germany, Japan, Netherlands, Sweden, and the United Kingdom. Significantly, Germany and Sweden actually experienced *negative* average growth in health spending's share of GDP during this period.

The U.S. Spending Trajectory

But, one might say, health spending is a highly desirable "good" that is naturally correlated with national wealth. If people can afford more medical care, they will buy it. As the world's wealthiest nation, with a per-capita income 30 percent higher (on a purchasing power parity basis) than Germany's in 1990,[15] the U.S. might be expected to have the highest levels of health spending. However, once again the data reveal a disproportion. When analysts plot per-capita health spending against per-capita income, the two are nearly parallel for all other developed nations; but the U.S. floats well above the slope relating these two variables. "In 1991, U.S. [yearly health care] expenditures of $2,868 were almost $1,000 above the amount that would be predicted based on the average relationship found for the 24 [OECD] countries," observe George J. Schieber and Leslie M. Greenwald of the U.S. Health Care Financing Administration and Jean-Pierre Poullier of the OECD.[7]

The proportion of gross domestic product, or GDP, is often used to characterize a nation's health expenditures, because this index implicitly captures the priority placed on health care and avoids the comparison issues raised by monetary indices. In 1991, the latest year for which international comparisons were avail-

Table 9-2

National Per Capita Health Spending in U.S. Dollars, 1985-1991

Currency conversions using purchasing power parities

Nation	1985	1986	1987	1988	1989	1990	1991	Compound annual rate of growth
Australia	$ 998	$1,072	$1,112	$1,171	$1,225	$1,310	$1,407	5.9%
Canada	1,244	1,364	1,461	1,558	1,666	1,811	1,915	7.5
France	1,083	1,135	1,193	1,295	1,415	1,528	1,650	7.3
Germany	1,175	1,215	1,287	1,409	1,412	1,522	1,659	5.9
Japan	792	839	916	992	1,092	1,119	1,307	8.7
Netherlands	931	990	1,046	1,101	1,176	1,286	1,360	6.5
Sweden	1,150	1,165	1,240	1,303	1,390	1,455	1,443	3.9
United Kingdom	685	739	795	858	912	985	1,043	7.3
United States	**1,711**	**1,824**	**1,962**	**2,146**	**2,362**	**2,601**	**2,868**	**9.0**

Source: Schieber et al., 1993.

able in late 1993, the U.S. spent 13.2 percent of its GDP on health care. Canada, the next highest-spending country, devoted 10 percent of its GDP to health care. No other nation spent more than 9.1 percent (see Table 9-3).

But it is the expenditure trend that lends urgency to the U.S. debate, not any given absolute level. As a percentage of GDP, U.S. health spending rose at an annual rate of 3.9 percent between 1985 and 1991[7] — three times the average of the eight other developed nations during that period. Schieber and his colleagues calculate that nominal U.S. per capita health spending grew 70 percent faster than nominal per capita income during that period, increasing the divergence between America and the rest of the developed world. (Other nations also saw their health spending outpace GDP growth, but by far less.)

And while the annual growth rate in U.S. health spending is expected to abate somewhat during the latter 1990s, it is still projected to mount steadily — absent significant health care reform — until, in the year 2000, health's share of GDP reaches nearly 19 percent (see Table 9-4). This will further compromise the nation's ability to invest in other priorities, such as education or physical infrastructure; it will sabotage efforts to reduce the federal deficit; and it will continue to erode workers' wages, half of which were already eaten up by increasing health insurance costs between 1973 and 1989.[13]

Table 9-3

International Trends in Health Spending

As a percentage of gross domestic product (GDP), 1985-1991

Nation	1985	1986	1987	1988	1989	1990	1991	Compound annual rate of growth
Australia	7.7%	8.0%	7.8%	7.7%	7.8%	8.2%	8.6%	1.9%
Canada	8.5	8.8	8.9	8.8	9.0	9.5	10.0	2.7
France	8.5	8.5	8.5	8.6	8.7	8.8	9.1	3.6
Germany	8.7	8.6	8.7	8.8	8.3	8.3	8.5	-0.4
Japan	6.5	6.6	6.7	6.6	6.6	6.7	6.8	0.8
Netherlands	8.0	8.1	8.3	8.2	8.1	8.2	8.3	0.6
Sweden	8.8	8.5	8.6	8.6	8.6	8.6	8.6	-0.4
United Kingdom	6.0	6.1	6.1	6.1	6.1	6.2	6.6	1.6
United States	**10.5**	**10.7**	**10.9**	**11.1**	**11.5**	**12.2**	**13.2**	**3.9**

Source: Schieber et al., 1993.

Is it possible to deflect this trajectory? Clinton's health reform proposal aims to reduce the national increase in spending by the year 2000 from the projected 18.9 percent to 17.3 percent of GDP. Given the inexorable rise in U.S. health spending in recent decades, this has widely been criticized as unrealistic.

But in an international context, Clinton's target looks more feasible. His goal would permit, over the entire decade, a 3.9 percent increase in the GDP devoted to health care. This target, the Brookings Institution's Joseph White notes, is larger than the growth in GDP share in Australia, Canada, France, Germany, Japan, and the U.K. during the two decades from 1971 to 1991.[3] Germany, in fact, actually held health care spending to 12 percent below GDP growth between 1985 and 1991, without any discernible reduction in the volume or quality of care.

COMPARATIVE HEALTH CARE "INPUTS": NO ANSWER TO THE MYSTERY

One of the most intriguing aspects of comparative health system studies is the lack of a clear and consistent relationship between a national system's spending levels and its capacity — personnel, equipment, and physical facilities — or the rates at which capacity is used. To be sure, there are some correlations between such "inputs" and spending. A nation with more doctors for a given population will generally spend more than one with fewer. Technical equipment, once in place, generates its own utilization and associated costs. Yet some nations with the highest capacities and utilization rates have managed to keep costs in line.

Table 9-4

Actual and Projected U.S. Health Expenditures

	1980	1985	1990	1991	1992	1993*	1995*	2000*
Total health expenditure ($ billions)	$250	$423	$675	$752	$832	$912	$1,089	$1,631
Avg. annual growth in health spending from previous year (%)	12.7	11.1	9.8	11.4	10.7	9.6	9.3	8.4
Health spending as % of GDP	9.2	10.5	12.2	13.2	14.0	14.6	15.7	18.9

* Projected

Source: Congressional Budget Office, March 1993.

The U.S., which is more restrained in such traditional measures as hospital admission rates, lengths of stay, and inpatient beds per 1,000 population, seems captive to uncontrollable medical inflation rates (see Table 9-5).

Much more comparative research needs to be done on the *content* of medical practice and health care to untangle such mysteries. There are some clues, but at this point they are only clues. For instance, hospital care in the U.S. is clearly much more intensive than in any other nation. Americans are admitted to the hospital less frequently than citizens of most developed nations, implying that they are sicker when hospitalized. Their stays are far shorter and they are ministered to by more personnel than in the other developed countries (except Australia). These U.S. traits are markers of greater intensity of care and higher — undoubtedly the world's highest — hospital costs. Nonphysician hospital personnel are better paid in the U.S., contributing to these costs.

Table 9-5

Inpatient Hospital Capacity and Utilization in Nine Nations

Data are from 1990 unless otherwise noted

Nation	Beds per 1,000 population	Bed days per capita	Admission rate (% of population)	Average length of stay (days)	Occupancy rate (%)	Employees per bed
Australia	9.8[a]	2.9[a]	23.0[a]	12.9[a]	82.4[a]	3.9[a]
Canada	6.6[a]	2.0	14.1	13.9[a]	84.9[b]	2.4[b]
France	9.7	2.9	23.3	12.3	80.4	1.1
Germany	10.4	3.3	20.9	16.5	86.5	1.3[a]
Japan	15.8	4.1	8.3	50.5a	83.6	0.8
Netherlands	11.5	3.7	10.9	34.1	88.5	2.1
Sweden	12.4	3.5	19.5	18.0	84.2	1.9[c]
United Kingdom	6.4	2.0	15.9[b]	14.5	80.6[d]	2.6[c]
United States	**4.7**	**1.2**	**13.7**	**9.1**	**69.5**	**3.4**

a 1989
b 1988
c 1987
d 1986
Source: Schieber et al., 1993.

High Technology: American Fetish, Japanese Obsession

Up-to-date comparative data are surprisingly sparse on the capacity of high-tech equipment such as cardiac surgery units, organ transplantation programs, magnetic resonance imagers, and CT scanners. The U.S. depends much more on such technology than nearly any other nation, and considerably more than Canada or European nations, another index of the high intensity of American care.

The U.S. General Accounting Office (GAO) concluded in 1992 that new technology and its rapid diffusion was the single most important factor responsible for a 63 percent increase in U.S. hospital costs between 1980 and 1989.[16] In addition to the price of new equipment per se, the GAO analysis noted that technology drives up the number and wage scales of the hospital labor force. Hospitals have a strong incentive to add new technologies in their drive to compete for physicians and patients, while physicians are driven by both remuneration and potential malpractice liability to order more tests and procedures than may be medically justified.

More than half the 50-year increase in U.S. medical spending can be attributed to technological change, Harvard University economist Joseph P. Newhouse argued in an influential 1992 article.[17] The technology factor dwarfs such commonly cited contributors as aging, increased insurance coverage, increased national income, and increased numbers of physicians, Newhouse believes. Furthermore, technology appears to be a major driving factor in other developed nations' growth in per capita health spending. "Whatever is behind the medical expenditure rise appears to be common across countries," Newhouse writes. "The advance in medical technology is, of course, one such common factor."[17]

While Americans' attraction to medical technology is unquestioned, Japan's example helps illustrate Newhouse's point. Expensive medical equipment has become a "high-tech fad" in the Land of the Rising Sun.[18] Despite government efforts to restrain diffusion of technology, "proliferation of many 'big-ticket' items has continued almost exponentially" in recent years, write John C. Hornberger, MD, Matthew Holt, and Aki Yoshikawa. "Many small and medium-sized hospitals now have expensive devices. Even Japanese clinics are becoming technology-intensive. . . . It is safe to say that, in general, Japanese doctors like high-tech gadgets."[18]

As early as 1982, Japan had more CT scanners (2,120) than all of Europe. Unlike the situation everywhere else but the U.S., even very small Japanese hospitals may have MRI scanners (see Table 9-6). Considering that Japan has about twice the U.S. number of hospitals for half the population, the availability of these and other expensive technologies in Japan is remarkable. But even more remarkable is the fact that Japan manages to support this high-tech arsenal with health expenditures less than half the U.S.', apparently through low unit costs.

Doctors: It's Not Just the Numbers That Count

The outward signs of physician capacity and utilization do not suggest that the U.S. is particularly out of line. It is true, and often commented upon in the

Table 9-6

MRIs in U.S. and Japanese Hospitals, 1990

Percentage of hospitals with MRIs and Japan/U.S. ratios

	Japanese hospitals	U.S. hospitals	Japan/U.S. ratio
Total	7.3%	15.6%	0.47
20-49 beds	1.3	1.0	1.30
50-99	3.4	4.3	0.79
100-299	6.9	17.5	0.39
300-499	14.1	37.3	0.38
500+	39.5	48.3	0.81

Source: DI Okimoto and A Yoshikawa. Japan's Health System: Efficiency and Effectiveness in Universal Care, 1993.

U.S., that the number of American physicians per capita has grown rapidly — more than 50 percent between 1970 and 1990, a trend that is expected to continue beyond the turn of the century.[19] However, in international perspective, the U.S. physician complement — 2.3 doctors per 1,000 population — is about average for developed nations, and Americans see their doctors less often than their counterparts in most comparable countries (see Table 9-7).

A major difference, which contributes greatly to disproportionate U.S. medical costs, is that American doctors are much more likely to be specialists, their incomes are the world's highest, and they practice a more expensive style of medicine than physicians in other societies. "The proportion of the physician work force in medical subspecialties (such as cardiology and gastroenterology) doubled between 1970 and 1990," notes Philip R. Lee, MD, deputy secretary of the U.S. Department of Health and Human Services.[19]

The intensity of services provided to U.S. patients appears to be generally higher than in other developed nations, and service intensity has grown rapidly in recent years (see Table 9-8). A study by the U.S. Physician Payment Review Commission shows that the volume of services provided to Medicare enrollees increased by 33 percent, or 7 percent annually, between 1986 and 1990. "To put this in perspective," Lee says, "these figures suggest that if this rate of increase continued until the year 2000, the average enrollee would receive twice as much medical care as was received in 1990." Parallel data from the Blue Cross-Blue Shield Associa-

Table 9-7

Physician Complements and Annual Patient Contacts

All data from 1990 unless otherwise noted

Nation	Physicians per 1,000	Annual physician contacts per capita
Australia	2.0*	8.8
Canada	2.2	6.9
France	2.7	7.2**
Germany	3.1	11.5***
Japan	1.6	12.9***
Netherlands	2.5	5.5
Sweden	2.9	2.8
United Kingdom	1.4	5.7**
United States	**2.3**	**5.5**

*** 1986**
**** 1989**
***** 1988**
Source: Schieber et al., 1993.

tion suggest that volume intensity has increased at least as rapidly among the privately insured.[19]

Pharmaceutical utilization is the exception to the general rule that American patients are treated more intensely than those of other nations. Patients in many developed nations, such as Germany and Japan, are much more likely to leave their physicians' offices with a pharmaceutical prescription in hand (see Table 9-9)

The drastic U.S. imbalance of specialists and generalists, interacting with an open-ended, fee-for-service-based reimbursement system and technological overcapacity, seems to be at the root of America's general service intensity problem, rather than any one of these factors in isolation. That imbalance has been the subject of much hand-wringing among U.S. medical educators for at least two decades. In 1984, Columbia University medical economist Eli Ginzberg diagnosed the position of American medical education as "very vulnerable" and predicted: "We could be in one hell of a mess in 10 years."[20] Ginzberg was right, but such Cassandra-like warnings did not alter the federal government's medical training policy, with its strong incentives to specialize. The problem is well-recognized by

Table 9-8

Medicare Volume Increases per Enrollee for Selected Services, 1986-1990

Service	Avg. annual rate of change	Percent of total Medicare volume increase
MRI scans	57.4%	1.1%
Angioplasty	29.0	0.8
Upper GI endoscopy	12.0	1.4
Echocardiogram	25.6	1.6
Cataract lens replacement	7.7	5.8

Source: Physician Payment Review Commission, 1993.

the Clinton Administration, which is the first to propose using the federal government's considerable financial leverage to limit specialty training and bolster generalist output. However, those proposals face an uphill battle whose outcome cannot, in late 1993, be foreseen.

Administrative Costs: The Consensus Problem

Arguments are endless about whether the U.S., compared to other nations, has too many of some things (subspecialists, malpractice attorneys, high-tech facilities) or too few of others (generalists, community-based alternatives to institutionalization, incentives to be price-conscious). But virtually everyone agrees that the complex American system of health insurance, government health programs, and charity care imposes an inordinate administrative cost burden.

High administrative costs afflict all parts of the system:

- health insurance, through costs associated with marketing, risk selection, claims processing, utilization review, and profits.
- hospital administration, due to the complexities of billing multiple (and multiplying) payers with different rules and forms, to utilization review, to the need to determine patients' coverage and the benefits to which they are entitled, to complex hospital cost structures designed to maximize reimbursement, and to high administrative salaries.

Table 9-9

Drug Prescriptions in the U.S. and Germany, 1990

Number of separate Rx medicines per capita

	Number of Rx drugs per person
United States	6.4
Germany	19.8

Source: Neel JR in Knox, 1993.

Table 9-10

Per Capita Cost of Health Care Administration U.S. vs. Canada, 1987

Category	Spending per capita	
	U.S.	Canada
Insurance administration	$106	$17
Hospital administration	162	50
Nursing home administration	26	9
Physicians' overhead and billing expenses		
Expense-based estimate	203	80
Personnel-based estimate	106	41
Total costs of health care administration		
High estimate	497	156
Low estimate	400	117

Source: Woolhandler and Himmelstein, 1991.

- physician practices, through the need for personnel to bill (and re-bill) multiple payers, deal with different utilization review and pre-approval rules, determine patient eligibility, and the like.
- patients, who must deal with confusing paperwork generated by each encounter (for the two-thirds of Americans who are outside prepaid health plans), sort out complex coverage rules, and argue with insurers and providers about what they are entitled to.

Steffie Woolhandler, MD, and David U. Himmelstein, MD, of Physicians for a National Health Program, which advocates a single payer system like Canada's for the U.S., calculate that administrative costs consumed between 19 and 24 percent of all U.S. health spending in 1987, or $400-$497 per capita.[21] By their estimate, Canada spent between 8.4 percent and 11.1 percent on health care administration that year, or $117 to $156 per capita (see Table 9-10).

Large U.S. hospitals employ nearly three times more administrative personnel per bed than their Canadian counterparts, and they spend 4.2 times more per bed on administration, according to one comparison by Roger S. Hunt, senior vice president of the Northwestern Health Care Network in Chicago, who has been a hospital administrator in both systems (see Table 9-11).

If U.S. administrative costs could be reduced to Canadian levels, the U.S. General Accounting Office calculated in 1991, the U.S. could save $67 billion a year — enough to extend health insurance to America's 37 million uninsured residents with about $3 billion left over.[22] Others have challenged the GAO's assumptions; John F. Sheils, Gary J. Young, and Robert J. Rubin of the consulting firm Lewin/ICF estimate that U.S. administrative savings in the insurance, physician, and hospital sectors would total $46.8 billion under a Canadian-style system.[23]

Despite such assumption-sensitive disagreements, few dispute the U.S.' higher administrative costs compared to other developed nations'. The net cost of private health insurance in the U.S. (administration, profits, and premium taxes) ranges from 5.5 percent to 40 percent of premiums, depending on the size of the insured firm,[24] with an average of 14.2 percent in 1990.[25] By comparison, Britain's National Health Service spends 2 percent to 5 percent on administration,[26,27] and German sickness funds' administrative costs average from 4.5 percent to 5.5 percent of revenues.[28]

Ominously, America's health administrative costs are rising rapidly from their already-high levels. Uwe Reinhardt of Princeton University points out that program administration and the net cost of private health insurance represented one of the fastest-rising components of U.S. health expenditures during the 1980s, climbing more than 180 percent between 1980 and 1987[29] (see Table 9-12). The General Accounting Office estimated in 1992 that administrative costs grew at an average annual rate of 7 percent for the median U.S. hospital during the 1980s, accounting for about 13 percent of hospital operating cost increases between 1980 and 1988.[16]

Subjective Measures: The Ultimate Test

Indices such as percent-of-GDP and comparative utilization rates are valuable measures of health system performance. But perhaps the truest indicator is

Table 9-11

Hospital Administrators in the U.S. and Canada Employees and Cost per Bed, 1991

	U.S. Hospital		Canadian Hospital	
Department	FTEs/100 occupied beds	Cost/ occupied beds	FTEs/100 occupied beds	Cost/ occupied beds
Medical records	9.4	$4,418	8.1	$3,246
Finance	8.5	6,420	4.0	1,485
Billings and collections	8.3	7,215	2.0	592
Utilization review	2.1	941	0.3	136
Information review	15.7	12,976	2.2	2,100
TOTAL	44.0	$31,970	16.6	$7,559

Values in U.S. dollars. Based on 1991 budget comparison of 700-bed U.S. urban teaching hospitals and 1,200-bed Canadian two-hospital system.
FTE = full-time equivalent.

Source: Hunt R. Northwestern Healthcare Network, 1993, from Canadian Coordinating Office for Health Technology, 8/92; and American Hospital Association, Hospital Statistics, 1992-93

how well a system satisfies the people whom it is intended to benefit. By this index, the U.S. health *system* fails more strikingly than by any other measure, even though 85 percent to more than 90 percent of Americans consistently report they are satisfied with the quality of the care they get.

The most comprehensive international assessment of public satisfaction with health care was a 10-nation survey published in 1990 by Robert J. Blendon of Harvard School of Public Health, and his colleagues (see Table 9-13) Nearly 90 percent of Americans said they thought the U.S. health care system needed fundamental changes or complete rebuilding, about twice the proportion who were comparably dissatisfied in Canada and West Germany. Even in the United Kingdom, which spent only 37 percent as much as the U.S. at the time of that

Table 9-12

Growth in Selected U.S. Health Expenditures, 1980-1987

Category	Percent change 1980-1987
National health expenditures	+101.5 %
Health services and supplies	+104.5
Hospital care	+ 91.6
Physician services	+119.4
Program administration and net cost of private health insurance	+181.5

Source: Reinhardt, 1992.

Table 9-13

Public Views of National Health Care Systems Opinions in 10 Nations, 1990

Nation	Minor changes needed	Fundamental changes needed	Completely rebuild system	Per capita health expenditure (U.S. dollars)
Canada	56%	38%	5%	$1,483
Netherlands	47	46	5	1,041
West Germany	41	35	13	1,093
France	41	42	10	1,105
Australia	34	43	17	939
Sweden	32	58	6	1,233
Japan	29	47	6	915
United Kingdom	27	52	17	758
Italy	12	46	40	841
United States	**10**	**60**	**29**	**2,051**

Source: Blendon et al., 1990.

poll, the percentage who said they were seriously dissatisfied was only three-quarters as large.

While more recent international surveys have not been done, a national U.S. survey performed in late 1993 also found that 84 percent of respondents felt the American system needed "fundamental change" or "complete rebuilding."[30]

Physicians' opinions provide a different reflection of health system performance. An in-depth survey of doctors in the U.S., Germany, and Canada, published in 1993, found American doctors to be the most dissatisfied[31] (see Table 9-14). Only 23 percent felt the U.S. system works well, compared to 33 percent of Canadian physicians and 48 percent of German doctors. Asked to name the most serious problems in their medical practices, American physicians were most concerned about patients who can't afford needed care (73 percent) and excessive payment delays or disputes (78 percent); German doctors were most concerned about a shortage of competent nurses (77 percent) and limits on the time they can spend with patients (58 percent); and Canadian doctors mentioned a nursing shortage (56), patients who insist on unnecessary care (53 percent), and a limited supply of well-equipped facilities (50 percent).

THE ERA OF HEALTH SYSTEM REFORM: STRUGGLING WITH COMMON PROBLEMS

Beset by intrinsic medical cost pressures, aging populations, economic stagnation or recession, and a sense that health care providers and institutions are insufficiently accountable to the people they are set up to serve, most developed nations are reforming their health systems.

In all such countries, health care occupies a large and growing place on domestic political agendas. It is at once a symbol of a society's commitment to help those in need; a major supplier of jobs and an economic "great white hope" for spawning future biomedical enterprise; and a budgetary drain that threatens to smother other pressing social needs, such as education, economic development, and infrastructure replacement. No other social enterprise is so fraught with its peculiar combination of necessity, emotion, symbolism, hope, and headaches.

The daunting complexity of the health care enterprise has long made politicians wish it could operate more or less on automatic pilot. But it is becoming evident to policymakers in most developed nations that it demands continual monitoring and management. The health care financing structures set up in most nations decades ago — in Germany in 1883, in Britain in 1948, in Canada during the 1960s — have proved durable. In fact, most such national health systems are remarkably workable in light of the vast changes in the "product" they are supposed to deliver. The proof of their success is their popularity, at least everywhere other than in the U.S.

The national health systems of developed nations have provided structures that have not only spread the benefits of medicine to entire societies, but have

Table 9-14

How Doctors Rate Their Health Systems

Physician attitudes in the U.S., Germany and Canada, 1992

	U.S.	Germany	Canada
Doctors' overall rating of their respective health care systems (% who agree)			
Works well	23%	48%	33%
Fundamental changes needed	68	46	63
Complete rebuilding necessary	9	6	4
Major problems are...			
Access to care for indigent patients	55	5	1
High cost	38	32	11
Administrative burdens/bureaucracy	12	25	9
Would advise a career in medicine	37	33	26
Serious problems in doctors' medical practice (% who mention)			
Patients who can't afford needed care	73%	15%	25%
Excessive payment delays/disputes	78	39	24
External review of clinical decisions	53	43	28
Limited supply of well-equipped facilities	14	20	50
Patients insisting on unnecessary care	42	49	53
Limits on time spent with each patient	35	58	44
Shortage of competent nursing staff	54	77	56
Limits on length of hospital stay	57	29	30

Source: Blendon et al., 1993.

given societies ways to set priorities and limits. No nation is seriously considering "completely rebuilding" its health system, as the pollsters so frequently ask. Except perhaps in the United States, "health care reform" means repair, retooling, refinement, experiments in incentive-changing. It does not mean abandoning cherished principles or structures, but rather attempting to make them work better.

What follows are brief summaries of how several societies are reforming their health systems to meet new challenges, with suggestions on how these experiments may be relevant to the U.S. reform debate.

CANADA: SQUEEZING MORE OUT OF A GENEROUS SYSTEM

Whether or not the U.S. adopts — or evolves toward — a single payer health financing system like Canada's, there are strong reasons to pay close attention to the way America's northern neighbor copes with its health care problems in the 1990s. Canada's style of medicine is the most "American" in the world, from its second-most-expensive spending pattern to the way its doctors are trained and the settings in which they practice. (In its virtually total reliance on fee-for-service, Canada might be said to resemble an America of an earlier day, as U.S. physicians increasingly practice in systems with a variety of payment mechanisms other than the pure fee-for-service model. However, fee-for-service medicine is still the dominant mode and determinative influence in both nations.) Although Canadians' medical expectations differ from Americans', there is considerable overlap; Canadian patients and physicians can't help knowing, and being influenced by, the medical standard of care south of the border.

Canada offers a good example of a health care system that must bend to external economic pressures. This is a relatively recent phenomenon. "The term 'cost control' didn't come into provincial governments' lexicons until the mid-1980s," observes Catherine Fooks, director of research services for the Ontario Premier's Council on Health, Well-Being and Social Justice and the Premier's Council on Economic Renewal.[32] Then two trends collided: Health care spending increased at rates parallel to those in the U.S., and the Canadian economy turned sharply downward. "The health care system was not behaving any differently," Fooks explains. "It was the general economy that was changed." Canada's persistent economic downturn and generous social welfare programs have brought it the highest per capita public debt relative to GDP of any OECD nation —- just under $20,000 for every Canadian man, woman, and child in 1993.[33]

The worsening situation resulted in a faltering federal commitment to health care. By 1990, mounting deficits forced Parliament to limit federal health care transfer payments to the 10 provinces. Growth in the federal contribution was pegged to growth in the overall Canadian economy, a rate well below health care inflation.

The increasing stringencies are felt throughout Canada. Although individual provinces have responded in differing ways and degrees, the major steps include:

Ceilings on gross physician billings. All doctors' fees in many provinces are reduced when these ceilings are exceeded, and individual physicians may also be subject to prorated fee reductions that can be as much as 25 percent below usual fees. Total payments to Ontario physicians in 1993-94 were expected to be almost 5 percent below the previous year. "Average physician gross incomes in Canada are falling, and the declines will continue," reports Ralph Sutherland, MD, an Ontario health policy consultant.[34]

Expanded roles for non-physician health professionals. Ontario, the largest province, is moving to empower nurses, nurse-practitioners, midwives, physiotherapists, and others to practice independently and bill the provincial health plan for services.[34] This is expected to increase competition for patients among health professionals, and some speculate it will lead to unemployment or underemployment among Canadian physicians.

Restrictions on numbers and types of doctors. Medical schools, which like other university-level schools in Canada are provincial institutions, have recently started to restrict enrollment. The University of Ontario medical school, the nation's largest, cut entry-level slots by 22 percent in 1993.

Ontario, which, in contrast to the situation south of the border, even has a surplus of family practitioners,[35] in 1993 became the first province to put strict limits on where new physicians are permitted to practice. In order to obtain a billing number from the Ontario Health Insurance Plan, new doctors trained outside the province must agree to practice in an underserved area.[34]

Tighter budgetary controls on hospitals. Canadian hospitals have lived with prospectively negotiated global budgets for some years — and many hospital administrators prefer them for the leverage the system gives them in intramural hospital battles. However, since 1990, provincial governments are no longer making up the deficits that result when hospitals overspend their annual budgets.

Furthermore, provincial health plans are getting much tougher in their annual negotiations with hospitals. Ontario hospitals, which got only a one percent increase in funds in 1992, were cut 5 percent in 1993.[32]

It is not yet clear whether the 1990s stringencies will further depress Canada's complement of medical technology, already considerably below the U.S.' (see Table 9-15) However, they are clearly forcing considerable thought about how to stretch available resources further and more attention to research on what medical interventions are truly effective, as well as cost-effective. For example, Ontario and British Columbia have found that they could sharply reduce their queues for open-heart surgery — a sore point that has garnered a disproportionate share of attention south of the border — by computerizing the waiting lists and making sure that waiting patients were referred to available surgical slots in a more timely manner.[36]

Canada's rising health care costs are "forcing us to go back and look at things that were in medicine for a long time," comments the Center for Health Services and Policy Research's Evans. "We are getting away from the business-as-usual model — which is that if you just yell loud enough, you'll break through the consensus that costs need to be controlled."[37]

GERMANY: AN ALIGNMENT OF ECONOMIC TROUBLES

German health care has been characterized in the past two decades by periodic reforms. While within Germany these course corrections have usually been considered only partial successes, the readiness to reform has almost certainly been a factor in that nation's achievement in holding health spending in line with

Table 9-15

Medical Technology in the U.S. and Canada, 1991-92

	Canada		United States	
Technology	Number of hospitals with units	Units per million pop.	Number of hospitals with units	Units per million pop.
Cardiac catheterization	49	1.84	1,457	5.80
CT scanner	200	7.46	3,633	14.42
Lithotripsy	11	0.41	370	1.47
MRI	32	1.20	1,036	4.11
Radiotherapy	127	4.79	969	3.84
Open-heart surg.	33	1.24	867	3.44
Organ transplant	28	1.08	555	2.20

Source: Hunt R. Northwestern Healthcare Network, 1993, from Canadian Coordinating Office for Health Technology, 8/92; and American Hospital Association, Hospital Statistics, 1992-93.

economic growth. But in prosperous times, nations can afford some slack in health care cost control. The real test comes when economies sour and other priorities compete for resources with health care.

An alignment of such forces lies behind Germany's ambitious Health Care Structural Reform Law of 1993. Like Canada, Germany's economy fell on hard times in the early 1990s, resulting in soaring unemployment rates. By 1993, even blue-chip employers such as Daimler-Benz and Volkswagen were laying off thousands of workers. At the same time, the collapse of the Communist bloc presented an historic opportunity to reunite Germany. The immediate expense of absorbing East Germany will undoubtedly taper off eventually, but in the short term, reunification has proved to be an expensive victory. Germany's federal government and institutions in the western states, including the sickness funds, were obliged to subsidize the rebuilding of the new eastern states, where 30 percent or more of the population was without work and unable to pay monthly contributions into the statutory health insurance system. Meanwhile, familiar inflationary forces in health care did not take a holiday.

The "contribution rate" — the percentage of gross wages that German workers must pay for health insurance — is a closely watched barometer. The stability of this rate is a central concern of politicians, employers, and union leaders alike. Between 1991 and 1992, the contribution rate rose one percentage point, from 12.2 to 13.2 percent. Spending by the statutory sickness funds, which insure 90 percent of the German population, rose nearly twice as fast as the funds' revenues in 1991 and 1992. This increase, coupled with economic and reunification pressures, was enough to precipitate a rare consensus among Germany's three main parliamentary parties that something had to be done. The result, the *Gesundheitsstrukturgesetz*, or health care structural reform law, has been called the most sweeping revision of the German health care system in the past 50 years.

Strengthening the Center

The 1993 reform appears to mark a decisive swing of the pendulum toward more centralized control of health spending and away from the traditional German emphasis on self-government and self-restraint among health insurers and providers. While Germany has been well-served by its blend of central goal-setting and autonomous regional bargaining as a way to control costs, the latest reform employs sterner measures. Global budgets, previously employed only for ambulatory physician services, were extended to hospitals, dental care, pharmaceuticals, and sickness fund administrative outlays. Moreover, these new budgets were capped for three years, with non-negotiable increases that may not exceed the expected growth in sickness fund revenues — which, in turn, reflect general economic growth.

Among other major features:

Physicians are put at risk for their prescribing habits. Germans are prescribed twice as many medications as Americans and one-third more than the European average. To rein in excess utilization, doctors are held liable for the first 280 million deutschmarks of pharmaceutical spending in excess of the prospectively set budget, with drug companies responsible for the second 280 million. This is the first time German doctors have been held financially liable for health spending beyond their own fees.

The measure, which was fiercely fought by German physicians, had its intended effect: Prescription drug sales plummeted by 21 percent in the first six months of 1993. In addition, Germany intends to reduce by one-third the number of pharmaceutical products that will be reimbursed.

Hospitals will no longer be guaranteed their full operating costs but will be paid on a prospectively based system resembling American DRGs (diagnostic-related groups). The aim is to reduce excessive hospital lengths of stay produced by long-established per-diem payments, which give hospitals a strong incentive to keep patients as long as possible.

Sickness funds will be opened to competition. Except for white-collar workers, Germans have been restricted in their choice of insurers. In 1993, about half of all German workers could choose,[38] but even their choice was limited. To encourage sickness funds to keep their costs (and workers' compensation rates) low, Germans will be able to choose freely among the 1,150 sickness funds beginning in 1996. To prevent cherry-picking and other forms of risk selection, policymakers will devise a risk compensation mechanism that will shift money from sickness funds with disproportionate numbers of older or sicker patients to those with younger, healthier subscribers.

The number of new physicians admitted to ambulatory care practice will be limited. Between 1993 and 1998, new doctors will be unable to set up practices in oversupplied areas. Beginning in 1999, the total number of doctors entering outpatient practice will be limited by a formula related to population need. This is a radical departure from Germany's *laissez-faire* philosophy toward the right to practice medicine.

Physicians' practices will be monitored more closely. Ambulatory care doctors will be at risk of having their fees reduced if they exceed regional utilization norms by 25 percent (compared to the previous 40 percent), and sanctions will be harsher.

The working-out of these measures should command the attention of U.S. policymakers, since many address problems common to both nations. "The United States should carefully monitor Germany's past experience and current reforms using global budgets, physician fee schedules, and constraints on resource growth as they unfold over the next three years," concluded a 1993 General Accounting Office report on the German reforms.[38]

Debating Market Forces

In the mid-1990s, Germany expects to have a lively debate about the extent to which "market forces" can or should be introduced into the statutory sickness fund system. Should German patients, accustomed to nearly first-dollar coverage of a very generous range of benefits, be made more price-sensitive through higher copayments? Should the benefit package be stripped down, carving out a niche for private supplemental insurance? (Heretofore, this has been an all-or-none choice; higher-income Germans have had to choose between statutory insurance and private insurance.) Neighboring Holland, which has been attempting to inject more competition into its complicated sickness fund system since 1987, has put some of these American-inspired reforms on hold because many believed market-oriented changes were undermining fairness — in the Netherlands, as in Germany, a primary value.[39]

Clearly, Germany has considerable room for medical economizing, not just in the pharmaceutical area. But there was no consensus in late 1993 as to how much the nation should rely on central controls, how much on competition, and how much on fostering "personal responsibility." Of course, that question is also very much at the heart of the U.S. debate about health care cost control.

BRITAIN: SOCIALIZED MEDICINE MEETS MANAGED COMPETITION

When in late 1987 Prime Minister Margaret Thatcher announced her program for reforming the National Health Services, critics there and in the U.S. assumed it meant "privatizing" the 40-year-old government-run health system — more emphasis on private health insurance, a greater market niche for private service providers, the encouragement of a two-tiered system of care, more user fees, and other developments hostile to the notion of a universal, progressively funded, and fair health system.

Not so, say the Tory ministers and managers who are now several years into the reforms launched by Thatcher and carried forward by her successor, John Major. Their aim, they insist, is not to dismantle or undermine the NHS but to make it more responsive and to enhance "value for money."

Cutting expenditures or their rate of increase, that quicksilver goal of most other developed nations' health reform policies, is not even the principal aim, they say. The British health service is already one of the developed world's cheapest, spending only about one-third per person as much as the U.S. It has also been efficient by many standards; for instance, its unit costs actually declined in recent years, while unit costs in most comparable countries have risen. In addition, health sector employment has risen only one percent since 1980, by far the lowest rate among 15 OECD nations with comparable data.[27]

However, the NHS has had conspicuous flaws, in particular its limited access to technology and unresponsiveness to patient demand, symbolized especially in notorious waiting lists for much elective care. The objective of the reform is to address these flaws without spending considerably more. "There was a serious concern that we couldn't handle the need by increasing the budget, because it would need such an increase that the economy couldn't stand it," explains Brian Mawhinney, the British Health Minister.[26]

From "Administration" to "Management"

A central feature of the British reforms is to separate the roles of health care *purchaser* from that of health care *provider*. Instead of a centrally determined budget that is merely administered by NHS officials from regional offices, the reform aims to decentralize decision-making as much as possible, challenging regional health authorities to manage within their budgets as shrewdly as possible. This involves the authority to contract selectively for specific services, driving the best possible bargain to meet the health needs of their region. "This presents significant challenges to a health care delivery model that grew up in a no-risk world," observe Marsha Regenstein and Sharon Silow-Carroll of the Economic and Social Research Institute in Washington DC.[6]

The reform attempts to create "internal markets" within the NHS to foster competition. Among other things, this permits NHS money to "follow the patient," giving providers a strong incentive to offer the most efficient, responsive, and highest-quality care. "You cannot trust hospitals to provide a balanced package of services. There are too many vested interests," explains Sir Duncan Nichol, the NHS' chief executive. "We are trusting purchasers to do it by giving them the money. We took money lying in hospitals and passed it to purchasers on a resident basis, using a formula that is weighted by age, sex, and mortality (as a proxy for morbidity)."[27]

To implement this new philosophy, the reform law:

- offered hospitals, ambulance services, and some community services the option of self-government as NHS Trusts, with control over their own capital assets and freedom to negotiate the terms and conditions of their operations;
- introduced a voluntary funding scheme for general practitioners, who comprise 90 percent of the public's contact with the NHS and account for 20 percent of its spending, in which GPs with large practices (initially over 9,000 registered patients, subsequently reduced to 7,000) to become "fundholders"; this permits them to bargain and contract with hospitals, hospital-based specialists, and other providers to meet their patients' needs;
- issued a new Patient's Charter promising, among other things, the right to be given "detailed information on local health services, including quality standards and waiting times, to be guaranteed admission for treatment within two years, and to have any complaint about NHS services investigated";
- set new national performance standards, such as immediate triage for patients arriving in emergency departments, no more than 30 minutes' wait in outpatient departments, and ambulance response times not exceeding 14 minutes in urban areas and 19 minutes in rural areas.[27]

The System Responds

According to NHS officials, the first three years of the reform has produced demonstrable measures of increased efficiency and responsiveness. They include:

- Hospital inpatient activity grew by more than 7 percent in the first year, versus an historical rate of 2 percent, resulting in an additional 1.3 million patients being treated in 1991 and 1992, with the new autonomous Trust hospitals outperforming those managed under the old system.
- While waiting lists are undiminished — about one million patients nationally, or about three months of NHS throughput — the length of time patients wait has allegedly been reduced, with 50 percent of elective patients seen within five weeks, 70 percent within three months, and 98 percent within one year. "Sure this is still too long," Nichol acknowledges, "but it is not the horror story it was before."[27]
- Hospital specialists are emerging from their former isolation to conduct clinics in larger GP practices.

- GPs have shown enthusiasm for becoming Fundholders, which permits them to manage their patients' care more effectively and plow savings back into improvements in their practice (but not in doctors' pocketbooks). By April 1994, officials expect that one-third of the population will be covered by Fundholding practices.

In addition, patient flow has changed, which is having large impact on some institutions. Some of the nation's leading teaching institutions in London are threatened by loss of patients and revenues, and some are considered likely to merge. Meanwhile, private, non-NHS hospitals are bidding for contracts. Still, Mawhinney says, criticism of the government for trying to "dismantle" or "privatize" the NHS has abated. "We don't want to privatize the NHS," the health minister says. "No one accuses us of that any more."[26]

Beyond Medical Care

In addition to reforming health service delivery, Britain has embarked on an ambitious program to identify which services are more effective in improving the health of individuals and communities. This effort, launched with publication of a 1992 White Paper called "The Health of the Nation," has initially targeted five national targets:

- Reducing death rates for coronary heart disease and stroke by 40 percent in the under-65 population and 30-40 percent for those aged 65 to 74 by the year 2000;
- Reducing death rates for breast cancer, cervical cancer, and lung cancer by 15 to 30 percent by early in the next century;
- Cutting suicide rates by 15 to 33 percent (depending on the population group) by 2000;
- Reducing the incidence of gonorrhea by 20 percent and the rate of pregnancies among females under age 16 by 2000; and
- Reducing accidental deaths by 25 to 33 percent by 2005.

The government has also decided to devote 1.5 percent of the NHS budget for health services research, in an attempt to target resources more effectively. "There is rationing in our system, there always has been, there probably always will be," Nichol says. "Wherever you start, you come back to the question of what you are discarding when you squeeze — and that's a problem for all health systems."[27]

LEARNING FROM THE "REFORM EPIDEMIC"

One of the striking aspects of the virtual pandemic of health reform in developed nations is that the fever can strike no matter where a country finds itself on the spectrum of health spending. High-spending nations such as Canada and Germany are engaged in reforms of ambitious sweep, but so is the low-spending United Kingdom. Ironically, the biggest spender of all is dithering over therapeutic options for its ailing system — radical surgery, conservative medicine, or perhaps a homeopathic tincture of competition?

One lesson to be drawn is that money, important as it is, is not the whole story. Policymakers and citizens alike are unhappy with their health care arrangements for diverse reasons, perhaps best summed up as a growing sense that throwing more money at health providers will certainly not buy better health, in societal terms. Uncontrolled medical inflation without better management, in fact, may actually make health *care* worse, in the sense not only of more expensive but less responsive, more impersonal and less humane, more meddlesome and less realistic in the public expectations it engenders.

It's Management, Stupid

Robert Evans points out that a typical response of health care providers and their defenders to this growing malaise is to blame external pressures for uncontrolled medical inflation — forces such as aging of the population, technological advances, and unquenchable public expectations. All these explanations are false, Evans notes, "and they reverse the conclusions of all Canadian commissions and most European reforms: more management, not more money."[10]

This conclusion is a painful lesson for Americans, who distrust authority, especially government authority. As political scientist James Marone of Brown University points out, Americans habitually yearn for technical-appearing solutions to complex social problems. "We don't like politics and don't trust politicians, so we look for solutions that operate automatically without any human interference," Marone says. "It's a really old dream in the U.S. There is a whole series of smarter mousetraps and tricks for solving problems, from the free market to DRGs, that are set up with the implicit hope that they will operate automatically, and in a fairly mechanistic fashion."[40]

The concept of managed competition explicitly recognizes that market forces in health care will never operate in the automatic fashion, that health care markets need to be structured, monitored, kept honest, and — according to the Clinton Administration, the Thatcher/Major governments, and current reformers in Germany, the Netherlands, and Sweden — subjected to the external discipline of budget limits. For this reason alone, the course of health reform in those European nations is worth Americans' close attention, because no one really knows whether the theories of managed competition will test out in large-scale national experiments, once they are sullied by real-world, hands-on implementation. (Theorists, of course, can always disown such experiments by saying that the theory, as they envisioned it, was never really tested.)

It is important to understand, however, that managed competition, to use the term loosely, is often not intended by reformers in other nations to control costs. It is more often used as a tool to increase provider accountability, responsiveness, and flexibility (as in Britain); and to counter tendencies toward unfairness (as in Germany's upcoming experiment in free choice among sickness funds, whose contribution rates have been disturbingly divergent). The words of Sir Duncan Nichol, certainly no left-winger, are cautionary: "If you are seriously interested in cost control, you will not get there without a global budget. Price and volume controls alone will not suffice."[27]

Richard Saltman of Emory University, discussing Sweden's recent reforms — which include elements of competition, freer patient choice, and allowing the money to follow the patient as in Britain — notes a pattern among OECD nations' health reforms: "Most of the 24 OECD nations are trying to use market incentives on the production side of the system, where the services are actually delivered. Nobody has succeeded in installing market mechanisms on the financing side. The Netherlands stopped its experiment on the financing side — competition among multiple payers — because they decided it would destroy solidarity."[41]

A NEW GAME, AN OPEN FIELD

Apart from these overarching issues, other nations are in the midst of trying many reform strategies, many of which are, at last, on the table in America. Canada and Germany are trying to gear medical training to population needs, in terms of both numbers and specialty mix. This is a complex task that will clearly benefit from transnational communication and research.

Pharmaceutical spending is a growing issue in many countries. Often overshadowed in the past by the bigger-ticket spending components (hospitals, physicians, high technology), prescription drug expenditures are being tackled head-on by Britain and Germany. The U.S., where the issue has been neglected largely because most people do not yet have prescription drug coverage, can piggyback on these efforts and perhaps even use them to build appropriate safeguards into drug benefit programs when they are adopted for Medicare or inserted into a national minimum benefit package for the under-65 population.

Virtually all nations are examining their health care benefit packages, trying to prune away "non-essential" services. This is another challenging exercise that leads directly to the task of investigating medical outcomes, health outcomes, patient expectations, cost-effectiveness, and cost-benefit analysis. The U.S. is a world leader in this realm and could both teach and benefit from other nations' attempts to examine what works and what doesn't in health care.

Similarly, the U.S. is far ahead of other nations in health delivery system innovations. As Britain and Sweden are demonstrating — and Canada, Germany, and Japan might do well to heed — capitated payment and risk contracting for providers' services can be engrafted into widely different financing systems. This lesson may circle back to these shores, in fact. Joseph White of the Brookings Institution thinks the Clinton health security proposal, with its eclectic every-idea-under-the-sun approach, might evolve toward "an amalgam of Germany and Hawaii," in which group- or staff-model HMOs would compete with an all-payer regulated fee-for-service system." That development, White notes, could be the best of both worlds; or it could, at least in the short term, "produce a multi-tier system in which both doctors and patients would be subject to more vehement regulation of care by private insurers than today."[3]

The point, however, is that health reform today is a new game on an open field. The ideas and recombinations are multiplying, and ideology seems less important than it used to. In this spirit of pragmatism and experimentation, learning from successes and failures across national borders may prove not only valuable but indispensable.

REFERENCES

1. Kennedy Sen. EM. Personal communication, June 28, 1991.
2. Knox RA. At Last, a New Idea Supplants the Old One of Choice. *Boston Globe*, September 23, 1993: 15.
3. White J. Controlling the Costs of Health Care: International Experience. Testimony before the U.S. Senate Finance Committee, October 13, 1993.
4. Rodwin VG. American Exceptionalism in the Health Sector: The Advantages of "Backwardness" in Learning from Abroad. *Medical Care Review* 44 (1), 1987: 119-152.
5. Schwartz LL and MW Stanton. Social Problems That Escalate America's Health Care Costs. *The Internist*, July-August, 1992: 16.
6. Regenstein M and S Silow-Carroll. *Market Reforms and Regulation: Lessons From Europe's Health Care Systems.* The Economic and Social Research Institute, forthcoming in 1993.
7. Schieber GJ, J-P Poullier, LM Greenwald. Health Spending, Delivery, and Outcomes in OECD Countries. *Health Affairs* 12 (2), Summer 1993: 122.
8. Knox RA. *Germany's Health System: One Nation United, with Health Care for All*. Faulkner & Gray, 1993: 283.
9. McGinnis JM and WH Foege. Actual Causes of Death in the United States. *Journal of the American Medical Association* 270 (18), November 10, 1993: 2208.
10. Evans RG. Testimony before the U.S. Senate Finance Committee, October 13, 1992.
11. Lohr KN, K Yordy, PF Harrison, and AC Gelijns. Health Care Systems: Lessons from International Comparisons. *Health Affairs* 11 (4), Winter 1992: 239-341.
12. Mechanic D. Can the U.S. Learn from Other Health Care Systems? Keynote address, conference on "Can New England and the U.S. Learn from Other Health Care Systems?" Boston MA, October 21, 1993.
13. Reischauer RD. Testimony before the Subcommittee on Health, Committee on Ways and Means, U.S. House of Representatives, March 2, 1993.
14. Commonwealth Fund/Kaiser Family Foundation, 1993.
15. Wicks EK. *German Health Care: Financing, Administration, and Coverage.* Health Insurance Association of America, 1992: 16.
16. General Accounting Office. *Hospital Costs: Adoption of Technologies Drives Cost Growth.* GAO/HRD-92-120, 1992.

17. Newhouse JP. Medical Care Costs: How Much Welfare Loss? *Journal of Economic Perspectives* 6 (3), Summer 1992: 3-21.

18. Hornberger JC, M Holt, and A Yoshikawa. *Japan's Health System: Efficiency and Effectiveness in Universal Care*. Faulkner & Gray, 1993: 191-212.

19. Lee PR. Current Trends in Health Care Costs and Health Insurance Coverage. Testimony before the Subcommittee on Health of the U.S. House Ways and Means Committee, January 26, 1993.

20. Knox RA. Medical Education in the Future. *Health Affairs* 4 (2), 1985: 119.

21. Woolhandler S and DU Himmelstein. The Deteriorating Administrative Efficiency of the U.S. Health Care System. *New England Journal of Medicine* 324, May 2, 1991: 1253-58.

22. General Accounting Office. *Canadian Health Insurance: Lessons for the United States*. GAO/HRD-91-90, 1991: 65.

23. Sheils JF, GJ Young, and RJ Rubin. O Canada: Do We Expect Too Much from Its Health System? *Health Affairs* 11 (1), Spring 1992: 7-20.

24. Danzon PM. Hidden Overhead Costs: Is Canada's System Less Expensive? *Health Affairs* 11 (1), Spring 1992: 24.

25. Levit KR, HC Lazenby, CA Cowan, and SW Letsch. National Health Expenditures, 1990. *Health Care Financing Review* 13 (1), Fall 1991: 36-37.

26. Mawhinney B. Personal interview with Brian Mawhinney, M.D., M.P., British Minister of State for Health, November 8, 1993.

27. Nichol D. Britain's National Health Service: Will Competition Make It More Efficient? Speech at International Health Policy Forum: "Global Lessons in Cost Containment: The New Worldwide Drive to Restrain Health Spending." Washington DC, November 16, 1993.

28. Altenstetter C. The German Health Care System. Address by Christa Altenstetter of City University of New York, at a conference on "Can New England and the U.S. Learn from Other Health Care Systems?" Boston MA, October 22, 1993.

29. Reinhardt UE. The United States: Breakthroughs and Waste. *Journal of Health Politics, Policy and Law* 17 (4), Winter 1992: 653.

30. Kaiser/Commonwealth Fund Health Insurance Survey, a nationwide poll of 2,000 adults over age 18 conducted August 6-30, 1993, and published November 10, 1993.

31. Blendon RJ, K Donelan, R Leitman, A Epstein, JC Cantor, AE Cohen, I Morrison, T Moloney, C Koeck, and SW Levitt. Physicians' Perspectives on Caring for Patients in the United States, Canada, and West Germany. *New England Journal of Medicine* 328 (14), April 8, 1993: 1011-16.

32. Fooks C. International Cost Comparisons: Canada. Address at a conference, "Can New England and the U.S. Learn from Other Health Care Systems?" Boston MA, October 22, 1993.

33. Fulton J. Speech at International Health Policy Forum: "Global Lessons in Cost Containment: The New Worldwide Drive to Restrain Health Spending." Washington DC, November 15, 1993.

34. Sutherland R. Practicing Medicine in Universal Health Systems. Speech presented at International Health Forum: "Global Lessons in Cost Containment: The New Worldwide Drive to Restrain Health Spending." Washington DC, November 15, 1993.

35. Vayda E. Preventive and Primary Care in English-Speaking Canada. Talk at conference on "Can New England and the U.S. Learn from Other Health Care Systems?" Boston MA, October 22, 1993.

36. Naylor DC (1991) and R Evans (1993). Personal interviews.

37. Evans R (1993). Where in the World Are Health Costs Headed? Speech at International Health Policy Forum: "Global Lessons in Cost Containment: The New Worldwide Drive to Restrain Health Spending." Washington DC, November 15, 1993.

38. General Accounting Office. *1993 German Health Reforms: New Cost Control Initiatives*. GAO/HRD-93-103, 1993: 14.

39. Kirkman-Liff B and DW Light. Personal interviews, 1993.

40. Marone J. Personal interview, November 17, 1993.

41. Saltman R. Talk at conference on "Can New England and the U.S. Learn From Other Nations' Health Systems?" Boston MA, October 22, 1993.

CHAPTER 10

The Lobbyists Line Up

Richard M. Sorian

With an issue as complex as health reform, it is no wonder that scores of interest groups are weighing in. In fact, the debate over health reform could be the biggest exposition of lobbying since the Tax Reform Act of 1986 unleashed so many high-paid lobbyists that the hallway outside the Senate Finance Committee hearing room was dubbed "Gucci Gulch."

As legislators debate health reform they will be inundated with advice from everyone from anesthetists to zoologists. Anticipating action on reform, health-related political action committees (PACs) poured a record $15 million into congressional campaigns in 1992. While it is simplistic to assume that such largesse will buy any group what it wants on reform, lobbyists' influence is undeniable.

Congress has always made use of interest groups in the legislative process. In the period before the mid-1970s, trade associations and other groups often provided the bulk of the staff work performed on Capitol Hill. Understaffed members of Congress would often ask lobbyists to write bills for them to introduce. Amendments to those bills would be written by opposing groups.

That pattern began to change in the 1970s as Congress increased its staff in response to President Nixon's tendency to abuse executive power. Lawmakers began hiring experts on various issues, including health care, to counter the growing White House staff. Naturally, many of these new congressional staffers came from the interest groups. Today, Capitol Hill and the so-called "K Street Corridor," home to many of the trade groups in downtown Washington, perform like a revolving door, with Hill staffers going to work for associations and private sector lobbyists filling the vacancies left in Congress.

Congress still depends on interest groups for information. But lawmakers also rely on such groups for lobbying support. It's not unusual for Presidents and members of Congress to ask such groups to launch a "grassroots" campaign for or against a piece of legislation. The amount of coordination that goes on in this game is not well known to the public but is a vital link to the legislative process.

This reliance on interest groups to aid the process is not as sinister as it may sound. After all, such groups have the expertise legislators need to make sound decisions. Who knows better than a hospital lobbyist how such facilities operate? How they would respond to certain changes in the rules? Or how such changes might affect hiring patterns, profit margins, and other matters of importance? Naturally such expertise carries with it a bias, but it's not that difficult to separate the chaff from the wheat.

This chapter profiles the various interest groups that will lobby Congress on health reform. It is in no way an exhaustive list — such an effort would fill the pages of a book twice this size — but it provides a comprehensive look at the groups that have the greatest probability of affecting the course of health reform.

THE PROVIDERS

Physicians

Perhaps no other segment of the health care industry stands to win or lose as much under health reform as do physicians. As reform reshapes the health care delivery system, its financing system, and its patient flow, all physicians will see their profession change. As a result, medical lobbyists will have a critical role in the shaping of a final bill.

Physicians have seen their lobbying apparatus nearly torn asunder during the 1980s. Known previously for its nearly impenetrable unity, the profession fell victim to a Washington strategy of divide and conquer.

Once Congress got a handle on Medicare hospital costs, lawmakers turned their attention to the physician side of the equation. Limits on inpatient payments led to a bulge on the outpatient side of the ledger. While much of that money went to outpatient facilities, a great deal found its way into doctors' wallets.

Congress began pressuring physicians' income in the mid-1980s. Absent any tested way to establish a prospective payment system, Congress chose instead to freeze Medicare fees for periods of time. But that only exacerbated doctors' tendency to increase the volume of services provided to offset the losses on a per-case basis. To counter that, Congress chose to reduce specific fees that had become too high. Most of those cuts were aimed at specialists, including ophthalmologists who performed cataract surgery, proctologists who treated prostate problems, and cardiologists who performed bypass surgery.

The unevenness of these changes led some specialty groups to cut special deals with the Congress, thus ending the unity that had protected all doctors. That's not to say that a unified profession wouldn't have felt the sting of attempts to rein in health care costs. But the ability to divide the doctor lobby bodes poorly for the big fight to come on reform.

The American Medical Association (AMA)
Founded: 1847
Membership: 287,000 individuals
Executive Vice President: James S. Todd, MD
Political Action Committee: American Medical PAC
Key issues: Cost controls, Medicare cuts, malpractice reform, antitrust

The proverbial 800-pound gorilla of the medical lobby, the AMA wields enormous clout — just not as much as it thinks it does. It is the largest group representing physicians' interests, yet it represents less than half of the medical profession, a fact that AMA's opponents like to cite frequently.

From the 1940s through the 1970s, AMA had the kind of power that few lobbies have ever had — and none do today. During those years AMA could, and did, stop legislation in its tracks, thwarting everyone from Harry Truman to Jimmy Carter on health reform. Its opposition to government-provided insurance kept any such program off the books for 20 years and resulted in enormous compromises in the final Medicare bill that affect that program even today.

AMA was not shy about flexing its muscles, spending its money, or even stretching the truth. Though members called Medicare "socialized medicine," physicians remain one of the best-paid professions in the country, earning an average net income of $170,000 in 1992, with one in every four dollars doctors earn coming from the program.

Today's AMA is a much different creature than the group that fought Medicare. It's even a different creature than the group that fought the Reagan-Bush cuts of the 1980s. Set aside are the confrontational tactics that earned the AMA a bad name. In their place is an inclusive approach that calls for negotiation with Congress.

Much of that is the result of the transition to power of AMA Executive Vice President James Todd, MD, who took over the organization in 1989. While he had been being groomed for the job by his predecessor, James S. Sammons, MD, Todd took the helm earlier than expected when Sammons resigned after the revelation of some financial misdealings. Sammons had been an AMA leader cut from the old mold. Crusty, abrasive, and sometimes downright rude, he wielded absolute authority over the medical lobby. Under Sammons, AMA's negotiating strategy could be summed up as: "Just say no. And if they didn't hear you, say no again."

For a time, that tactic worked, and AMA gained a reputation as a powerhouse. But the approach began to wear on members of Congress, and in the mid-1980s it backfired. In the 1986 congressional election, Sammons ordered AMA's political action committee to "spend what it takes" to defeat Democratic Reps. Andrew Jacobs Jr. of Indiana, and Fortney "Pete" Stark of California. Both men had irritated Sammons and the AMA brass by proposing limits on doctors' ability to bill their Medicare patients above and beyond Medicare's fee limits. The ploy failed miserably and alienated the two Congressmen and many of their peers. And both Jacobs and Stark were on the powerful House Ways and Means Committee, the latter serving as its Health Subcommittee Chairman.

By the time Sammons left in 1989, Stark was barely speaking to the AMA's lobbyists. In fact, when he would schedule hearings on Medicare policy, Stark would sometimes "forget" to invite an AMA witness. Todd, who had served an apprenticeship under Sammons, wanted to change that relationship and made it clear that *his* AMA would be more cooperative.

On reform, there was a lot of room for agreement. Before he stepped down, Sammons had created something he called "Health Access America," a coalition of health care groups looking for a solution to the growing problems of insurance coverage and health costs. When it was unveiled in 1989, the proposal was quickly derided as an AMA attempt to deflect attention away from its oppositionist tendencies. The plan did not contain any significant cost containment proposals and sought to guarantee doctors' independence from government regulation.

But the AMA plan also contained elements that, four years later, would show up in President Clinton's plan. AMA endorsed requiring employers to pay for health insurance for their workers. It backed creation of a standard benefits package for all Americans. And it proposed sharply expanding Medicaid to cover more of the poor.

Despite AMA's support on those core elements of the Clintons' plan to expand access to all Americans, during the early months of the Clinton Administration, the AMA was locked out of the discussions going on at the White House. After a public objection to its exclusion — and a lawsuit filed by a separate group representing doctors — AMA gained access to the White House Task Force and to the First Lady. In June, First Lady Hillary Rodham Clinton went to the AMA's House of Delegates meeting in Chicago to offer an olive branch.

Aside from their areas of agreement, AMA will fight the Clintons on several key issues: cost containment, malpractice reform, and physician autonomy. On that last point, the doctors' group has made some headway: One of the key changes made to the September draft of the Clinton plan was dropping alliances' right to limit the number of fee-for-service plans.

American College of Physicians (ACP)
Founded: 1915
Membership: 77,000 individuals
Executive Vice President: John R. Ball, MD
Political Action Committee: None
Key issues: Cost controls, Medicare cuts, primary care

A major factor in the undermining of AMA's leadership among physicians is the presence of the American College of Physicians. Always a bit of a rebel, ACP has angered many of the other physician lobbies with its embrace of the Clinton plan, including tight cost containment.

Because it represents many lower-paid primary care physicians, ACP's positions often depart from the more money-conscious positions of the AMA and other groups. Its leader, John Ball, enjoys playing on the national scene and realizes that for his group to have much of a say it has to depart from the party line.

ACP's early 1993 endorsement of global budgeting upset other physician groups but bought tremendous access to the Clinton team. When the organization endorsed the Clinton plan in mid-September, it clinched itself a prime seat at the lobbying table.

American Academy of Family Physicians (AAFP)
Founded: 1947
Membership: 73,000 individuals
Executive Vice President: Robert Graham, MD
Political Action Committee: None
Key issues: Cost controls, primary care, universal coverage

Like the ACP, AAFP prides itself on taking a different tack from the AMA. Nearly all of the academy's members are primary care physicians, so its liberal positions on many issues are not surprising.

Graham, who served at the Department of Health and Human Services in the Carter and Reagan Administrations, has strong connections to Washington. He uses them to gain access to Capitol Hill and the executive branch of government. That, in turn, gives the AAFP an inordinate amount of say on key issues. In 1989, AAFP strongly supported enactment of Medicare's resource based relative value scale (RB-RVS), which hiked primary care fees relative to those paid to specialists. Since then, his group has helped to win approval of larger Medicare fee increases for primary care doctors.

American Society of Internal Medicine (ASIM)
Founded: 1956
Membership: 26,000 individuals
Executive Vice President: Alan R. Nelson, MD
Political Action Committee: None
Key issues: Primary care, health work force, cost controls

Like the ACP and the AAFP, the ASIM is driven by a desire to improve the status and the reimbursement of primary care physicians. While smaller in number than the other two groups, it is strengthened by its presence in Washington DC. ASIM also played a critical role in the development and passage of Medicare's resource based relative value scale.

On reform, the group has been generally more supportive of the Clinton plan than AMA and other national groups. However, because ASIM leader Alan Nelson is a former president of the AMA, the two groups have better relations than some others. ASIM has stopped short of full endorsement because of concerns about the degree of cost containment but is expected to be an ally of reform.

American College of Surgeons (ACS)
Founded: 1913
Membership: 52,000 individuals
Executive Director: Paul A. Ebert, MD
Political Action Committee: None
Key issues: Cost controls, Medicare cuts, malpractice reform, specialty care

Like the AMA, the ACS tends to look out for its members' pocketbooks first and foremost. However, historic tensions between the two groups often result in a parting of the ways. Part of that is due to AMA's need to represent a broad section of physicians — including surgeons and primary care doctors — while ACS simply represents only the cutters.

That tension has led to public disagreements on such issues as the enactment of Medicare's RB-RVS and the congressional debate over volume controls on Medicare cases. ACS strongly opposed passage of the RB-RVS and broke ranks with the AMA to support volume controls with the proviso that separate controls be set for surgeons. That move helped break the stalemate on Capitol Hill and led to enactment of the Medicare Volume Performance Standard. It also has left bitter feelings between AMA and ACS.

ACS has been cautious regarding the Clinton reform plan. It doesn't like the continuing emphasis on primary care but seems sensitive about appearing too greedy.

Nurses

American Nurses Association (ANA)
Founded: 1896
Membership: 200,000 individuals
Executive Director: Shirley A. Girouard, RN
Political Action Committee: ANA PAC
Key issues: Reimbursement of nurses, state scope of practice laws, universal coverage.

Health care reform may mark the culmination of years of growth in the power of the nursing lobby. Nearly dormant during the Reagan-Bush years, nurses have become a power to reckon with in the Clinton Administration. Some of that comes from the group's historic support of Democratic candidates in losing causes. And a big part of it comes from the ANA's early endorsement of the Clinton-Gore ticket during the 1992 campaign.

Until the 1992 Presidential campaign, nurses have not been very active politically. ANA President Virginia Trotter Betts has been included in the Administration's inner-circle discussions over health reform and has been a prime public spokesperson for the President's plan. ANA endorsed the Clinton proposal in mid-September of 1993.

Along the way, nurses received several key concessions. First, the bill calls for elimination of state restrictions on nurses' scope of practice. That would wipe out state statutes that prohibit nurses from prescribing drugs and performing other functions reserved for MDs. Second, it calls for direct reimbursement by Medicare and private insurers of services performed by physician assistants, nurse practitioners, and other advanced practice nurses. And, finally, it calls for a doubling of federal support for the training of nurses, nurse practitioners, and licensed practical nurses.

Hospitals

From the mid-1970s until near the end of the 1980s, hospitals were a powerhouse in the national debate over health care financing and health reform. Their 1979 victory over President Jimmy Carter on hospital cost containment gave the industry a dragon-slayer reputation. But that image dissipated in 1983, when President Ronald Reagan rolled over the industry in passing Medicare's prospective payment system. Hospitals had to accept limits on their Medicare payments as a result of the failure of the industry's voluntary effort to control its costs in the wake of Carter's defeat.

Hospitals' concessions, however, ended up diminishing their lobbying power. First, the success of the new Medicare system proved that hospital costs could be controlled — albeit for only one payer — and that there was waste in the system. And the fact that the new system did not wreak havoc on the quality of hospital care or on the sector's employment level gave lawmakers heart for future efforts.

So hospitals enter the national reform debate in a weakened state. After nearly a decade of the prospective Medicare payment system, hospitals' profit margins have shrunk — although the industry still manages a decent 4-to-6 percent margin on total business — and the amount of excess capacity has increased (an average of 40 percent of beds are unoccupied).

The new Medicare system also helped to break down industry unity among hospitals. When they were fighting the common enemy — Carter — hospitals were skilled in fighting as a team. But when Reagan pressed for a system of payment that rewarded some providers and penalized others, unity was replaced by infighting. Throughout the mid-1980s, hospitals battled each other instead of the government in Washington. Southern hospitals battled northern hospitals. For-profit hospitals fought against nonprofit hospitals. Urban hospitals feuded with rural ones. All the infighting weakened the industry for its battles against regulation.

Another factor diminishing the power of the hospital industry has been the decreased influence of the for-profit sector and its lobbying arm. When the 1980s began, for-profit medicine seemed to be the thing of the future. Profit-making hospitals were expected — or feared — to take over the whole industry. Some in Congress railed against this eventuality and even threatened legislation. The for-profits, while comprising a minority of the industry, were considered the toughest fighters.

At the same time, competitive pressures — and perhaps some old-fashioned greed — led many nonprofit hospital administrators to imitate their for-profit brethren. The competitive nature of those hospitals led some local governments to question whether nonprofits should retain their tax exemption. In some cases, hospitals performed little or no charity care while spending millions on advertising.

While a few of the worst offenders did, indeed, lose their blanket exemption, states stopped short of stripping the entire field of that right.

American Hospital Association (AHA)
Founded: 1898
Membership: 6,000 facilities; 50,000 individuals
President: Richard J. Davidson
Political Action Committee: American Hospital Association PAC
Key issues: Cost controls, Medicare cuts

As the largest of the hospital groups, AHA has the greatest influence over national policy. However, that wasn't always so. Until recently, because of the sharp divisions among hospitals, AHA was not considered a true voice for its members. But as those differences have subsided, AHA has risen again, though not to the level of power it enjoyed in the 1970s.

AHA has the advantage of representing one of the largest employers in many congressional districts. In 1991, hospitals employed more than 4.2 million individuals in the U.S. So, the threat of job losses is perhaps the greatest tool hospitals can wield, and AHA isn't shy about using it.

Since 1991, AHA has been led by Richard Davidson, the former president of the Maryland Hospital Association. He brought to the job a plan to get out ahead of reform by advocating change before the President and Congress did it for him. Davidson pushed the AHA to support what he called community care networks, composed of hospitals, physicians, and insurers that would cooperate instead of compete. So strong was Davidson's dislike of the competition of the 1980s that he banned the word "industry" from his association's jargon. Instead, it was the hospital "community."

And Davidson sent some early signals to Congress that AHA planned to be more of a player in the debate over health reform. Davidson moved his office from Chicago to AHA's Washington headquarters, just down the block from the U.S. Capitol.

During the Clintons' work on health reform, Davidson and the AHA remained fairly quiet, choosing not to criticize the President and First Lady. That earned Davidson a prominent place in the Rose Garden during a ceremony held on September 23, 1993, the day after the President unveiled his strategy in a speech to a joint session of Congress. Davidson stopped short of endorsing the Clinton outline, but his positive comments earned him points at the White House and may strengthen AHA's role in the debate. But the AHA's chumminess with the White House also led to a backlash against Davidson from his more conservative members. They are convinced that the only way to get anything tangible under reform is to withhold an endorsement until the last minute.

Federation of American Health Systems (FAHS)
Founded: 1966
Membership: 1,400 hospitals and health systems
Executive Director: Michael D. Bromberg

Political Action Committee: Federation of American Hospitals PAC
Key issues: Cost controls, Medicare cuts

Until recently, FAHS was the powerhouse in hospital lobbying. Led by Michael Bromberg, widely considered one of the best lobbyists of any kind in Washington, the group had an inordinate amount of influence over federal health policy, even though it only represented the for-profit or proprietary segment of the industry.

Part of that clout came from the knowledge of the issues that Bromberg and his staff brought to the fight. Some of it came from Bromberg's own broad network of contacts in Congress and the Republican White House. And part of it came from the proprietary hospitals' influence in southern states that happened to be represented by well-placed lawmakers.

During the 1970s and 1980s, when lawmakers were cutting final deals, it was FAHS that was consulted last. That gave the group incredible influence. In the mid-1980s, when the AHA was foundering, Bromberg's group was the de facto spokesperson for hospitals in Washington.

But by the end of the 1980s, the group's influence had waned. Part of that was due to the fact that many of the specific issues that energized the for-profit group and kept its membership united had gone away. And part of it seemed to coincide with Bromberg's decision to slow his pace. George Bush's defeat in November 1992 depreciated FAHS' clout considerably as well.

Still, with 1,400 well-placed members, among them a half-dozen extraordinarily influential CEOs, FAHS will have a seat at the table and, more than likely, one at the final meetings to decide the details of reform. The group remains adamantly opposed to government-imposed price controls, whether they are applied directly on providers or via insurance premium limits.

Catholic Health Association of the United States (CHA)
Founded: 1915
Membership: 700 hospitals, 300 nursing homes
President: John E. Curley, Jr.
Political Action Committee: None
Key issues: Cost controls, Medicare cuts, abortion

While representing only a small fraction of the industry, CHA manages to have a great deal to say about the course of major health legislation. Some of that influence comes from the placement of member hospitals in key parts of the country. Part of it comes from Catholic hospitals' charity work and their general reputation as the "white hats" of health care.

Like Davidson's AHA, John Curley's CHA made a point of supporting the Clintons' health reform work. The organization's embrace of many of the Clinton concepts of reform such as universal coverage and an employer mandate will give it more clout than otherwise would be the case. But expect CHA to stand firm on cost controls and the issue of mandatory abortion coverage

THE INSURERS

Health Insurance Association of America (HIAA)
Founded: 1956
Membership: 300 companies
President: Willis D. Gradison, Jr.
Political Action Committee: Health Insurance PAC
Key issues: Insurance reform, limits on choice, cost controls

Insurers have been painted as the villains in the health reform debate. For the most part, the image is based in fact. During the 1980s, insurers stepped up their efforts to weed bad risks from the insurance pool. At the same time, premium hikes imposed in the latter part of the decade helped to fuel the cost explosion that in turn fueled the reform debate.

Like most industries affected by reform, the insurance clique is split. Large companies with significant managed care portfolios are supportive of Clinton's proposal to regulate insurance policies and require nearly all customers to go through monopolistic purchasing alliances. But small insurers recognize that these policies would mean the end to many of them and would certainly reduce the profits of the rest.

HIAA now represents primarily the interests of the small insurers. That caused the "Big Five" insurance firms — Aetna, Cigna, MetLife, Prudential, and Travelers — to leave HIAA and create their own organization, dubbed the Alliance for Managed Competition.

With little left to lose, HIAA launched a preemptive strike against the Clinton plan with a series of expensive television ads that began airing before the President's plan was made public. The ads portray a middle-class couple worrying about limited choice of physicians and the danger of cost caps on insurance. The campaign drew an angry retort from Hillary Clinton, but the resulting publicity may have been just what the insurers wanted.

Group Health Association of America (GHAA)
Founded: 1959
Membership: 1,100 individuals
President: Karen Ignagni
Political Action Committee: Group Health Association of America PAC.
Key issues: Managed care, administrative simplification

Reform's emphasis on managed care could be a bonanza for the already muscular group health industry. The promise of a new flow of cash-paying customers is promising. At the same time, like others that would benefit from the new system, managed care firms worry that new federal rules will sap them of their flexibility and their profitability.

GHAA begins the debate with a new leader. In 1993, the group's long-time president, James Doherty, retired. He was replaced by a bright young woman from the labor movement. Before joining HIAA, Karen Ignagni had been a high-ranking official in the AFL-CIO after spending her early career on Capitol Hill. She brings the group a new, fresher image and improves its relations with labor groups.

Blue Cross and Blue Shield Association
Founded: 1946
Membership: 69 organizations
President: Bernard R. Tresnowski
Political Action Committee: None
Key Issues: Insurance reforms, cost controls, paperwork reduction

As the reform debate begins, the Blues are a troubled organization, suffering from bad publicity about plan failures, allegations of fraud, and rising costs. Still, because they insure nearly 70 million Americans, the Blues will be a key player in the debate over reform and, specifically, in the discussion of insurance reforms.

The Blues stand to benefit from several elements of reform. First, because the plans have been, for many Americans, the insurer of last resort, the Blues have had a disproportionate number of bad risk members. That will change if the risks are spread out as proposed by all the major reform bills, including Clinton's. Second, by reforming insurance rules to require the use of community rating and open enrollment, reform could force other insurers to play under the same rules now enforced on the Blues.

The organization is a strong proponent of reform and could be used to counter the opposition of traditional indemnity insurers represented by HIAA and the Alliance for Managed Competition.

THE CONSUMERS

Consumer groups have historically played a supporting role in national debates over health care. While consumer pressure led to many of the earlier debates over health care, the consumer movement had not yet coalesced into effective lobbying organizations. Nothing could be further from the truth today. In fact, the rise of health reform on the national agenda can be traced to consumer groups pressuring politicians to pay attention to the rising cost of health care and the lack of security Americans felt about their coverage.

Like other sectors, consumer groups aren't unified in their position on reform. A large number favor a government-run single payer model of reform. Others are supporting a mixture of government and private solutions. But nearly all these groups agree on one thing: the status quo must go.

The American Association of Retired Persons (AARP)
Founded: 1958
Membership: 33 million plus
Executive Director: Horace Deets
Political Action Committee: None

Key issues: Prescription drug coverage, long term care, out-of-pocket costs

Because of its size and its research capacity, AARP is the most influential of the consumer groups involved in health reform. But the size of the organization sometimes works against it, particularly when AARP's leaders can't get a clear reading of their members' desires.

The organization was bloodied in the 1989 fight to repeal Medicare's catastrophic insurance benefits. AARP had supported enactment of those benefits just a year earlier but had misread its membership's willingness to pay for the benefits they got. When a senior citizen grassroots rebellion cropped up, AARP ran for the hills.

Still, the group has managed to retain its clout but is much more hesitant about using it. Going into the health reform debate, AARP insisted on two things: a prescription drug benefit for the elderly and at least a start toward a long term care policy. It got both. As a result, AARP helped to organize and fund a consumer coalition in favor of reform.

AARP remains concerned about the Clintons' plan to use Medicare savings to finance a big chunk of reform. Still, the betting is that AARP will support the Clinton plan, an endorsement that strengthens the chances of passage.

Families U.S.A

Founded: 1981

Membership: 225,000

Executive Director: Ronald Pollack

Political Action Committee: None

Key issues: Universal coverage, costs controls, consumer involvement

One of the earliest and most uncritical supporters of the Clinton effort has been Families U.S.A., a group created by the former Villers Foundation to advocate for health care reform and to represent the poor. An extremely active group, Families is quick to issue a report or hold a press conference to keep the pressure on for health reform. During the 1992 campaign, Families barely disguised its support of Bill Clinton's health reform plan, even issuing a somewhat questionable report favoring the Democrat's proposal just before the election.

With Clinton in power, Families has been on the inside of much of the debate over reform. The group's Executive Director, Ronald Pollack, is an experienced Washington hand and has been an unofficial adviser to the White House Health Reform Task Force.

Families can be counted on to keep the drumbeat going with town meetings, demonstrations, letter-writing campaigns. As the Health Security Act moves through Congress, Families will exert pressure to make sure universal coverage stays in the bill.

Consumers' Union

Founded: 1936

Membership: not a membership organization

President: Rhoda Carpatkin

Political Action Committee: None

Key issues: Universal coverage

Since the reform debate began in earnest, Consumers' Union has been strongly advocating a single payer system modeled after the Canadian system. It has been very effective in organizing at the grassroots level and keeping the pressure on for reform at town meetings and the like.

With its somewhat singular fixation on single payer, it is not clear how effective Consumers' Union will be in the debate over a public-private mix of reforms. Where the group will play a role is exerting pressure for states' freedom to design a single payer system at the local level.

BUSINESS

Because of its impact on the nation's employers, health reform is a critical issue for business groups. Traditionally, such organizations have hung together on issues of national importance. And business' opposition to health reform in the 1960s and 1970s was a key factor in the inability to enact such legislation.

Today, business is divided on the question of health reform. Small firms tend to oppose it, because they fear the cost of having to insure their workers. Large business is much more supportive of reform because of the rising cost of their insurance coverage. And, large businesses feel that the presence of so many firms that do not insure their workers results in a significant shift of costs to large firms.

National Federation of Independent Business (NFIB)

Founded: 1943

Membership: 570,000 individuals

President: S. Jackson Faris

Political Action Committee: National Federation of Independence Business Free Enterprise PAC.

Key issues: Employer mandate, insurance costs

Clinton's embrace of an employer mandate to cover two-thirds of the uninsured puts the small business community square in the middle of health reform. NFIB, which is the largest representative of small firms, is adamantly opposed to such a mandate and has vowed to do whatever it takes to fight it.

But, like other sectors, small business is divided. Those small firms that do buy insurance for their workers recognize that reform would cut their costs dramatically. And some of those that don't buy coverage for their workers see that it has reduced their competitiveness with those that do. Still, a core group of firms believe that the government has no right to order them to spend money on insurance.

National Association of Manufacturers (NAM)

Founded: 1895

Membership: 12,500 individuals

President: Jerry J. Jasinowski

Political Action Committee: None
Key issues: Cost controls, employer mandate, universal coverage

NAM will be a powerful participant in the reform debate. During the formulation of his plan, President Clinton actively courted the group of large employers to support his proposal. That attempt did not entirely succeed — NAM issued a statement critical of the far-reaching nature of the Clinton proposal — but it has kept the group out of the opposition camp.

NAM's somewhat ambiguous position is the result of being pulled in opposite directions on certain key issues. For example, since large businesses tend to insure their workers, the employer mandate that angers so many small firms doesn't produce the same reaction. In fact, since large companies tend to pick up the costs incurred by uninsured workers as a result of cost-shifting, an employer mandate could save the big firms some money. At the same time, Clinton's dependence on regulation to control cost increases upsets the corporate world, which tends to prefer market forces. And NAM isn't happy with the power that would be given to the new Health Alliances, fearing that would eclipse employers' ability to control utilization and costs.

Still, the manufacturers' group has more in common with the Clinton team than it does with the small business community. With some modifications — particularly a reduction in bureaucracy — the Clinton plan could attract strong support from NAM and groups like it. The group is pushing to change Clinton's proposal to only allow firms with more than 5,000 workers to set up their own alliances; NAM would like to see that number dropped to 1,000.

Chamber of Commerce of the United States
Founded: 1912
Membership: 200,000 individuals and businesses
President: Richard L. Lesher
Political Action Committee: National Chamber Alliance for Politics
Key Issues: Health costs, employer mandate

Like the NAM, the Chamber of Commerce has mixed feelings about health reform. After years of rejecting an employer mandate as a means to deal with the uninsured, the group now supports the idea. But the Chamber remains concerned about the level of regulation in the Clinton plan. It doesn't like the notion of powerful health alliances taking away business' role in negotiating for health benefits.

The shift in big business' position on reform stems from the continuously rising cost of insurance and the fact that firms that don't insure their workers are at a competitive advantage to those that do. Reform could create the kind of even playing field that large companies prefer.

Despite its generally positive feelings about reform, the Chamber has to be careful about how closely it aligns itself with the Clinton White House. When Chamber lobbyists gave the President's economic policies a positive review, the Republican party lit into the group and pushed it to oppose elements of the Clinton plan.

LABOR

Labor unions have pushed hard for employer-funded health insurance for workers for years and not surprisingly have been aggressive supporters of health reform. In fact, much of the current private health insurance system was shaped by union-management negotiations. Beginning in the mid-1940s, unions began to demand health benefits as an alternative to wage increases (which were limited by post-War wage controls).

In the 1980s, as union power fell precipitously, health care benefits became the focus of labor-management negotiations. Several major strikes centered on the question of whether unions would agree to "give back" some of their health benefits. Labor won most of those fights, but in return gave up wage increases, and earnings fell behind the cost of living.

In the current debate, unions are after several things. First, they want universal coverage. Second, they want government-enforced cost containment so that employers won't continue to demand reductions in benefits to cut costs. And, finally, unions want to protect the benefits they have negotiated.

Clinton gave labor almost everything it wanted. The employer mandate approach to universal coverage is very popular among unions. The comprehensive benefit package would result in better benefits for some workers (although there is concern about contracts that have better benefits than the President proposes). And Clinton rejected the call for a cap on the tax exemption for health benefits.

American Federation of Labor and Congress of Industrial Organizations (AFL-CIO)

Founded: 1955
Membership: 14,100,000 individuals
President: Lane Kirkland
Political Action Committee: Committee on Political Education (COPE)
Key issues: Universal coverage, cost containment

As the largest umbrella labor organization, AFL-CIO leads labor's efforts in health reform. It is a strong supporter of the Clinton plan and plans to independently promote its passage around the country.

AFL-CIO President Lane Kirkland has been trying to push health care reform to the top of the national agenda for nearly 20 years. In 1992, he conditioned labor's support for any Presidential candidate on a promise of health reform.

During the formulation of the Clinton plan, AFL-CIO was consulted and listened to on a string of issues. Labor's opposition to a cap on the tax exemption for health insurance benefits led the White House to scrap that measure. And unions' demand for a broad benefit package — one that would at least match the majority of the existing plans that have been negotiated — contributed to the comprehensiveness of the standard benefit package in Clinton's plan.

While labor's support for reform is almost a "given" in Washington, it will be an important factor around the country. Local unions can organize rallies and letter-writing campaigns to show support for the Clinton plan.

Service Employees International Union (SEIU)
Founded: 1921
Membership: 1,000,000 individuals
President: John J. Sweeney
Political Action Committee: COPE
Key Issues: Health worker conditions, health sector jobs, cost controls

As the largest union representing health care workers, SEIU will have a critical voice in reform. Among its concerns are the conditions under which hospital workers work; the size of the health care work force; and, like other unions, universal coverage and cost controls.

The union's president, John Sweeney, wears two hats. As president of SEIU, he represents one of the largest member unions in the country. And as chairman of the AFL-CIO's health care committee, he speaks for labor as a whole on issues related to health reform.

OTHERS

Pharmaceutical Manufacturers Association (PMA)
Founded: 1958
Membership: 109 companies
President: Gerald J. Mossinghoff
Political Action Committee: Pharmaceutical Manufacturers Association Better Government Committee
Key issues: Price controls, new prescription drug benefit

As the prescription drug industry's main representative, PMA is under the gun to fight off attempts to regulate drug prices. The group is known for its ability to halt legislation but is not so well known for an ability to draft alternatives. In order to get its way now, it might be as necessary to do the latter as it is the former.

PMA members stand to benefit from the much broader drug coverage in Clinton's plan. By including outpatient drugs in the standard benefit package and creating a new Medicare drug benefit, the Clintons are offering drug makers more than 70 million new insured customers.

At the same time, drug makers are very leery of plans to require discounts for Medicare — drug companies already cut their prices for Medicaid and most managed care companies. And they are sure to keep fighting Clinton's proposal to rein in prices on new "breakthrough" drugs.

The relationship between the Clinton Administration and the PMA has been bad from the start. The President and First Lady used drug makers as a punching bag as they pursued broader efforts on childhood immunization. Later, the White House softened its criticism of the industry, but relations remain very poor.

The National Governors' Association (NGA)
Founded: 1908
Membership: 55 governors
Executive Director: Ray Scheppach
Political Action Committee: None
Key issues: State authority, Medicaid reform

Always a player, NGA's hand is significantly strengthened by the presence of one of its own in the White House. A past chairman of NGA, President Clinton has made it clear that governors and state legislators must have a say in health care policy.

The Clinton reform plan reflects that commitment by giving states a large role in shaping reform at the local level. Should Clinton's blueprint become law, states will gain a great deal of power in the health care field. State flexibility also is reflected in the streamlined waiver process established for states that want to set up a single payer model of reform. That move pleased both the NGA and the consumer groups pressing for a Canadian model of health care.

The Jackson Hole Group
President: Paul Ellwood, MD
Political Action Committee: None
Key issues: Level of competition, level of regulation, universal coverage

As the proponent of a "pure" version of managed competition, the Jackson Hole Group will be a significant voice of moderation in the national debate. The Group, a loose amalgamation of academics, insurers, hospitals, physicians, and others who have been gathering informally in Paul Ellwood's Wyoming home for years, embraces many of the concepts that the Clinton plan includes. But it opposes some of the President's more regulatory additions to its blueprint, in particular the use of insurance premium caps and an employer mandate on insurance purchase.

Group members can be expected to work with moderates like Rep. Jim Cooper of Tennessee (D) and Sen. John Breaux of Louisiana (D), who have introduced legislation more closely following Jackson Hole's managed competition model.

CHAPTER 11

Congress: The Players and the Process

Richard M. Sorian

Before any health plan can become law, it must wend its way through a complex and arcane congressional process. Most pieces of legislation are referred to two committees (one in the House of Representatives and one in the Senate). But health reform is under the jurisdiction of at least a dozen separate panels. Each has the power to slow or even stop the legislation's progress; all will in some way change the face of the plan.

This chapter traces the likely course of health reform through the legislating process — first through the House and then through the Senate. Because reform includes changes in the tax code, the Constitution requires that it begin in the House. The stamp each committee will leave on the bill depends on a number of factors. Most important are the personalities and agendas of the full committee and subcommittee chairs, the legislative turf that each panel controls, the knowledge and skills of the key staff members, and the presence of lawmakers who, for one reason or another, have staked a prominent position in the debate.

For both houses, the chapter divides the committees of jurisdiction into two categories: major committees that deal with the core of the legislation, and minor committees that have jurisdiction over only a small element of the legislation.

THE HOUSE

In the House, there are three major committees with jurisdiction over health reform. Two of them — Ways and Means and Energy and Commerce — are quite familiar to those who deal with the Congress on health matters; the third — Education and Labor — is a relative newcomer to the debate.

The Committee on Ways and Means

By virtue of its jurisdiction over the tax code, Social Security, welfare, trade, unemployment compensation, and Medicare, no House committee has a broader power base than the 38-member Ways and Means Committee. Because of House rules, Democrats have a wider majority on Ways and Means than on other committees. The 2-to-1 ratio of Democrats to Republicans gives Chairman Dan Rostenkowski unusual influence over the panel and the House as a whole.

Ways and Means' jurisdiction includes Medicare Part A (which covers hospital reimbursement issues) and, jointly with Energy and Commerce, Part B (which covers physician, outpatient, and durable medical equipment issues). Because of its jurisdiction over the tax code, Ways and Means also must vote on much of the financing of health reform, including higher taxes on cigarettes, a surtax on large businesses, as well as Medicare spending cuts.

A jurisdictional fight between Ways and Means and Education and Labor over the enforcement of an employer mandate may dog the House leadership throughout the reform debate. If, as President Clinton proposes, enforcement is handled by the Labor Department, then Education and Labor retains influence over that portion of the plan. If, however, Ways and Means succeeds in switching enforcement to the Treasury Department, then it regains jurisdiction.

Because Ways and Means includes a number of senior members from major cities, urban health care issues (e.g., teaching hospital payments, public hospitals, and disproportionate share facilities) rank high on members' agendas.

The Chairman. Since 1981, Ways and Means has been headed by Illinois Democrat Dan Rostenkowski, a product of the Chicago Democratic machine. During the 1980s, Rostenkowski exerted tremendous influence on health care legislation, helping to shape the 1983 Medicare prospective payment system law, the 1986 Consolidated Omnibus Budget Reconciliation Act (COBRA), and the 1989 budget bill that reformed Medicare's physician payment system.

Like all good politicians, Rostenkowski is best in one-on-one situations where he can bring members in line with a deft combination of courtship and intimidation. With his control over the tax code, Rostenkowski can promise nearly any member something for his or her district in return for a key vote for or against a piece of legislation. As a result, Rostenkowski's legislative defeats can be counted on the fingers of one hand (although some of them, like repeal of Medicare's catastrophic health insurance program, are quite prominent).

If there's any threat to "Rosty's" influence over health reform, it's the legal cloud that's hung over him all through 1993. Federal prosecutors have been investigating whether he traded part of his office allotment of stamps for cash. Whether or not Rostenkowski can prove his innocence in the case may not matter. Under Democratic House rules, committee chairmen must surrender their leadership positions while under indictment. (They can reclaim their posts if the indictment is dropped or the lawmaker is found not guilty, but this often takes several years.)

If Rostenkowski were to be indicted, under current rules, the chairmanship would automatically go to Sam Gibbons, a Florida Democrat who has spent much of his 30-plus years in the House waiting in the wings for one or another senior member to step aside. While Rostenkowski tends to lead through savvy negotiating and sheer political force, Gibbons is more of a "go along to get along" type who probably wouldn't hold much sway with the often divided members of the committee or the House. If Gibbons replaces Rostenkowski at the helm, it is likely that other senior Democrats on the panel — Charles Rangel of New York, J.J. (Jake) Pickle of Texas, and Richard Gephardt of Missouri — will gain influence and power over its workings.

The Ranking Republican. Leading the Republican minority is Bill Archer of Texas, an economic conservative who has shown a willingness to work with Rostenkowski on certain issues but generally hews to an oppositionist line. His first strong foray into health reform was a November campaign to get the employer-mandated health insurance premium in Clinton's plan labeled a tax by the Congressional Budget Office and put on the federal budget. That one failed. Archer will attempt to advance the House Republican leadership's health reform plan through amendments in committee, but the Democrats have him outnumbered and his impact is expected to be minor.

The Health Subcommittee. The Subcommittee on Health is likely to be the focal point of much of the early wrangling on reform. Its ideologically diverse membership includes single payer advocates as well as hard-core managed competition fans. Fear of gridlock at the subcommittee level has led Rostenkowski to suggest that he may bypass the subcommittee and work on reform at the full committee level.

At the helm of the subcommittee is Fortney (Pete) Stark of California. Since he took over that slot in 1985, Stark has been a productive and influential chairman whose major roadblock to true power has been his mercurial personality and often outrageous statements. He once called former Health and Human Services Secretary Louis Sullivan, an African American, "a disgrace to his race" for supporting his Administration's health policies. As is frequently the case, Stark was forced to apologize and his stature was eroded. While such statements gain him the headlines he seemed to relish they diminish the respect among his colleagues and his influence on major issues.

Still, Stark is credited with widening the jurisdiction of his panel far beyond Medicare, allowing him to draft legislation that affects the whole health care system. In 1986, for example, Stark pushed through a bill making it a federal crime for a hospital to transfer an uninsured patient for non-medical reasons. In that same bill was a law allowing laid-off workers to extend their group-rate insurance for up to 18 months (since extended to 29 months).

Subcommittee Ranking Republican William Thomas of California rose to the senior subcommittee slot in 1993 upon the retirement of Bill Gradison of Ohio, who quit to become president of the Health Insurance Association of America. Many on and off the Hill regard the loss of Gradison and the ascendancy of the acerbic Thomas as a setback for reform. While Gradison was seen as a knowledgeable and temperate legislator who could work with Stark, Thomas knows less about health care than about how to make partisan strategy. Like Archer, Thomas will try to amend the Clinton plan in committee but to little avail.

Key Players. Ways and Means is stocked with members who are knowledgeable and active on health care issues. Among those sure to have a major say on reform are Democrats J.J. Pickle of Texas, Barbara Kennelly of Connecticut, Michael Andrews of Texas, Sander Levin of Michigan, Benjamin Cardin of Maryland, and Jim McDermott of Washington. Republicans to watch include Nancy Johnson of Connecticut and Fred Grandy of Iowa. Andrews, Johnson, and Grandy teamed up behind a "purist" managed competition bill late in 1993 and will try to drag the Clinton proposal to the right.

Key Staff. Ways and Means employs some of the best health staffers on Capitol Hill. At the full committee level, Rostenkowski is assisted by Janice Mays, his chief counsel and staff director. While Mays is more schooled in tax law than health policy, Rostenkowski relies on her political judgment. Full committee Republicans get their counsel from Anne Labelle, a former official in the Reagan and Bush administrations who also served on the staff of Senator Orrin Hatch of Utah when he was the senior Republican on the Senate Labor and Human Resources Committee. Labelle is trained as a dentist and an economist.

On the Health Subcommittee, Stark relies on staff director David Abernethy, who joined the chairman shortly after he took control of the panel. A veteran of New York State politics (he served as a key adviser to Governor Mario Cuomo), Abernethy also had previous experience on Capitol Hill as a staff assistant to the late Representative Tim Lee Carter, a Kentucky Republican. Abernethy is considered one of Congress' chief experts on hospital payment issues and on capital reimbursement.

Stark gets his advice on physician payment issues from Jamie Reuter, a former staffer with the Congressional Research Service of the Library of Congress. Reuter helped push through the 1989 law altering Medicare's physician payment system.

The Energy and Commerce Committee

The jurisdiction of this 44-member committee is so wide it has been described as covering everything that "moves, burns, or is sold." Because of that sweeping agenda, it could touch virtually any area of health reform it has a mind to. Currently, the panel oversees the Public Health Service, the Food and Drug Administration, the Title X family planning program, the Maternal and Child Health program, Medicaid, and Part B of Medicare, which it shares with the Ways and Means

Committee. In addition, the panel can legislate changes over such diverse issues as preventive health, hospital construction, clinical lab regulations, managed care regulation, substance abuse, biomedical research, medical education, mental health, community and migrant health centers, medical device regulation, medical ethics, and orphan drug development. And that's just in health care.

Energy and Commerce also exerts influence over the entire insurance industry, so it will handle reform of that part of the health system as well.

The Chairman. At the helm since 1981 has been the often-intimidating and legislatively skillful John Dingell (D-MI). Dingell succeeded his father, John Sr., in the House and has faithfully introduced his Dad's national health insurance bill in each Congress since. While known chiefly for his efforts to ease the impact of environmental laws on his home state's auto industry, Dingell also has put his imprint on health policy, including sponsorship of laws stiffening federal regulation of clinical laboratories and nursing homes. As chairman of the committee's Oversight and Investigations Subcommittee, Dingell also plays a role in keeping the bureaucracy and its constituents honest with well-publicized hearings into such things as health fraud and indirect medical research costs at universities.

The Ranking Republican. The Senior Republican member of the committee, Carlos Moorhead of California, rose to that seat in 1993 upon the retirement of Norman Lent of New York. This is Moorhead's first shot at leadership after 20 years in the House, and he's had little impact on health. While he has one of the most conservative voting records in the House, Moorhead is known chiefly as a conciliator, so he might try to cut a deal with Dingell.

The Subcommittee on Health and the Environment. Since 1979, the Energy and Commerce Subcommittee on Health and the Environment has been headed by the energetic Rep. Henry Waxman (D-CA), one of the most liberal members of the House and one of its most effective legislators. With a powerful political base in California, Waxman built a strong following in the House that enabled him to fight many of the reductionist Reagan-Bush health care policies. Now with health reform at the top of the national agenda, he has the chance that has evaded him so far — to fix the health care system instead of plugging its holes. While his support for an employer-based system has sometimes swayed — he sponsored a single payer bill with Dingell in 1992 — Waxman is sure to be at the center of the deal-making over the Clinton plan.

On the Republican side, 1993 marks the beginning of what is likely to be a long tenure for Thomas Bliley of Virginia as the ranking minority member of this key subcommittee. After more than a decade of service on the panel, Bliley was ready to take the slot when William Dannemeyer of California quit to run for the Senate. While both men are conservatives, Bliley gets along much better with Waxman than the acerbic Dannemeyer. As a result, he may be able to cut some deals on reform. His Virginia district requires him to fight tobacco tax increases, but Bliley otherwise is free to bargain.

The Subcommittee on Commerce, Consumer Protection, and Competitiveness. New regulations on the insurance industry fall under the sway of the Commerce Subcommittee, chaired by Cardiss Collins of Illinois, who represents many of the poorest neighborhoods in Chicago and makes sure those who have the least get the best deal they can in Washington. Elected in 1973 to replace her husband after he died in a plane crash, Collins has spent a great deal of time on issues like Medicaid eligibility expansion and insurance reform.

A relatively new member of the House, ranking Republican Cliff Stearns of Florida, was elected in 1988 and is known for his fiscal conservatism. The owner of several motels and restaurants, Stearns questions the use of an employer mandate to broaden insurance coverage of the working uninsured.

Key Players. Energy and Commerce's broad public health domain has stocked the panel with members who are interested in health care issues. Among Democrats: Ron Wyden of Oregon, Jim Cooper of Tennessee, and retired physician Roy Rowland of Georgia. Among Republicans: Michael Bilirakis of Florida and Scott Klug of Wisconsin.

Key Staff. Dingell depends on staff director Alan Roth for political advice and health counsel Donald Shriber for health policy recommendations. Moorhead depends on legislative assistant Stacey Windham.

On the Health Subcommittee, Waxman has one of the deepest staffs on the Hill starting with chief of staff Karen Nelson — an expert on Medicaid, among other things — Andreas Schneider and Michael Hash on Medicaid and Medicare, Timothy Westmoreland and Ruth Katz on public health programs, William Schultz on prescription drug issues, and Ripley Forbes on a series of substance abuse programs. Republicans rely on a small but talented staff headed by Mary McGrane and Howard Cohen.

On the Consumer Subcommittee, Collins' staff director is David Schooler; Stearns relies on minority counsel Dennis Wilson.

The Education and Labor Committee

Clinton's decision to build an employer-based reform program has thrust this committee deep into health policy for the first time. The committee has had jurisdiction over the ever-controversial Employee Retirement Income Security Act of 1974, which governs self-insured employers. Under reform, ERISA likely will be amended to give states more leeway over regulating self-insured employers and to change the rules for what will come to be known as "corporate alliances."

But the 44-member panel is aggressively moving to establish control over other large pieces of reform. Late in 1993, it released a detailed breakdown of 13 areas of the Clinton plan it said it should control. On the list: the employer mandate, establishment of health alliances, the creation of the National Health Board and its authority to impose duties on players in the system, the integration of workers' compensation into health reform, changes in retiree health benefits, expansion of worker retraining programs, creation of school-based health clinics, application of cost controls on corporate alliances, and all matters enforced by the Department of Labor.

The Chairman. An able legislator on issues involving labor unions and government education programs, William Ford (D-MI) has headed the panel since

1991. He is famous for saying labor unions "elected me and keep me in office," so he is expected to work closely with the AFL-CIO and the home-state United Auto Workers on health reform. Another close working partner ought to be Dingell, as the two are old friends and political allies.

The Ranking Republican. Having squeaked into his ninth term in the House in a three-way race in 1992, William Goodling of Pennsylvania is a slightly weakened ranking GOP member. In the past, Goodling and Ford have worked together on many issues. Health reform — a new issue to both — may not be so easy. Goodling will be pressed by the conservative Republican House leadership to oppose the Clinton employer mandate, but with only 15 votes in the committee he may have a hard time having much impact.

The Labor-Management Relations Subcommittee. When Subcommittee Chairman Pat Williams of Montana talks, benefits managers all over the country listen. Subtle shifts in the policies endorsed by this panel — which in recent years have dealt primarily with the rights of plaintiffs in disputes over health and other benefits claims — can cost employers millions. Williams last year survived the toughest reelection bid of his tenure when he held on to the newly unified single district in his state. He'll work on ERISA and the employer mandate before the full committee gets a crack at it. A liberal on most issues, Williams can be expected to stick with Clinton despite pressure from small business owners back home.

Ranking Republican Marge Roukema of New Jersey, generally a moderate on social legislation, is a critic of the Clinton employer mandate. She may push for some early compromises on that issue.

Key Staff. Ford may rely on staff director Patricia Rissler for political advice, but the key staffer on this panel is Phyllis Borzi, who works as a counsel on the Labor-Management Relations Subcommittee and is considered Congress' foremost expert on ERISA. Russell J. Mueller is the chief minority staffer.

In addition to these three major committees, at least four other House committees will have a crack at the reform legislation. Each is likely to have a limited time to ponder the bill so they, unlike the major committees, will have less ability to halt reform in its tracks.

The Judiciary Committee

This 35-member panel has been at the center of much of the great social change of our time — from civil rights to abortion to Watergate — and it will have a seat at the health reform table as well. Judiciary will play a key role in reforming the nation's malpractice laws — or not, as the case very well may be. Traditionally opposed to federal intervention into tort reform, the panel will have to confront the growing consensus that malpractice is a key cost driver in medicine. Judiciary also will oversee changes in the antitrust laws designed to make it easier for doctors and hospitals to share expensive high-tech equipment or form networks. Additional responsibility could come in strengthening penalties for health care fraud.

The Chairman. At age 71 and after 41 years in the House, cigar-smoking Jack Brooks of Texas is the second most senior member of the body and one of its greatest characters. He's also a born legislator with a solid grip on his committee. Since taking the panel's helm in 1989, Brooks has left his mark on civil rights and other issues. He's a staunch opponent of malpractice tort reform and could be a major stumbling block to that portion of the bill.

The Ranking Republican. Brooks' GOP counterpart is the gentlemanly Hamilton Fish of New York, the owner of one of the more prestigious names in politics. He counts among his relatives a governor, a U.S. Senator, a Secretary of State, and a Congressman. But this Fish proves that nice guys often do finish last. Despite his 25-year tenure, Fish isn't often influential on issues, legal or otherwise. But when he chooses to team up with Brooks — as he did in 1989 on the Americans with Disabilities Act — he can help push through legislation.

The Subcommittee on Civil and Constitutional Rights. Before it's all over, it's likely this panel will have it out over abortion and its place in the new health care system. Facing off are two of the most diametrically opposed panel chiefs in the Congress. Don Edwards (D-CA) is one of the House's best minds on legal issues. As chairman of the subcommittee since 1971, Edwards has played a central role on the national debates over civil rights, abortion rights, fair housing, and the Voting Rights Act. The pro-choice Edwards can and often does decide what will or won't emerge from the panel and from the full committee.

Serving opposite Edwards — and opposite is the operative word — is Henry Hyde (R-IL). Considered as knowledgeable and as respected as Edwards, Hyde is as conservative as Edwards is liberal. Known nationally for his opposition to abortion, Hyde is known in the House for his intellectual honesty; for example, he favors programs assisting poor families as a logical extension of opposing abortion. While the Chairman and Ranking Republican clearly disagree on abortion and several other issues, they find surprising agreement in other areas and work well together.

Key Staff. Brooks relies on general counsel Jonathan Yarowsky, while Fish seeks advice from minority chief counsel Alan Coffey Jr. Edwards' chief staffer is Catherine LeRoy, and Hyde relies on Kathryn Hazeem.

The Veterans' Affairs Committee

This 35-member committee will have its hands full integrating the existing veterans' health system into the newly reformed system. Because vets jealously guard their government-run hospital system, rolling them into a broader reform plan was never seriously considered. But the panel won't be looking for the status quo. Top priorities are streamlining the convoluted requirements for eligibility to the veterans' system and securing Medicare reimbursement for eligible veterans at VA facilities. Clinton also has proposed spending $2 billion to improve the quality of VA facilities, so the panel will have some decisions to make about how to spread that money around.

The Chairman. One of the most conservative Democrats in the House, G.V. (Sonny) Montgomery of Mississippi has headed the committee since 1981. Initially, he worked to protect veterans from budget cuts aimed by Presidents Reagan and Bush. He's also known for his advocacy of legislation to assist active military members, including sponsorship of the G.I. Education Law of 1985, which provides education assistance to new recruits. Montgomery and President Clinton don't see eye-to-eye on many issues, including the budget. As a result, Montgomery hasn't tried to exert his seniority on the Armed Services Committee to become chairman of that panel. Instead, he will stick to veterans' issues.

The Ranking Minority Member. One of the quieter members of the House, Bob Stump of Arizona holds the senior GOP seat on Veterans' Affairs, where his conservative politics match Montgomery's well. A former Democrat (he switched parties in 1981 after voting with President Reagan on his budget and tax cuts), Stump favors reform of the VA health system as part of overall national reform.

The Subcommittee on Hospitals and Health Care. One of only two physicians in Congress, Roy Rowland of Georgia brings real-life expertise to medical issues. As chairman of the Hospitals and Health Care Subcommittee, he has protected veterans' facilities while holding their administrators to a tough line on quality. Rowland also holds a senior seat on the Energy and Commerce Committee and on its Subcommittee on Health and the Environment, so he'll have some crossover effect on reform.

Meanwhile, ranking Republican Christopher Smith of New Jersey came to Congress as a kind of Johnny-One-Note lawmaker, pressing his strong anti-abortion views. Now, 16 years later, Smith is more of a mainstream legislator with an impact on a broad array of issues, including veterans' health care.

Key Staff. Montgomery is served by chief counsel and staff director Mack Fleming, while Stump relies on minority counsel Carl Commentator. Rowland's counsel is Ralph Ibson, and Smith is advised by Christina Alvarado.

The Committee on Armed Services

With 56 members, the committee is one of the largest and most important in the House. On health care matters, however, it has been relatively silent, maintaining the status quo in the military health system. The committee will consider both proposals to integrate the military's medical care system into the new national system and plans to cut spending on CHAMPUS and other programs to fund part of the reform plan.

The Chairman. One of the most liberal members of the House, Ronald Dellums of California became chairman of this conservative committee in 1993 following the appointment of Les Aspin as Secretary of Defense. Dellums is a leading member of the Congressional Black Caucus and an advocate of a single payer health system.

The Ranking Republican. Floyd Spence of South Carolina has quietly served 22 years in the House; as ranking member of Armed Services he tries to keep the size of defense spending cuts small. His involvement in health issues is minimal, but his knowledge of the system was enhanced by his 1988 double-lung transplant surgery.

The Subcommittee on Military Forces and Personnel. With jurisdiction that runs from recruiting to medical care, this panel is likely to shape most of the full committee's thinking on armed services health issues. Its chairman is Ike Skelton of Missouri, a 17-year veteran of the House. A moderate Democrat on most issues, he has concentrated mainly on education benefits for those in military service.

Ranking Republican Jon Kyl of Arizona has taken a strong interest in military medical care over the years. He's been a keen participant in the effort to shift the Civilian Health and Medical Program of the Uniformed Services (CHAMPUS) to a managed care system. He's also widely expected to run for the U.S. Senate in 1994.

Key Staff. Staff director Marilyn Elrod heads a bipartisan group that advises all members of the panel.

The Committee on Post Office and Civil Service

This otherwise obscure committee has control over the Federal Employees Health Benefits Program (FEHBP), which is critical for several reasons. Managed competition advocates and other conservatives tout the program, which insures more than nine million federal employees nationwide, as a model of the competitive system they advocate. Meanwhile, Clinton has praised its accomplishments yet targeted it for extinction.

The Chairman. William Clay of Missouri, a former union activist and civil rights worker, has represented his St. Louis district since 1969. He also is the second ranking Democrat on Education and Labor, so he'll have a voice in several aspects of reform. Clay is a strong supporter of organized labor, including federal workers.

The Ranking Republican. John Myers of Indiana has served in the House since 1967 and is the fourth most senior Republican in the House. He's got a senior position on the key Appropriations Committee and could shift to the ranking slot on that panel if Joseph McDade of Pennsylvania is convicted of corruption charges.

The Subcommittee on Compensation and Employee Benefits. By virtue of its jurisdiction and its chairs, this subcommittee is likely to have a disproportionate impact. Chairwoman Eleanor Holmes Norton of the District of Columbia joined Congress in 1991 and has quickly emerged as a key liberal voice. While the DC Delegate doesn't have full voting rights on the floor (she can vote but if her vote decides an issue a recount can be requested), Norton has full power in committee. Since her district includes the largest number of federal workers in the country, she is a key voice on their benefits.

Norton's counterpart, Constance Morella, lives only a few miles away in suburban Maryland and shares many of the Chairwoman's views on federal workers. Elected to Congress in 1986, Morella is one of the few moderate Republicans left in the House.

The Key Staff Members. Clay depends on staff director Gail Weiss, while Myers relies on minority staff director Joseph Fisher. Norton's staff chief is Cedric Hendricks; Morella's staff director is Curtis Thayer.

The Committee on Small Business

With small business issues central to the health reform debate, this 45-member panel will hold considerable sway. The panel will consider the impact on small business of the proposed employer mandate and other issues.

The Chairman. John LaFalce of New York has been a key voice on small business issues before and after he became committee chairman in 1987. In 1989, for example, he led the effort to repeal a law barring employers from discriminating among employees on health benefits. On reform, however, he's a single payer advocate and generally sympathetic to the notion of an employer mandate.

The Ranking Republican. Jan Meyers of Kansas is a moderate House Republican who has moved quickly up the ranks. She became the senior GOP member of the Small Business Committee in 1992, only seven years after joining the House. She has been a member of a working group on health reform.

Key Staff. LaFalce's staff director is Donald Terry; Meyers gets her counsel from Stephen Lynch.

Other House members who will have an impact on the course of health reform include the following:

Majority Leader Richard Gephardt. Keenly interested in health care issues, Gephardt's views have metamorphosed in his 16 years in the House. When he entered, Gephardt was what was then called a neo-conservative, meaning he differed from the traditional liberal social and economic policies of the Democratic party. Time — and liberals' electoral defeats — drew Gephardt and the party closer together. When the Missouri Democrat ran a respectable race for the Democratic Presidential nomination in 1988, he became a national figure and was easily elected Majority Leader in 1989 when Tom Foley became Speaker of the House. Gephardt will keep the heat on all House committees to keep reform moving. Once it's on the House floor, the Majority Leader will be in charge.

House Speaker Thomas Foley. Since taking power in 1989, Foley has shown little of the hard-edged ruthlessness many believe is needed to get a massive effort like health reform through. Foley prefers to get along with his Republican and conservative Democratic opponents, but Gephardt tends to keep him on target.

Minority Leader Robert Michel. Poised for retirement after the 103rd Congress, Michel represents the best — and worst — of traditional moderate Republicanism. He'd rather cut a deal than cut a colleague down to size, but after more than 37 years in the minority has left this Illinois Republican with little to show for his legislative talents. And, since the mid-1980s, he's been challenged by the ultra-conservative, ultra-combative wing of his party led by Minority Whip Newt Gingrich of Georgia.

Minority Whip Newt Gingrich. One of the keenest minds and sharpest tongues in Congress, Gingrich tends to squander those talents on partisan bombast. Yet he's almost certain to win the Minority Leader slot after Michel retires. He leads a minority committed to making the majority as uncomfortable as possible. On health reform, the Gingrich coalition sees a problem that's been exaggerated being addressed with socialistic solutions. His preference would be to use government tax rules to allow Americans to save money for the health bills. Critics say what Gingrich really wants is the status quo and a defeat for Bill Clinton.

THE SENATE

Only slightly less complex than the House, the Senate has two major committees that must consider health reform and a handful of minor committees that will take a look at part of it. Ultimately, Senate rules that allow unlimited debate and unrestricted amendments make committee jurisdiction less important than in the House. The real action usually takes place on the floor.

The Committee on Labor and Human Resources

This 17-member panel has a long history of involvement in the great social events of the nation. In the 1960s, it was the site of much of the Great Society legislation. Today, it will play a major role in considering health reform. Unlike other committees, Labor and Human Resources does not have a health subcommittee, but Chairman Edward Kennedy's passion for health reform puts the issue at the top of the panel's agenda.

The panel will consider everything from the employer mandate to public health infrastructure. Kennedy is known to stretch his jurisdiction as far as he can, so the panel may get into other issues as well. Its politics are decidedly liberal, and it's likely a plan that could pass Human Resources couldn't win a majority in the Finance Committee. Watch for Kennedy and ranking Republican Nancy Kassebaum to cut some of the key early deals in the lawmaking process.

The Chairman. Edward Kennedy of Massachusetts has often been called "Mr. Health" for his sponsorship of major health legislation and his career-long commitment to improving health care delivery and public health. In the 1960s and 1970s, he was an advocate of a form of national health insurance that would be referred to today as single payer. In fact, when President Jimmy Carter made the last attempt at national reform, Kennedy stymied the bill because it didn't go far enough. In the Reagan years, however, Kennedy grew more pragmatic, adopting the play-or-pay approach to reform that utilizes the current private sector system. Now with another Democrat in the White House, Kennedy appears committed to doing whatever it takes to get a bill through.

The Ranking Republican. Nancy Landon Kassebaum of Kansas took the senior GOP seat in 1993 when Orrin Hatch of Utah gave it up to take a similar post on the Judiciary Committee. Kassebaum is considered a moderate on social issues and may work well with Kennedy. But she will be hemmed in by the requirement that she follow marching orders from the GOP leadership.

Key Players. On the Democratic side, Kennedy often looks to Barbara Mikulski of Maryland and Tom Harkin of Iowa to carry the liberal agenda. Also watch for Harris Wofford of Pennsylvania — the midwife of health reform — and Paul Wellstone of Minnesota — a single payer advocate — to be involved. Republicans Dan Coats of Indiana, Dave Durenberger of Minnesota, and Orrin Hatch of Utah also will be very active.

Key Staff. Kennedy relies heavily on health staff director David Nexon, a veteran of Capitol Hill and a former staffer with the Office of Management and Budget. Staff director Nick Littlefield will also pitch in with political advice and deal with the Senate leadership. Kassebaum depends on her staff director Susan Hattan and on health policy coordinator Andrew Patzman as well as Martin Sieg-Ross and Jane Williams.

The Committee on Finance

On par with the House Ways and Means Committee, the 20-member Finance Committee has the broadest and most significant jurisdiction in the Senate, ranging from tax and trade law to Medicare, Medicaid, Social Security, and welfare programs. A seat here is considered a prize. While Finance has two subcommittees to handle health care issues (Health for Families and the Uninsured and Medicare and Long-Term Care) they only hold hearings; all legislative action is at the full committee level.

The Chairman. New York's Daniel Patrick Moynihan took the helm in 1993 upon the selection of Lloyd Bentsen as Treasury Secretary. One of the brightest and most eccentric members of the Senate, Moynihan traditionally has limited his health policy role to issues affecting New York state. However, with that state's large number of hospitals and burgeoning Medicaid program, those interests have overlapped many of the items on the national reform agenda. Still, Clinton isn't sure how far he can trust Moynihan to carry the reform ball; that's why so much of the President's bill is designed to place primary jurisdiction in Kennedy's committee.

The Ranking Republican. Like Ways and Means' Rostenkowski, Bob Packwood of Oregon spent much of 1993 under a cloud. A Senate investigation into charges of sexual harassment could bump Packwood from power — either directly or indirectly by tying him up for much of the year. On health issues, Packwood is considered somewhat moderate but more than willing to follow orders from Minority Leader Robert Dole of Kansas, who also holds a seat on the Finance Committee. If Packwood should be forced out or aside, William Roth of Delaware would take his place. Either way, Dole would be the real power.

Other Key Players. The presence of Majority Leader George Mitchell of Maine, who formerly chaired Finance's Health Subcommittee, is important. Mitchell wants reform to happen and will keep a close eye on Moynihan. Also very active are Jay Rockefeller of West Virginia, who chaired the Pepper Commission on Comprehensive Health Reform in the late 1980s; Max Baucus of Montana, on rural health issues; David Pryor of Arkansas, on drug pricing; Donald Riegle of Michigan, on Medicaid; and Thomas Daschle of South Dakota and John Breaux of Louisiana, who both favor a purer form of managed competition. Active Republicans include Dole; John Chafee of Rhode Island, whose Republican reform bill has won many supporters; Dave Durenberger of Minnesota; and Hatch of Utah.

Key Staff Members. Moynihan relies on staff director and chief counsel Lawrence O'Donnell for political advice and senior health counsellor Faye Drummond for policy matters. Paul Offner, a former state legislator and Ohio Medicaid director, is a key Democratic staffer on Medicaid. An expert on health issues, minority staff director Edmund Mihalski recently announced he is leaving the committee.

The Committee on Commerce, Science, and Transportation

A 20-member committee that rarely figures in major debates, Commerce will be a player in health reform as it considers changes in insurance rules. It may also work on consumer information standards, new uses of telecommunications in medicine, and how health plans are allowed to market themselves.

The Chairman. South Carolina's Ernest Hollings has served in the Senate for 27 years and has built a strong reputation as an economic conservative (he coauthored the now-infamous Gramm-Rudman-Hollings law requiring automatic spending reductions to balance the budget) and a social moderate. One of the more colorful members of the Senate — he once called Howard Metzenbaum of Ohio "the Senator from B'nai B'rith" — Hollings also is a gifted legislator. He's particularly adept at bottling up legislation he dislikes in his committee.

The Ranking Republican. John Danforth of Missouri is one of the most respected members of the Senate because of his intellect and his moral suasion. An ordained minister and scion of the family that created Ralston Purina, Danforth often has acted as if he did not worry about the political ramifications of his acts, just whether they were right or wrong. In health care, Danforth is known for raising issues like the right to die and the use of living wills. He will retire at the end of 1994.

Key Staff. Hollings' chief counsel and staff director is Kevin Curtin; Danforth relies on Jonathan Chambers, his minority staff director.

The Committee on Judiciary

This 18-member panel has seen more than its share of bad publicity in recent years with its herky-jerky approval process for judicial nominees. Still, the committee is considered a key part of the Senate, and its members are among the brightest legal minds in government. With similar responsibilities as its House counterpart, the Judiciary panel will write the parts of reform dealing with malpractice and antitrust. Clinton may find the Senate panel more open to the former and less so to the latter.

The Chairman. Joseph Biden of Delaware has led the Judiciary Committee since 1987. A member of the Senate since 1973 (elected when he was barely past the statutory minimum age of 30), Biden is considered one of the Senate's best orators, but his leadership skills have not been polished.

The Ranking Republican. Orrin Hatch of Utah started his Senate career in 1977 as one of the most conservative members of the body. His advocacy of smaller government and opposition to most of organized labor's agenda helped cement that reputation. In the 1980s, however, Hatch began to change as he spent six often awkward years as chairman of the Committee on Labor and Human Resources. When he found that fronting Ronald Reagan's health policies gained him nothing but grief and criticism, Hatch began to work with Edward Kennedy of Massachusetts and improved his reputation. In 1993, Hatch switched from the senior GOP slot on Labor and Human Resources to the same spot on Judiciary. He'll have something to say about health reform on both committees as well as from his seat on Finance. On Judiciary, watch for Hatch to push for caps on malpractice awards.

The Subcommittee on Antitrust, Monopolies, and Business Rights. With hospitals and doctors pleading for more liberal antitrust rules that would allow them to share resources, this panel now has a key role in health. But providers haven't found an ally in Chairman Howard Metzenbaum of Ohio. Further emboldened by his impending retirement, Metzenbaum remains an activist Senator with a liberal bent. As Chairman of this key subcommittee, Metzenbaum could prove to be a tall hurdle for antitrust changes sought by the medical and hospital profession. He has declared war on doctors, who he says come to Congress "with blood on their hands" when they ask for antitrust relaxation. His opposition may be one reason that Clinton may seek to make most of his antitrust changes via regulation instead of legislation.

Ranking Republican Strom Thurmond of South Carolina is one of the most colorful throwbacks in Congress. An arch-conservative who started his long career as a Democrat, Thurmond is known mainly for his opposition to everything from civil rights legislation to liberal judicial nominees. Still, his courtliness allows him to maintain good relations with most of his colleagues. Metzenbaum is not one of them.

Key Staff. Biden's chief counsel is Cynthia Hogan, while Hatch relies on Sharon Prost. Metzenbaum seeks counsel from Gene Kimmelman on antitrust matters, while Thurmond's minority general counsel for those issues is Patty Vaughan.

The Committee on Small Business

This 21-member committee is rarely in the spotlight but could have a lot to say about health reform because of the impact of an employer mandate on small firms.

The Chairman. Dale Bumpers of Arkansas is one of the Senate's biggest Clinton boosters. Another former governor of Arkansas, Bumpers is also one of the most respected members of the Senate thanks to his thoughtfulness and good manners. He will probably serve as one of Clinton's lead blockers in the Senate.

The Ranking Republican. Larry Pressler of South Dakota, one of the least impressive members of the Senate, may have hung on to his seat as long as he has (since 1978) because of a lack of decent challengers. Still, he is a strong voice for small business, which makes up a large segment of his state's business community.

Key Staff. Bumpers' chief of staff is John Ball; Pressler depends on Thomas Hohentnaner in a similar role.

The Committee on Veterans' Affairs

This 12-member committee has exerted more influence over broad health policy since it came under the leadership of its new chairman, Jay Rockefeller of West Virginia. The panel will look at the effect of reform on veterans' health care programs and the potential to integrate some of those benefits into the broader alliances.

The Chairman. Jay Rockefeller of West Virginia became one of the Senate's leading voices on health reform after chairing the Bipartisan Commission on Comprehensive Health Reform, known as the Pepper Commission, in the 1980s. Rockefeller brings that same spirit to the Veterans' Affairs Committee, where he has worked to protect VA health programs, particularly those in his small, mostly rural state.

The Ranking Republican. Frank Murkowski of Arkansas is rarely heard in the public discourse over most issues but is a leading voice on veterans' health care. Elected to the Senate in 1980, he soon became chairman of this committee. During his six-year tenure, Murkowski showed surprising skill in warding off proposals to pare benefits. He now works closely with Rockefeller.

Key Staff. Rockefeller's majority chief counsel and staff director is James Gottlieb; Murkowski's staff is headed by John Moseman.

The Committee on Governmental Affairs

This 12-member panel oversees the FEHBP and will mark up parts of the bill that affect that program's nine million participants. The committee also has a hand in new federal agencies or major shifts in departmental organization, so creation of a new National Health Board might also fall under its influence.

The Chairman. John Glenn of Ohio is best known as a former astronaut, but he's a competent legislator as well. As chairman of the Governmental Affairs Committee, Glenn doesn't often get the kind of juicy issues that make headlines, but he is considered a key voice on the Senate floor on a number of issues.

The Ranking Republican. Delaware's William Roth is known best for his advocacy of tax cuts but isn't known for much else. If he somehow winds up replacing Packwood at the top of the Finance Committee Republicans, his seat here would go to Ted Stevens of Alaska, one of the Senate's testiest members.

Key Staff. Glenn's staff director is Leonard Weiss; Roth relies on Franklin Polk.

Other Major Players

In the Senate, where rules allow for unlimited floor debate and consideration of as many amendments as Senators can concoct, the leadership of both parties will have to take charge. Mitchell and Dole can either decide to work together and iron out the major differences between the parties on the bill, or work against one another and stymie the legislation altogether. The odds favor the former. Both men are experienced legislators and, perhaps more importantly, both are steeped in the detail of health care policy and legislation.

Others to watch for include Republican Sen. Phil Gramm of Texas, a sharp-tongued critic of the Clinton plan who is positioning himself for a possible 1996 run for President; Democratic Sen. Robert Kerrey of Nebraska, who has made health reform one of his priority issues; and Jesse Helms, a Republican from North Carolina who is expected to fight the abortion benefit.

Craig Havighurst contributed to this chapter.

CHAPTER 12

The End of the Health Reform Journey

Cathy Tokarski and Janet Firshein

Despite the high priority that President Clinton has attached to reforming the nation's health system and the public's clamoring for change, passage of a comprehensive law that provides health insurance to all Americans and controls costs is fraught with obstacles.

Clinton has all but staked his Presidency on the passage of health reform, but his ability to marshall congressional forces behind him has yet to materialize. The former Arkansas governor, who was elected to office in 1992 without a majority of the American public behind him and without a clear mandate to govern, has been forced to compromise — even backtrack — on major first-year initiatives. But Congress' November 1993 passage of the controversial North American Free Trade Agreement could signal a change in perception about Clinton's ability to lead.

While Clinton has made universal, guaranteed health coverage a non-negotiable principle of health reform, members of his own party — perceived as the group most willing to act — aren't falling into lockstep. Roughly 90 Democrats have signed on to a bill that would create a single payer system, which Clinton clearly opposes. Another group, more philosophically aligned with the President, is pushing a "pure" version of managed competition that Clinton says fails to pass the universal coverage test.

To get a health reform bill passed, Clinton will have to court and win GOP support. Republicans, most of whom recognize the political urgency of health reform, are also staking out their own turf. In the Senate, a group of moderates have crafted a plan that features many of the same elements found in the Clinton bill. But significant differences remain. And the more conservative wing of the Republican Party has introduced less sweeping proposals that could win wider support depending on how well Clinton builds his base of consensus.

An election-sensitive Congress will listen carefully to the American public. Voters will ultimately decide if the benefits of sweeping health reform are worth the price. While the notions of universal access and security resonate among many, the public's desire for sweeping social change could wane as the detailed costs and trade-offs are made clear. If, as many suspect, a general tax increase is needed to pay for the Clinton plan, support for a major overhaul could rapidly disappear.

As voters listen to the health reform pitch of the Clinton Administration, industry lobby groups will turn up the volume on campaigns of their own. Unlike the health industry of the past, the majority of doctors, hospitals, insurers, and drug makers today acknowledge that a major restructuring of the health system is needed and is inevitable. While the Administration and Congress try to craft a health reform law that could drastically affect the future of the health care industry, lobbying groups will continue to pour millions of dollars into efforts to sway public opinion in their direction.

COMPETING STRATEGIES, COMMON GOALS?

For nearly three years, Rhode Island Republican Senator John Chafee and his GOP colleagues have met every Thursday morning to debate health policy dilemmas and solutions. On September 15, 1993, the 23-member Senate Republican Health Care Task Force that Chafee commands unveiled its health reform strategy. The measure, expected to be introduced in legislation in early 1994, is widely regarded as the chief alternative that is likely to serve as the basis for a bipartisan compromise.

The Health Equity and Access Reform Today, which has drawn the support of a diverse range of Republicans, including Senate Minority Leader Robert Dole (R-KS), Sen. Nancy Kassebaum (R-KS), and Sen. Orrin Hatch (R-UT), would provide universal access to insurance for all Americans by the year 2000, two years beyond the Clinton timetable of 1998.

Unlike Clinton, who believes coverage and cost control must go hand-in-hand, the Senate GOP team is pursuing a "pay-as-you-save" strategy that would phase in insurance protection for everyone as savings are accrued.

So committed are the team members to that strategy that the plan would require the Congressional Budget Office (CBO), which tallies the budgetary effect of all legislation, to annually assess whether the changes proposed would yield the necessary savings to allow universal access within the GOP timeframe. If the program is on track, coverage would be phased in according to schedule. But if the anticipated savings fail to emerge, then the phase-in to universal coverage would be delayed until Congress and the White House found alternative financing mechanisms. The GOP argues that the Clinton plan, with its adornment of new and expensive benefits, takes a "buy now, pay later" route.

Moderate Republicans believe that a radical overhaul of the current system is unnecessary; they do agree, however, that comprehensive reform is needed. Like Clinton, their plan would set broad federal guidelines to guide states, including creation of a standard benefit package.

The Chafee group envisions a restructured health delivery system based on the "managed competition" model, in which accountable health plans, including managed care networks, would compete for consumer business. Their plan also would drastically revamp today's troubled health insurance market by abolishing risk selection; provide for administrative streamlining to cut paperwork; attempt to prune outlays for defensive medicine through medical malpractice reform, including a cap on non-economic damages; ease federal antitrust restrictions on hospitals and doctors to encourage efficiency and reduce duplication; and place a greater emphasis on preventive and primary care.

In contrast to Clinton, the GOP strategy shies away from drastic federal intervention and relies more on the market to enforce the structural and behavioral changes required for reform to succeed. Like the supporters of "pure" managed competition, the Chafee cohort also supports a tax on health benefits, and has proposed a limit on tax deductions for benefits beyond a guaranteed standard package. Tax cap supporters say the current system is perverse because an uninsured individual gets no tax break, while a person who has a "Cadillac" health plan enjoys an exemption worth thousands of dollars. Making people pay taxes on benefits beyond a standard package, says Chafee, would make the tax code fairer, sensitize consumers to the cost of health care services, and yield revenue to the federal government that could be used to help expand access.

One of the biggest deviations from the Clinton plan is the Senate GOP's repudiation of a federal mandate on all employers to provide health insurance to their workers. Fearful that a mandate on business would wreak havoc on the economy and trigger a massive loss of jobs, the Chafee plan advocates a mandate on individuals as a way to broaden coverage. Backers have yet to adequately explain, however, how such a policy could be enforced.

The GOP also disavows giving alliances regulatory powers or creating a national health board with the authority to put limits on health insurance premiums. The Chafee proposal would allow, not force, small employers (defined as those with up to 100 employees) and individuals to form an alliance or insurance purchasing network to boost their market leverage.

To help low-income persons buy health insurance, the GOP plan would offer vouchers to uninsured individuals ineligible for Medicaid. These vouchers, to be given to individuals in families with incomes up to 250 percent of the poverty line, would be equal to the value of a health plan and would be phased in over five years, with the poorest receiving assistance first.

Like Clinton, the GOP looks to tap Medicare and Medicaid as the source of funds for this benefit. The plan proposes to squeeze $210 billion from both programs over five years by cutting their annual growth rate to 7 percent by 2000. They also propose to raise funds by forcing wealthier beneficiaries to pay higher Medicare premiums, eliminating disproportionate share payments to hospitals that treat many uninsured, and cutting medical education payments. Medicaid spending would slow by eliminating disproportionate share payments to states and encouraging states to enroll more recipients in managed care.

THE MANAGED COMPETITION PLAN

Only one health reform bill (H.R.3222) has managed to draw a significant number of bipartisan supporters. Reps. Jim Cooper (D-TN) and Fred Grandy (R-IA) on October 6, 1993, introduced the Managed Competition Act of 1993, with 28 Democratic and 22 Republican cosponsors. Two weeks later in the Senate, John Breaux (D-LA) and Dave Durenberger (R-MN), along with Senators Sam Nunn (D-GA) and Joseph Lieberman (D-CT), tossed a similar measure (S.1579) in the legislative hopper.

Cooper, a champion of managed competition, was the first one to hatch the idea in legislative form in 1992. He says his approach is a political middle ground between Clinton's plan and the Senate Republican alternative.

Like the Senate GOP, the Cooper/Grandy managed competition group rejects employer mandates, global budgets, insurance premium caps, and creation of large, highly regulated health purchasing cooperatives. They also support eliminating the open-ended health insurance tax breaks employers now receive.

But unlike both Clinton and the Senate GOP, the managed competition camp does not make universal access a goal or even a key principle. In addition to disavowing an employer mandate, the group rejects a requirement for individuals to buy health insurance. The group wholeheartedly rejects giving states flexibility to design their own programs, mostly because they fear that deferring to governors will lead to creation of single payer systems.

The centerpiece of the managed competition legislation is its call for the establishment of regional health plan purchasing cooperatives (HPCCs) — state-chartered, nonprofit cooperatives within defined geographic territories — that businesses with fewer than 100 employees would have to join. Like the Clinton and GOP plans, HPCCs would give individuals and businesses greater clout in the marketplace and facilitate broader choice of health plans. The Cooper/Grandy bill would give states the option to raise the 100-employee threshold, but states could only shift half their populations into these new entities.

The bill also would provide strong tax incentives to encourage providers and insurance companies to form health plans, including linking businesses' deduction for health insurance premiums to the cost of the lowest-price plan offered in their region. Any additional benefits would be taxed to discourage "inflationary 'Rolls-Royce' health policies," the bill says.

Although the Cooper/Grandy bill rejects the establishment of a National Health Board, it would create a Health Care Standards Commission, whose recommendations would be approved or rejected by Congress. This commission would establish reporting and other consumer standards for health plans.

To widen access to care for low-income persons, the bill would replace the Medicaid program with a new federal program covering individuals and families with incomes of as much as 200 percent of the federal poverty level. Individuals and families with incomes that fall below the poverty line would be given a voucher to join a health plan with "nominal" cost sharing. Those with incomes between 100 percent and 200 percent of poverty would have to pay a portion of the insurance premium. Medicaid spending would be redirected to cover the cost of the new voucher program. To raise the additional $25 billion the congressional budget crunchers say is needed, the bill would raise $16 billion via a cap on tax benefits and $9 billion by reducing Medicare provider payments.

Cooper acknowledges that the bill would cover only 60 percent of the nation's 37 million uninsured. However, he says that about half of the remaining uninsured would be able to enroll on their own once wholesale insurance reforms are in place and coverage becomes more affordable. Reliance on an employer mandate is a "clumsy and expensive way" to expand access, says Cooper.

THE SINGLE PAYER SOLUTION

Introduced on March 3, 1993, by Rep. Jim McDermott (D-WA) and Sen. Paul Wellstone (D-MN), the American Health Security Act (H.R.1200/S.491) would provide health coverage to all U.S. citizens and legal aliens paid for by an as-yet unspecified amount in new income taxes levied on corporations and individuals. A separate, dedicated health security tax, derived as a result of the new tax rates, would fund the system.

The bill, which has approximately 90 cosponsors, would eliminate the private insurance industry and public health insurance programs such as Medicare and Medicaid. Unlike the Clinton bill, the single payer proposal does not rely on an employer mandate to achieve universal coverage. And while it would change how health care is paid for, the bill would not substantially alter today's health care delivery system.

One of the proposal's biggest selling features to consumers is its projected $67 billion that would be wrung from insurers' administrative overhead. The CBO predicted in a 1993 study that a single payer health system combined with global spending limits would cut $319 billion in health care spending between 1995 and 2000. McDermott, one of two physicians in the House, argues that single payer is the fastest route to universal coverage and would eliminate the confusion consumers face in trying to get care in today's system.

Under the bill, the federal government would collect the tax revenue that pays for health services and define the standard benefit package. Instead of the private insurance industry and various federal programs, a new health security trust fund would pay states for administering and delivering health services. Health services would remain in private hands, however. Health costs would be controlled through a federally established health budget.

To gain access to the system, individuals would receive a "health security card," which entitles them to a comprehensive array of inpatient and outpatient benefits; no cost-sharing is required for acute care services. In addition to traditional inpatient and outpatient coverage, the bill would cover preventive services, long term and chronic care services, home- and community-based care, prescription drugs, and substance abuse and mental health services. Health providers must be qualified by states to provide services. Doctors and other health practitioners would be entitled to fee-for-service payments but states would be encouraged to develop alternative payment methods such as global fees for outpatient procedures.

A National Health Security Board would establish and update minimum standards to ensure quality of services and to monitor efforts by states. It would also establish a health budget that would specify the total amount to be spent by the federal government and the states, then allocate those expenditures among states. Growth in per capita health spending will be linked to the increase in Gross Domestic Product. States would have to fund covered services from their coffers if they exceed their annual budget.

The bill also would fund increased primary care services in underserved urban and rural areas, prohibit state administrative expenses from exceeding 3 percent, and encourage electronic billing of medical claims.

THE LESS-IS-MORE APPROACH

For philosophical and political reasons, some Senate and House Republican conservatives are backing a far more limited approach to health reform. While support for their proposals isn't broad, especially in the Senate, the conservative lawmakers could win additional votes if Congress and the American public decide that the cost of comprehensive health reform far outweighs the benefits.

A proposal backed by 10 GOP Senators, including Phil Gramm (TX), John McCain (AZ), and Jesse Helms (NC), attempts to modify some of the economic distortions of the health care market and create new incentives for consumers to purchase insurance. The proposal features tax credits for the poor, limits on experience-rated health insurance premiums, and Medisave accounts.

It would provide $64.3 billion in tax credits over five years to people with incomes below 200 percent of the federal poverty line. Tax credits would enable poor Americans to purchase a catastrophic health plan with a $3,000 deductible and a package of preventive care benefits. People with preexisting medical conditions could not be denied coverage, but insurers could continue to use experience rating to price their health premiums. However, the federal government would purchase a catastrophic plan for individuals whose experience-rated premiums were more than 150 percent of the average premium in their area. That provision is expected to cost $21 billion over five years, Gramm estimates.

In addition to experience rating, insurers could charge different premiums based on health habits. "Individuals with moderate income who receive federal assistance will be required to pay more if they are overweight, smoke, drink excessively, or engage in other activities that are harmful to their health," the plan says.

A final cost, estimated at $64.3 billion, would be incurred by allowing self-employed individuals to claim the full cost of their health insurance as a tax deduction. The total five-year cost of the bill: $144.2 billion. Backers say this would be paid for by capping the federal share of Medicaid ($112.6 billion) and slowing the rate of Medicare's growth ($61.5 billion). Other elements of the proposal include paperwork simplification, malpractice reform, and an end to unspecified "impediments" to building small group purchasing pools.

In the House, 120 of the 176 Republicans have signed on to a bill called the Affordable Health Care Now Act of 1993. Its underlying philosophy: Pass those measures, such as insurance market and malpractice reform, around which broad consensus exists, and see what effect those changes bring.

The bill (H.R.3080) requires that employers offer but not pay for insurance for their employees. The bill attempts to make consumers more cost-conscious by allowing them to make tax-free deposits into Medisave accounts of up to $2,500 for individuals or $5,000 for families. Those choosing the Medisave route would be required to purchase a catastrophic health plan with a deductible of at least $1,800 for individuals or $3,600 for families. Interest accrued in the accounts would accumulate annually, but amounts withdrawn for non-medical purposes would be subject to a tax and a 20 percent penalty.

The House Republican plan would reform the insurance market by prohibiting preexisting condition exclusions. Insurers would be required to offer at least a standard plan and a catastrophic plan to all companies with two to 50 employees. Small businesses would be encouraged to pool their insurance purchases.

To help the poor, states would be allowed to set up Medicaid buy-in programs for people with incomes of up to 200 percent of the federal poverty line, and could enroll all Medicaid recipients in managed care plans without first obtaining a federal waiver. The bill would reform medical malpractice by requiring alternative dispute resolution systems and capping non-economic damages. It also would streamline paperwork, encourage electronic billing, and clarify antitrust provisions. The $4.7 billion, five-year cost would be covered by imposing a 10 percent co-insurance requirement for Medicare clinical lab services.

AREAS OF COMPROMISE

Despite the striking differences in the major proposals, several areas of compromise already exist. All plans favor reform of the insurance market to make coverage more affordable — especially to small businesses — and to prevent insurers from selecting only the healthiest individuals. Consensus also exists around proposals to guarantee insurance availability and renewability to enable individuals to switch jobs and retain insurance coverage.

Another area of common ground: administrative simplification. Every bill features a call for reduced paperwork and a common medical claims form to be submitted electronically. Eliminating the 1,500 claims forms now in use could yield anywhere from $7 billion to $30 billion in savings and would cut red tape that constrains providers and consumers.

Many areas of the country, notably California and Minnesota, have embraced managed care as the favored form of health care financing and delivery. But if the federal government, through health reform, puts the official "seal of approval" on managed care systems other states where HMOs and preferred provider organizations (PPOs) have been slower to take off would be sure to follow.

Virtually everyone agrees that the U.S. needs to emphasize primary and preventive health care and to train more health professionals to deliver this type of care. Currently, about 30 percent of all U.S. physicians practice primary or family medicine, compared to about 70 percent in other Western countries. While no dispute exists over the need to increase the supply of primary care practitioners, there is disagreement over how that goal should be reached.

A similar phenomenon exists over boosting health care services in underserved inner city and rural areas. Nearly every major health reform plan acknowledges that these gaps must be filled, but consensus diverges over how aggressive of a role the federal government should play.

AREAS OF DIFFERENCES

With a handful of issues ready for compromise, Clinton and the Congress must then go on to confront a much larger array of tougher, politically contentious questions that could make or break the success of comprehensive health reform.

Probably the most emotionally charged debate will revolve over whether an employer mandate is required to achieve universal coverage. While most Democrats believe that all Americans are entitled to health insurance, Republicans argue that the goal should be making insurance more affordable, thus widening access to coverage.

Clinton, however, says an employer mandate is the "fairest way" to ensure coverage for all Americans because it builds on the current employer-based system of health coverage and would not require a massive tax increase. But small business groups, chiefly the National Federation of Independent Business (NFIB) and National Small Business United (NSBU), will continue to argue that this approach will cost service-sector jobs, depress wages, and threaten U.S. competitiveness.

While Republicans remain opposed to an employer mandate, there have been signs in the past year that their opposition is beginning to thaw. In 1992, the U.S. Chamber of Commerce, which represents mostly small businesses, took a historic step in endorsing an employer mandate for the first time. The Association of Private Pension and Welfare Plans, which represents large and small businesses, also changed its stance in 1992 after long being opposed to a mandate. And medical and insurance groups, which have nothing to lose by backing the idea, have gone on the record endorsing expanded employer involvement.

To counter the predicted negative effects of an employer mandate, Republicans are advocating a mandate on individuals to purchase health insurance. This approach has not been rejected out of hand by Clinton, but he has said that it would be difficult to enforce, hard to administer, and would fail to achieve his goal of universal coverage. While the GOP appears committed to its individual mandate philosophy, members privately admit there is room for compromise if independent studies confirm that employment won't be adversely affected by an employer mandate.

Schisms within the small business community could hasten a change in heart among Republicans. While NFIB remains steadfast in its opposition, some of its 600,000 members concede that an employer mandate seems to be the only route for comprehensive reform and more affordable insurance coverage. Clinton's promise of a subsidy generous enough to help financially pressed firms pay for health premiums could win over those employers not philosophically opposed to a new government requirement. If Clinton can't win on the mandate issue, however, his goal of universal access becomes impossible without broad-based taxes.

The size and power of the regional health alliances or insurance purchasing cooperatives will be another political minefield. Clinton's plan would force employers with up to 5,000 workers to join alliances, thereby diminishing the cost-cutting success many large employers have seen in recent years. Although Clinton says he isn't wedded to the 5,000-employee cut-off, he argues that enrollment in alliances must be mandatory and they need to be large enough to prevent competition based on health risks.

That theory is not universally held. Republicans argue that the problem of insurance affordability resides within small businesses, not large ones. To solve this problem, they would encourage small employers to band together to enhance their ability to buy insurance at more affordable prices. By giving small businesses the chance to buy insurance at competitive rates, insurers would lower their prices, Republicans believe. Moderate Democrats, like Cooper, think small employers need assistance to pool their buying power but prefer a less sweeping mandate to achieve this goal.

Although business groups have been strong supporters of the Clinton health effort, they are universally opposed to the size of the health alliance proposed in his plan. That opposition will force Clinton to compromise. An outcry from Capitol Hill has led Clinton to weaken the powers of the alliances, shifting most of them to the states. Under Clinton's bill, alliances could only reject health plans with premiums that exceed 20 percent of the average in an area but they could not limit the number of fee-for-service plans.

It is doubtful, however, that the much smaller insurance pools proposed by Cooper and Grandy and the voluntary approach taken by the Senate GOP meet Clinton's criteria, thus setting the stage for a major skirmish.

While most provider lobbies support the direction of the Clinton bill, they remain adamantly opposed to his call for a cap on insurance premiums. They argue that cost controls, if set too rigidly, would distort the market and stymie innovation, not to mention put them at financial risk. Clinton officials say premium caps are the "linchpin" to cost control and that a national budget would serve as a "backstop" only if the premium caps are breached.

Republicans stand behind providers and insurers in their opposition to premium caps. Neither the Senate GOP or the Cooper/Grandy measures call for them, preferring instead to put their faith in a restructured market to eventually bring down the rate of increase in costs.

The single payer approach calls for a national health budget administered by states. States that breach their budget would have to find additional revenue to make up the difference. Single payer proponents were disappointed by Clinton's decision in early 1993 not to impose cost controls on the insurance and drug industries, an omission McDermott predicted would send premiums "through the roof."

Most conservative members also balk at the National Health Board's power to control insurance premiums through state alliances. Although the Clinton bill would make the seven-member Board accountable to the President, the presence of a powerful entity that controls the nation's health expenditures goes against the core beliefs of most Republicans. This is another area where Clinton will be forced to compromise, possibly by transferring the board's power over the health budget and other elements of the plan to the relevant agencies, such as the Departments of Health and Human Services, Treasury, and Labor.

SINGLE ISSUE BATTLES

While a very small element of the Clinton bill, a provision that calls for coverage of "pregnancy-related services" has touched off a firestorm of opposition among conservatives and moderate Democrats on Capitol Hill. More than 200 House members have vowed to vote against the Clinton bill if it retains abortion services as a covered benefit. Clinton argues that the benefit mirrors the trend among private insurers to cover abortion as a "pregnancy-related service." Nonetheless, some 20 years after the passage of *Roe v Wade*, which legalized a woman's right to an abortion, Congress and the American public remain deeply divided on the use of public monies to fund this service.

Pro-choice lawmakers, especially members of the Congressional Women's Caucus, will press to keep an abortion benefit in the final bill. On the other side of the political spectrum, House Republicans have suggested that abortion services be offered as a supplemental benefit paid for by individuals who choose this coverage. While this chapter in the ongoing abortion debate promises to be no less acrimonious than those that have preceded it, insiders say Clinton will not sacrifice health reform over a federally guaranteed abortion benefit.

Clinton's promises of a new prescription drug benefit, expanded home- and community-based care, and an early retiree health premium bail-out for big business has drawn fire even from reform advocates. On Capitol Hill, critics say that the addition of costly new benefits contradict Clinton's stated goal of lowering health care costs. But Clinton has little room to maneuver.

The powerful, 34 million-member American Association of Retired Persons has warned the President that the absence of a prescription drug benefit could cost that group's critical support. Faced with the fiscal reality of providing a costly long term care program, Clinton was forced to delay the home- and community-based benefit two years beyond what he had initially promised. He also has weakened provisions designed to help seniors protect their assets counted toward Medicaid eligibility for nursing home care.

The $12 billion proposal that promises to have the government pay 80 percent of health benefit costs for early retirees was also delayed by two years beyond its original projected schedule. Still, the large manufacturing companies that employ an aging work force can be counted on to fight to retain this provision. Should the Administration decide to drop this benefit when it begins negotiations with Congress, both business and elderly lobbies could have more to complain about.

Giving states the freedom to design their own health systems is a core belief for Clinton, himself a former governor. Governors have been major players in shaping the direction and content of the Clinton health reform plan. But now that the debate has shifted to Congress, state leaders will face resistance from some lawmakers opposed to increasing governors' powers over such things as using Medicare funds, drawing the boundaries of alliances, and setting up single payer systems.

While the Republicans generally favor letting states decide these matters, some Democrats do not, notably House Ways and Means Health Subcommittee Chairman Fortney "Pete" Stark (D-CA) and House Energy and Commerce Health Subcommittee Chairman Henry Waxman (D-CA). Managed competition leader Cooper also will resist overtures to let states chart a single payer path.

But Clinton is walking a fine line. To appease the large bloc of single payer advocates, he has made significant adjustments in his final bill, including mandatory participation in the regional health alliances. He also has added provisions to the final bill that would make it easier for states to implement single payer plans. For example, states that choose such an option would automatically be granted a waiver from the 1974 Employee Retirement Income Security Act. States' ability to enroll Medicare beneficiaries in single payer systems would be enhanced as long as benefits to this population remain the same or are improved.

THE MOVING FINANCING TARGET

Previous experience in forecasting the cost of government-sponsored health benefits has left lawmakers skeptical about the credibility of Clinton's financing projections. Just one week after the bill's October 27 introduction to Congress, Clinton and his aides were at work revising the financing estimates they used to develop the bill and clarifying what their reform proposal would cost the average American.

The only broad-based tax Clinton has proposed is one on tobacco products estimated to raise $65.3 billion. Support for a tobacco tax is generally high except among Southern lawmakers from tobacco-growing states. And public approval of a tobacco tax — seen as a way to deter smoking, particularly among the young — has grown significantly in recent years.

Clinton's proposal to wring $189.7 billion from Medicare and Medicaid will not survive. While other health reform bills propose cuts of similar magnitude, providers, states, and advocates for the poor claim such reductions will impair quality and limit access. Some policy observers believe Clinton's proposed Medicare and Medicaid reductions was done on purpose to force Congress, not the President, to suggest broad-based taxes to finance comprehensive health reform. But an election-sensitive Congress will resist taking that route. Consequently, both Clinton and Congress could be forced to scale back benefits or extend the plan's timetable for coverage.

The Administration's ability to build and retain support among small businesses hinges heavily on the integrity of the financing assumptions underlying federal subsidies for low-wage workers. The Administration estimates that it would cost the federal government $161.1 billion to help low-wage or unprofitable firms comply with its plan. HHS official Kenneth Thorpe, one of the Administration's chief budget estimators, says a generous financial cushion has been added to keep the subsidy from falling short.

But critics, including liberal Democrats, are attacking the proposal because the Administration is proposing to limit the federal government's contribution, and thereby, its financial exposure. While the move has generated enthusiasm among opponents of "open-ended" entitlements, congressional skeptics question who would be financially responsible to provide the guaranteed health coverage Clinton has promised if this limit is breached.

READING THE PUBLIC'S MIND

The economically, socially, and politically diverse American public is the most important group that Clinton and Congress must court. That challenge is daunting, as recent public opinion polls suggest. An October 1993 survey of 1,000 individuals conducted by the Henry J. Kaiser Family Foundation and Harvard University School of Public Health spotlighted the limited interest Americans have in major health system reform. Their keenest interest was reserved for reform's effect on their pocketbook. More than three-quarters (79 percent) wanted to learn more about how the Clinton plan would affect their out-of-pocket costs. A similar proportion (77 percent) were concerned about the plan's effect on the cost of health insurance premiums, and 73 percent said they wanted to know if the plan would require them to pay new taxes.

But questions about what impact health reform would have on the federal budget deficit or national health spending elicited less interest. Slightly more than half (56 percent) said they wanted to learn more about reform's effect on the federal budget, and only half (50 percent) said they cared about the impact on national health care spending.

More significantly, the key elements of most major reform plans were poorly understood by most Americans. While 59 percent of the respondents said they know what an HMO is, less than one-third (31 percent) claimed to know what managed care is and only 20 percent said they knew what managed competition means. Just one-quarter (25 percent) of the respondents said they know what single payer health care means.

"The public is still poorly informed and uninvolved," said Kaiser President Drew Altman. "Unless that changes, the spin controllers and special interests will dominate the debate."

EYES ON THE PRIZE

Unlike in decades past, all the right ingredients — presidential leadership, congressional activism, and public awareness — have combined to make comprehensive health reform a reality in 1994. The problems of unbridled cost increases and millions of uninsured and underinsured have only intensified. But this time, the missing factor — the willingness to compromise — may be within the nation's reach.

Still, it is easy to underestimate the sheer magnitude of undertaking comprehensive health care reform at a time when the American public holds the federal government — both Congress and the President — in low esteem and doubts its ability to administer high-quality public programs. At a time when the federal budget deficit stands at about $300 billion, Clinton will have a hard time convincing Americans that he can expand health coverage and control costs without further straining the federal budget. And Americans' resistance to new government programs, especially those perceived to favor the poor and unemployed, is an additional obstacle Clinton must overcome.

Orchestrating the drive to a final bill with a Democratic-controlled Congress that has yet to prove strong loyalty to the President could be one of Clinton's biggest hurdles. Upon unveiling his bill before Congress in October, Clinton proudly claimed "no pride of authorship," a nod to bipartisanship that may come to haunt him in 1994. Elected to office with just 43 percent of the popular vote, Clinton does not enjoy a mandate for action among the American public or among reform-minded members of Congress, many of whom have gone to pursue their own policy course. By November 1994, Congress will face re-election having promised to address health care's access and cost problems, but not necessarily under the Clinton Administration banner.

Failing to level with the American public about the potential benefits and trade-offs of health reform could incite a revolt reminiscent of the 1989 repeal of the Medicare Catastrophic Coverage Act. Congress had barely finished patting itself on the back for the expansion of benefits before a backlash among the elderly forced an unprecedented revocation just one year later. In 1993, voters are still clamoring for universal access and security, but their support for major social change could wane as the detailed costs and sacrifices are understood.

For both Clinton and the 103rd Congress, the political stakes are high. If Congress fails to act on promises it made in 1992, the public's retribution will be swift, and support for Clinton could erode beyond repair. Whether that scenario necessarily will play out depends greatly on Clinton's ability to persuade the Congress and the public to put aside their partisan differences and let him lead them into the brave new world of health reform.

APPENDIX

H.R.3600, S.1757 Health Security Act

Introduced Nov. 20, 1993, by Rep. Richard Gephardt (D-MO) and Sen. George Mitchell (D-ME)

Summarized by Roy Bredder

TITLE I — HEALTH CARE SECURITY

Title I of the bill would establish the basic health program sponsored by the Clinton Administration. It authorizes universal coverage, addresses coverage of families, specifies required benefits, establishes and defines the role of the National Health Board, specifies state responsibilities, defines the role of regional and corporate alliances, sets requirements for health plans, and establishes the responsibilities of the HHS Department, the Labor Department, and employers.

□ **Universal Coverage:** Eligible individuals would include all citizens or nationals of the U.S. under color of law, and long term nonimmigrants. Each eligible individual would be entitled to the program's comprehensive benefit package through the applicable health plan with which the individual is enrolled. Eligible individuals would have to enroll in an applicable health plan and pay required premiums. An individual could not disenroll from a plan until the individual is enrolled in another appropriate plan or becomes eligible for Medicare.

Nothing in the bill is to be construed as prohibiting: an individual from purchasing any health care services; an individual from purchasing supplemental insurance, consistent with the provisions of the bill, to cover health care services not included within the comprehensive benefit package; an individual who is not an eligible individual from purchasing health insurance, other than through a regional alliance; and employers from providing coverage for benefits in addition to the comprehensive benefit package.

The applicable health plan for a family would be the regional alliance health plan for the alliance area in which the family resides. For family members who are eligible to enroll in a corporate alliance health plan, the applicable health plan would be the corporate alliance health plan.

All members of the same family would be enrolled in the same applicable health plan. There would be coverage categories for individuals only, married couples without children, single individuals with children, and married couples with children. The bill includes a series of special enrollment rules for various categories of individuals and families, such as disabled, supplementary security income recipients, veterans who elect coverage under a health plan of the Veterans Department, active duty military personnel, and others.

Universal coverage for residents of states with single payer systems would be provided in accordance with the state plan.

□ **Benefits:** The comprehensive benefit package to be provided under the plan would consist of hospital services, services of health professionals, emergency and ambulatory medical and surgical services, clinical preventive services, mental health and substance abuse services, family planning services and services for pregnant women, hospice care, home health care, extended care services, ambulance services, outpatient laboratory, radiology, and diagnostic services, outpatient prescription drugs, outpatient rehabilitation services, durable medical equipment and prosthetic and orthotic devices, vision care, dental care, health educational classes, and investigational treatments. Detailed descriptions of each of these benefits are provided.

□ **Cost Sharing:** Each health plan would offer either lower cost sharing, higher cost sharing, or combination cost sharing. A plan with lower cost sharing could impose no deductible, would have an annual out-of-pocket limit on cost sharing of $1,500 for individuals and $3,000 for families, would require coinsurance of out-of-network services but otherwise would prohibit coinsurance, and would impose the copayments required for specified services under the bill. Out-of-network coinsurance amounts would be set by the National Board but could not be less than 20 percent.

Under a higher cost-sharing plan there would be an annual general deductible of $200 for individuals and $400 for families. Specific deductibles also would apply with regard to inpatient and residential mental health and substance abuse treatment, outpatient prescription drugs and biologicals, and dental care. No deductibles could be imposed for clinical preventive services, for prenatal care and one post-partum visit, or for prevention and diagnosis of dental disease. Higher cost-sharing plans would create a $1,500 out-of-pocket cost-sharing limit for individuals and a $3,000 limit for families. No copayments could be required. Coinsurance as specified for benefits under the bill would be imposed.

A combination cost-sharing plan would establish annual individual and family out-of-pocket limits of $1,500 and $3,000 respectively. Such plans otherwise would require different cost sharing for in-network items and services than for out-of-network items and services.

The bill contains a table of the copayments and coinsurance that would be imposed with regard to the various covered services. Individual payment amounts would be increased annually, generally in accordance with the increase in general health care inflation.

The National Board would assure uniformity in the application of the comprehensive benefit packages, could accelerate coverage of items and services that otherwise would not be covered until 2001, would specify and define specific items and services as clinical preventive services for high-risk individuals, would update periodicity schedules, and could promulgate regulations to assure that coverage is not provided for services unless they are medically necessary.

No state could restrict the practice of any class of health professionals beyond what is justified by the skills and training of the professionals. A health professional or health care facility could not be required to provide an item or service in the comprehensive benefit package if the professional or facility objects to doing so on the basis of a religious belief or moral conviction.

□ **State Responsibilities:** A state would be a participating state, for purposes of approval of the state's health care system, if the state meets several requirements. The state would have to submit a description of its plan to the National Board.

States would have to establish one or more regional alliances, certify health plans, assure the financial solvency of health plans, designate an agency or individual charged with coordinating state responsibilities, conform state laws to comply with later provisions of the bill relating to medical benefits under workers compensation laws, and carry out other responsibilities.

Specifics for each of these state responsibilities also are included in the bill. Alliances would be established in alliance areas. Each such area would have to encompass a population large enough to ensure that the alliance has adequate market share to negotiate effectively with health plans providing benefits in the area.

States would assure that amounts owed to alliances are collected and paid. States would assist in assuring that eligibility determinations are made on the basis of the best available information.

States would publish criteria for certification of plans. The criteria would relate to the quality of the plan, the plan's financial stability, the plan's capacity to deliver the comprehensive benefits, and to other characteristics of each plan.

States would assure that each eligible family has adequate access to enroll in a choice of regional alliance health plans, including adequate access to a plan whose premium is at or below the weighted average premium for plans in the regional alliance. States could require, as a condition of entering into a contract with an alliance, that one or more certified plans provide access to services of centers of excellence.

States could provide for adjustments to the risk-adjustment methodology and other financial incentives to regional alliance health plans to ensure that the plans enroll individuals who are members of disadvantaged groups. States also could provide extra services, such as outreach to encourage enrollment and transportation and interpreting services to ensure access to care, for certain population groups that face barriers to access because of geographic location, income levels, or racial or cultural differences.

Each state would establish a guaranty fund to provide financial protection to health care providers and others in case of failure of a regional alliance health plan. The health plans would pay up to 2 percent of premiums to finance this fund. States would have to assure that, in the event of the failure of a health plan, eligible individuals enrolled in the plan will receive continuity of coverage.

□ **State Single Payer Systems:** The National Board would approve the application of a state to operate a single-payer system if the Board finds that the system complies with the requirements of the bill. Such systems would have to be established under state law and be operated by the state. There would have to be mandatory enrollment in a health plan of all eligible individuals in each regional alliance area. States would have the option of enrolling Medicare eligible individuals and individuals who otherwise would enroll in a corporate alliance health plan.

The state would make direct payments to providers for services provided under the plan. Such payments could be on a capitated, at-risk basis based on prospectively determined rates. The system would have to provide the comprehensive benefit package required by the bill. Cost-sharing requirements of the bill could be reduced for any class of enrolled individuals or for any class of services, so long as cost sharing does not increase for other individuals or services.

Cost containment provisions would have to assure that per capita expenditures for covered benefits do not exceed the amount equivalent to the regional alliance per capita target premium as determined later in the bill. Other cost containment requirements would apply. Other requirements applicable to health plans generally under the program would apply to single-payer programs.

States would operate single-payer systems through use of a single, statewide alliance. Financing, at least in part, would have to include a payroll-based financing system that requires employers to pay at least the amount the employers would be required to pay if they were subject to the premium requirements set out later in the bill.

□ **Regional Alliances:** Regional alliances would be governed by Boards of Directors representing employers of employees who purchase coverage through the alliance and representing the employees who make such purchases. Health care providers, employees of, or persons with substantial ownership in or who receive substantial income from, health care providers, health plans, pharmaceutical companies, and medical equipment suppliers and similar health-related employers; persons who derive substantial income from the provision of health care; and individuals who are employees of or members of associations, law firms, or other entities that represent the interests of one or more health care providers, plans, or others involved in the health care field could not serve on the alliance board. Each alliance board would have a provider advisory board.

Corporate alliances would be those sponsored by large employers. Sponsors of multi-employer plans and rural electric cooperative and rural telephone cooperative associations could qualify as corporate alliances. Large employers are defined as those with more than 5,000 full-time employees. Employers whose primary business is employee leasing, the federal government, and state or local governments would be excluded from qualifying. Full-time employees of a large employer who sponsors a corporate alliance could enroll in a health plan offered by the alliance. The employer could exempt such employees who work in an establishment of the employer with fewer than 100 full-time employees.

All participants and beneficiaries of a multi-employer plan would be eligible to enroll in a health plan offered by the alliance. Full-time employees of rural cooperatives could enroll in corporate alliances established by the cooperatives. Certain welfare recipients, temporary or seasonal employees, and others would not be eligible to enroll in a corporate alliance.

Procedures for electing to establish a corporate alliance and for terminating the alliance for insufficient numbers of employees or for failure to meet the bill's requirements are set out.

□ **Alliance Responsibilities:** Regional alliances would negotiate a contract with any state-certified health plan for the enrollment of eligible individuals in the alliance area. Alliances also could enter into such contracts with any plan of the Veterans Affairs Department or with a Uniformed Health Services Plan of the Defense Department. An alliance would not have to enter into a contract with a plan if the proposed premium exceeds 120 percent of the weighted-average premium within the alliance or if the plan has failed to comply with requirements under prior contracts with the alliance.

Alliances would have to offer eligible enrollees a choice of health plans, including at least one fee-for-service plan. Each alliance would establish a fee schedule, negotiated with providers, applicable to such plans. As an alternative, states could establish fee schedules that would apply on a statewide basis. There is a specific provision, designed to circumvent antitrust laws, indicating that negotiation of fee schedules is considered to be permissible state action. Providers could not threaten or engage in any boycott. The fee schedules could be based on prospective budgeting.

□ **Enrollment:** Each alliance would assure that each eligible individual is enrolled in an alliance health plan. Each alliance would establish and maintain methods and procedures to assure such enrollment at the time each individual first becomes eligible, at the time an individual moves into an alliance area, and at the time of reach the age of individual eligibility. There would have to be procedures for point-of-service enrollment of individuals seeking service who are not enrolled.

Providers would have to notify the appropriate alliance in cases when an individual seeks services but does not present evidence of enrollment under an applicable health plan. The provider could seek payment for services form the alliance. The alliance would determine if the individual is eligible and enrolled. If the individual is eligible and enrolled, the alliance would notify the appropriate plan and forward the claim for payment. If the individual is not enrolled but is required to be enrolled, the alliance would record the individual's enrollment under a specific plan and forward the claim to the plan. Otherwise the point of service rules would apply.

If an individual is enrolled under a plan of another alliance or of a corporate alliance, the alliance involved would forward the claim to the other alliance and so notify the provider. If the individual is eligible to enroll under a plan of another alliance but has not done so, the alliance involved would forward the claim to that other alliance and would so notify the provider.

For point-of-service enrollment, an alliance would have to provide materials describing the health plans in the alliance within 10 days of being notified that an unenrolled individual has received services. The individual would have 30 days to enroll. If the individual fails to enroll, the alliance would enroll the individual in a health plan selected by the alliance on a random basis. Using the fee-for-service schedule by the alliance, the selected plan would reimburse the provider for the services that were provided.

The bill contains other, very specific, rules for enrollment of individuals. Examples include a provision allowing individuals who will reside in an area other than their assigned alliance area for a period of between three and six months to continue coverage under their existing health plan, in which case coverage in the temporary area would be limited to emergency services and urgent care; register with the alliance in the new area; or change enrollment in the previous alliance area to enrollment in a health plan that provides coverage on a fee-for-service basis.

Each regional alliance would hold annual open enrollment periods during which eligible individuals could choose among available health plans. Individuals could disenroll from a plan for cause at any time. Each alliance would establish enrollment priorities in the case of health plans that do not have sufficient capacity to enroll all eligible individuals seeking enrollment.

□ **Other Alliance Duties:** Each alliance would be responsible for issuing health security cards to eligible individuals. Information relating to costs of each health plan, characteristics and availability of health care professionals and institutions participating in each plan, restrictions on access, and a summary of the annual quality performance report would have to be provided by alliances to consumers. Marketing materials for health plans would have to be approved by the appropriate alliance. Each alliance would establish and maintain an office of an ombudsman to assist consumers.

Each alliance would carry out data collection activities, could not discriminate against health plans, and would coordinate enrollment activities with other alliances. Alliances could adjust payments to health plans or use other financial incentives to encourage plans to expand into areas that have inadequate health services. Alliances could take a variety of actions to assist in the development of new health plans in areas with inadequate health services. Alliances could not bear any insurance risk. The bill would require the National Board to promulgate standards to assure that employees and others with a specified relationship with a regional alliance do not engage in self dealing or other conflicts of interest.

□ **Negotiation and Acceptance of Bids:** Each regional alliance would provide information necessary to enable a health plan to submit to a premium bid. Such information would include demographic and other characteristics of the area, the uniform per capita conversion factor, the premium class factors, the regional alliance inflation factor, the risk-adjustment factors and reinsurance methodology and payment amounts to be used by the alliance in computing blended plan per capita rates, the alliance administrative allowance, and other similar information.

Alliances would calculate various components of the family share premium and components of the general employer premium. The amount to be paid with respect to each family would take into account the general family share, any income-related discount, and whether or not the family is a supplemental security income (SSI) family or is receiving aid to families with dependent children (AFDC).

Each alliance would be responsible for collecting all amounts owed the alliance. For employed individuals, the family share would be collected through employer withholding. For others, payment would have to be made prospectively.

□ **Payments to Health Plans:** Each alliance would compute a blended plan per capita payment amount for each health plan in the alliance. Each alliance would pay to each health plan, for each individual enrolled in the health plan, an amount equal to the net blended rate adjusted to take into account the relative actuarial risk associated with the coverage with respect to the individual.

The net blended rate is the blended plan per capita payment amount, as determined under later provisions of the bill, reduced by a consolidated set aside percentage and by any plan payment reduction imposed for the plan year. The consolidated set aside percentage would equal the administrative allowance percentage for the alliance plus 1.5 percentage points. The alliance administrative percentage could not exceed 2.5 percent. Alliances would pay the federal government an amount equal to the reduction in payments to health plans resulting from the consolidated set aside percentage. These payments would be used for academic health centers and graduate medical education.

There are extensive financial management requirements that would be imposed on alliances.

□ **Cost-Sharing Reduction:** Families enrolled in the AFDC or SSI programs, and families with incomes below 150 percent of the federal poverty line, would be eligible for cost-sharing reductions. No reductions would be permitted if it is determined that there are sufficient low-cost plans that are lower cost-sharing or combination cost-sharing plans to enroll the families that would qualify for reduced cost-sharing. The reduction in cost sharing that would be provided would be the amount necessary to reduce cost sharing to the level of a lower or combination cost-sharing plan. Additional reductions would be available to AFDC and SSI families. The alliance would pay the respective health plans for the cost-sharing reduction. Application and verification procedures for eligible families are included in the bill. Premium discounts also would be provided.

□ **Corporate Alliances:** Corporate alliances could offer enrollment in an appropriate self-insured plan or could negotiate with a state-certified plan to enter into a contract with the plan for the enrollment of eligible individuals. Corporate alliances would have to offer a choice or at least three health plans. There would have to be at least one fee-for-service plan and at least two plans that are not fee-for-service. Other enrollment related provisions for corporate alliances are basically the same as those that apply to regional alliances.

Premiums for corporate alliance plans would be community rated. They could vary only by class of family enrollment and by premium area. Premium areas would be designated by each corporate alliance. They would reasonably reflect the labor market areas or health care delivery areas served by the alliance.

Corporate alliances would make additional contributions towards the enrollment of certain low-income families. Many of the consumer information and related requirements applicable to regional alliances would be imposed on corporate alliances as well. Sponsors of large employer alliances would provided for the funding of benefits, the applicable solvency requirements, and compliance with any rules established by the Labor Secretary. For other corporate alliances, the employer would make payment of employer premiums under rules established by the alliance and consistent with rules of the Labor Secretary. Various ERISA requirements would apply to corporate alliances.

The Labor Secretary would serve as Trustee of any corporate alliance health plan that becomes insolvent. A corporate alliance health plan insolvency fund would be created. The fund would be financed from several sources, including assessments on self-insured corporate alliance health plans.

□ **Health Plans:** Self-insured plans and state-certified plans would have to provide the comprehensive benefit package specified in the bill. The plans would have to accept every eligible individual who seeks enrollment, up to the limits of the plan's capacity.

Health plans could not terminate, restrict, or limit coverage in any portion of the plan's service area for any reason, including nonpayment of premiums. Plans could not cancel coverage for any alliance-eligible individual until the individual is covered by another applicable health plan.

Plans could not exclude coverage of an eligible individual because of existing medical conditions, could not impose a waiting period before coverage begins, and could not impose a rider that serves to exclude coverage of particular eligible individuals. Plans could not engage in any form of discrimination.

Plans offering the lower cost-sharing schedule would have to apply the schedule to all items and services in the comprehensive benefit package. The plans also would have to offer enrollees the opportunity to obtain coverage for out-of-network items and services and could charge alternative premiums for individuals who obtain such coverage.

Health plans would have to establish premiums on the basis of community rating. There are requirements with respect to marketing activities by health plans and with respect to the provision of information relating to plan costs, providers, utilization control procedures, procedures to improve and assure quality of care, rights and responsibilities of enrollees, and information on the number of plan members who disenroll. Health plans would have to comply with the Social Security Act requirements relating to advance directives. Health plans would be required to have adequate grievance procedures.

□ **Arrangements With Providers:** Each health plan would have to have adequate arrangements with providers to assure the provision of all services covered by the comprehensive benefit package to enrollees. Each plan would have to cover emergency and urgent care services. Providers could not charge or collect more than the applicable payment amount. Providers could not bill patients directly but would submit charges to the applicable health plan.

State laws restricting plans that are other than fee-for-service plans would be preempted as would state laws relating to the corporate practice of medicine and to provider ownership of health plans. Health plans would have to meet financial solvency requirements and would have to comply with quality assurance requirements. Each plan would verify the credentials of practitioners and facilities, would ensure that all participating providers meet applicable state licensing and certification standards, would oversee the quality and performance of participating providers, and would investigate and resolve consumer complaints.

Each plan would disclose to enrollees the protocols used by the plan for controlling utilization and costs. Each plan would comply with confidentiality, data management, and reporting requirements.

□ **Supplemental Insurance:** Entities could offer supplemental insurance for coverage of items and services not included in the program's comprehensive benefits package. Excluded from the definition of supplemental insurance would be a cost-sharing policy, long term care insurance, disease-specific insurance, hospital or nursing home indemnity insurance, Medicare supplemental insurance, and accident insurance.

Supplemental policies could not provide coverage for items or services covered by the comprehensive benefits package. There could be no limitation on the individuals who could seek enrollment under such policies. The National Board would develop standards for the marketing of these policies. Standards are set out in the bill for the offering of cost sharing policies.

□ **Essential Community Providers:** Health plans would enter into a written provider participation agreement with electing essential community providers or enter into an agreement under which the plan will make payment to the provider as specified din the bill. Essential community providers are defined later in the bill. Standards for the participating provider agreement are included. Payments to providers without participating agreements would be made either on a fee-for-service basis or in accordance with Medicare payment methodologies.

The requirements with respect to essential community providers would apply only for the first five years of the program. After that period, the HHS Secretary would conduct studies regarding essential community providers, including studies of the definition of such providers, and would make recommendations to the Congress as to whether and to what extent, the essential community provider provisions outlined above should continue.

□ **National Health Board:** A seven-member National Health Board, to be appointed by the President with the advice and consent of the Senate, would be established.

The Board would have primary responsibility with respect to the interpretation and recommended revision of the comprehensive benefit package. It would administer the cost containment provisions of the bill. It would develop eligibility standards and have responsibility for a performance-based system of quality management. It would establish a national health information system, establish requirements for participating states and monitor state compliance with the requirements, develop premium class factors, develop a methodology for the risk-adjustment of premium payments, encourage the reasonable pricing of breakthrough drugs, establish minimum capital requirements, and set standards for health plan grievance procedures. The Board would prepare a comprehensive annual report to the President concerning the implementation of the program.

As noted earlier, the Board would review and approve state systems. It could impose sanctions on states that fail to meet conditions of compliance.

The bill would authorize federal planning grants to assist states in the development of health care systems. The HHS Secretary would implement and carry out the program in states that do not meet requirements, or fail to continue to meet requirements, for the state system.

The Board would be charged with developing premium class factors that reflect the relative actuarial value of the comprehensive benefit package of the class of family enrollment compared to such value of the package for individual enrollment. The Board also would develop a risk adjustment and reinsurance methodology. Extensive factors to be considered in developing these methodologies are set forth in the bill.

The Board would establish standards under which states could provide for an adjustment in the risk-adjustment methodology in order to provide a financial incentive for regional alliance health plans to enroll individuals who are members of disadvantaged groups. The Secretary would conduct and support research and demonstration projects to develop and improve the risk adjustment and reinsurance methodology. The Board would establish a 15-member technical advisory committee.

The Board would establish minimum capital requirements for regional alliance health plans. The minimum capital requirement would be $500,000. Additional capital could be required based on relevant factors with regard to each plan. The Board could request the National Assn. of Insurance Commissioners to develop model standards for the additional capital requirements. The Board also would establish standards for guaranty funding.

□ **HHS Responsibilities:** The Secretary would administer all aspects of the program except those delegated to the National Board. The Secretary would develop financial management standards and would perform periodic financial and other audits of regional alliances. The Secretary would establish an Advisory Council on Breakthrough Drugs. The advisory council would examine the launch prices of new drugs that represent a breakthrough or significance advance over existing therapies.

The Secretary would certify essential community providers. The categories of providers that could qualify as essential community providers are: migrant health centers; community health centers; homeless program providers; public housing providers; Indian health programs; AIDS providers under the Ryan White Act; maternal and child health providers; federally qualified health centers; rural health clinics; providers of school health services; and community practice networks.

The Secretary would establish standards for the certification of additional categories of health care providers and organizations as essential community providers. The bill includes procedures for the certification of essential community providers.

□ **Labor Department Responsibilities:** The Labor Secretary would ensure enforcement of requirements under the bill applicable to employers and the administration of corporate health alliances. Various specific requirements in this regard are identified.

□ **Employer Responsibilities:** Employers would assure compliance with payroll withholding requirements contained in later provisions of the bill. Employers would have to provide considerable information to employees concerning regional alliances and corporate alliances. Employers would have to provide specific, employee-identifiable information to alliances. Some of this information would have to be provided on a monthly basis.

TITLE II — NEW BENEFITS

□ **Medicare Outpatient Prescription Drugs:** Outpatient prescription drugs would be added as a benefit under Part B of Medicare. Most currently approved prescription drugs, biological products, and insulin would be covered. The benefit would not include coverage of any product that is intravenously administered in a home setting unless it is a covered home infusion drug. Home infusion drugs would have to be administered intravenously, subcutaneously, epidurally, or through other means using an access device that is inserted into the body and an infusion device to control the rate of flow of the drug. The drug would have to be administered in the home.

Home infusion drugs would be antibiotics that the HHS Secretary has not determined can generally be administered safely and effectively in a home setting and other drugs for which the Secretary has made a determination that they can be safely and effectively administered in the home. The Secretary would publish a list of covered home infusion drugs.

Coverage for outpatient drugs would begin after the eligible individual has paid a deductible of $250, increased annually to ensure that the same percentage of individuals each year will incur expenses equal to or greater than the deductible. Medicare would pay 80 percent of the payment basis for covered drugs for persons who have not met the out-of-pocket limit for drugs and 100 percent for those who have met the limit. The out-of-pocket limit would begin at $1,000 and would increase annually.

The payment basis for a covered drug would be the lesser of the actual charge for the drug or the applicable payment limit. In the case of multiple source drugs that have restrictive prescriptions and single source drugs, the payment limit would equal the lesser of the 90th percentile of the actual charges for the drug for the second previous payment calculation period or the amount of the administrative allowance plus the number of dosage units multiplied by the estimated acquisition cost.

For multiple source drugs that do not have restrictive prescriptions, the payment limit would equal the amount of the administrative allowance plus the number of dosage units multiplied by the unweighted median of the unit estimated acquisition cost. The estimated acquisition cost of a drug could not exceed 93 percent of the average manufacturer non-retail price for the drug. In the first year of the program the administrative allowance would be five dollars. This amount would increase annually in accordance with the increase in the consumer price index. The administrative allowance could be reduced with respect to covered drugs dispensed by mail order pharmacies.

The Secretary would establish programs to identify instances or patterns of unnecessary or inappropriate prescribing, substandard care with respect to drugs, potential adverse reactions, and appropriate use of generic products. The Secretary would establish standards for the prescribing of each covered outpatient drug and could establish a drug use review program.

In order for payment to be available for covered outpatient drugs, the manufacturer would have to enter into a rebate agreement with the Secretary. Based on information provided by the Secretary as to the number of dosage units of a drug that have been provided to eligible individuals, the manufacturer would provide a rebate to the Secretary equal to the greater of the difference between the average manufacturer retail price and the average manufacturer non-retail price or 17 percent of the average manufacturer retail price. No rebate would be required with regard to generic products. The bill includes other provisions for the determination of rebates for new drugs, for drugs marketed in certain other countries, and for other situations.

The bill contains extensive provisions relating to the qualifications of home infusion therapy providers, which would be certified. Payment for home infusion therapy services would be the lesser of the actual charges or the fee schedule to be established by the Secretary.

□ **State Long Term Care Programs:** States could establish plans for home and community-based services to individuals with disabilities. These plans would provide for an initial screening of individuals. There could be no income, age, or geographic limits on eligibility nor could there be limits based on the nature, severity, or category of the disability, the residential setting, other than an institutional setting, or other grounds specified by the Secretary.

Other plan requirements are stipulated. States could not subject consumer-directed providers of personal assistance services to licensure, certification, or other requirements the Secretary finds not to be necessary for the health and safety of individuals with disabilities. To the extent possible, individuals with disabilities would be able to choose the covered services they wish to receive and the providers who will provide them. States would have to ensure that the proportion of such services provided to low-income individuals is not less than the proportion of low-income individuals in the state.

Payment of providers could be on a fee-for-service basis, prepayment on a capitation basis, payment by cash or voucher to disabled individuals, or any combination of these. State plans would have to include quality assurance procedures. Administrative expenses could not exceed 10 percent of total expenditures.

Eligible individuals would be those: who require some assistance with at least three activities of daily living; who suffer from severe cognitive impairment or severe mental impairment, or both; who have severe or profound mental retardation; or who are children under six years of age who have a severe disability or chronic medical condition. A comprehensive assessment and a plan of care would be required.

Covered would be consumer-directed personal assistance services, case management, homemaker and chore assistance, home modifications, respite services, assistive devices, adult day services, habilitation and rehabilitation, supported employment, home health services, and any other care or assistive services determined by the state to be of help for individuals with disabilities. Personal assistance services are defined to include at least hands-on and standby assistance, supervision, and cuing with activities of daily living whether agency-administered or consumer-directed. Consumer directed services would be those provided by an individual selected by the individual receiving the services. Cost sharing on a sliding scale basis, according to income, would be required.

States would receive federal matching assistance for amounts expended under this program. The total federal budget for this program is specified in the bill. The limit would be $4.5 billion in the first year of the program and would increase to $38.3 billion by the eighth year.

□ **Medicaid Nursing Home Changes:** A National Long Term Care Insurance Advisory Council would be created. Among other duties, the Advisory Council would develop uniform terminology for use in long term care insurance policies, develop a standard format for such insurance, and advise as to whether federal standards should apply to premiums for such policies. The Advisory Council also would make recommendations as to whether federal standards are needed governing the terms and conditions insurers may place on eligibility to obtain improved coverage. The Council would make recommendations concerning the need for federal standardized sets of threshold conditions for payment of covered benefits.

Other recommendations would relate to dispute mechanisms, sales and servicing of policies, and possible regulation of the long term care aspects of continuing care communities.

The Secretary, after considering the recommendations of the Advisory Council, would be required to issue regulations to standardize formats and terminology of long term care policies, to require insurers to provide to customers and beneficiaries information on the range of public and private long term care coverage available, and to establish other appropriate consumer-related requirements. Detailed descriptions of the elements to be included in the regulations with regard to each of these areas are provided. Regulations also would be required with regard to a variety of coverage issues and other issues within the purview of the Advisory Council. The states would be required to establish programs to enforce the federal standards. No insurer could sell a long term care policy in a state that does not have such an enforcement program in effect.

The Secretary could make grants for the development and implementation of long term care information, counseling and other programs. The Secretary would conduct a demonstration program to test the effectiveness of various approaches to financing and providing integrated acute and long term care services for the chronically ill and disabled who meet certain eligibility criteria. The specifics of this program are included in the bill.

TITLE III — PUBLIC HEALTH INITIATIVES

□ **Work Force Priorities:** A National Council on Graduate Medical Education would be established. Approved physician training programs, which would be medical residency or other postgraduate programs, would ensure that the number of individuals enrolled is in accordance with the restrictions imposed by the bill.

The National Council annually would designate the number of individuals who could be enrolled in such training programs. At least 55 percent of the participants in these programs would have to be in programs in primary care. The National Council would make allocations among the medical specialties. Federal payments would be made to approved programs.

Special funding would be authorized for training of additional primary care physicians and physician assistants, training of underrepresented minorities and disadvantaged persons, nurse training, and training of health professionals and administrators in managed care, cost-effective practice management, continuous quality improvement practices, and provision of culturally sensitive care.

The Secretary of Labor would be given authority to carry out various job retraining programs to increase the supply of health professionals and other health personnel. A National Institute for Health Care Workforce would be established to make recommendations concerning all aspects of the needed supply of health care workers and regarding the impact of the health alliance system on health care workers.

□ **Academic Health Centers:** Federal payments would be made to academic health centers to assist with the costs that are not routinely incurred by other entities in providing health services but are incurred by the centers by virtue of their academic nature.

Regional and corporate alliances would ensure that the health plans of the alliances enter into sufficient contracts with eligible centers to ensure that enrollees in the plans receive the specialized treatment expertise of the centers. The HHS Secretary could make grants to eligible centers for the establishment and operation of information and referral systems to provide the services of the centers to rural regional and corporate alliance health plans.

□ **Health Research Initiatives:** The Director of the National Institutes of Health (NIH) would ensure that the Institutes conduct and support biomedical and behavioral research on promoting health and preventing disease, disorders, and other health conditions. The Administrator of the Agency for Health Care Policy and Research would conduct research on reform of the health care system.

□ **Public Health Functions:** Special funding would be provided to support core functions of public health programs. The core functions are defined as: monitoring and protecting the health of communities against communicable diseases and exposure to toxic environmental pollutants, occupational hazards, harmful products, and poor quality health care; identifying and controlling outbreaks of infectious disease and patterns of chronic disease and injury; informing and educating health care consumers and providers about their roles in preventing and controlling disease and the appropriate use of medical services; and developing and testing new prevention and public health control interventions.

Grants would be made to the states for the core health functions. The general categories of functions identified above are further defined in much greater detail.

□ **Health Promotion and Disease Prevention:** The Secretary could make grants for projects to develop and implement innovative community-based strategies to provide for health promotion and disease prevention activities for which there is a significant need. The Secretary annually would develop a statement of proposed priorities for these grants.

□ **Services Support:** Funds would continue to be available for support of community and migrant health centers. Funding would be provided for the development of qualified community health plans and qualified community practice networks. The health plans would be developed to provide the items and services included in the bill's comprehensive benefits package in one or more health professional shortage areas or to provide the items or services to a significant number of individuals who are members of a medically underserved population. A practice network would consist of a consortium of providers whose principal purpose is to provide services to the target populations of community health plans.

Loans and loan guarantees would be available to pay the principal and interest for the capital costs of developing qualified community health plans and networks.

Grants could be made to assist entities in providing enabling services such as transportation, community and patient outreach, patient education, translation services and other services the Secretary determines appropriate. Funding for the National Health Service Corps would be extended and increased. Special payments would be made to hospitals that experience a low-income utilization rate of at least 25 percent.

□ **Mental Health; Substance Abuse:** Supplemental formula grants would be available to the states for activities related to mental health and substance abuse. Funding could be used for enabling services, as described in the previous paragraph, with regard to mental health and substance abuse. The funds also could assist in improving state capacity to coordinate and monitor mental health and substance abuse services, provide incentives to integrate public and private systems for the treatment of mental health and substance abuse disorders, to carry out activities currently authorized under the alcohol and drug abuse and mental health block grants, and to provide technical assistance.

Loans and loan guarantees could be provided with regard to the capital costs incurred in the development of non-acute, residential treatment centers and community-based ambulatory clinics.

States would be required to submit plans to achieve integration of the mental health and substance abuse services of the state with those provided in the bill's comprehensive benefit package. The Secretary would establish a pilot program to demonstrate model methods of achieving this integration.

□ **School Health Education and Health Services:** An extensive financial assistance program would be established to assist school systems in the development and implementation of comprehensive school health education programs. Such programs would address locally relevant priorities. They would have to be sequential and age- and developmentally appropriate and would be provided from kindergarten through grade 12. The programs would have to provide comprehensive health education, including education concerning community health, environmental health, personal health, family life, growth and development, nutritional health, prevention and control of disease and disorders, safety and prevention of injuries, substance abuse including tobacco and alcohol use, and consumer health. Other requirements for these programs are specified.

Grants would be authorized for the development of school health service sites. Grants could be used to plan for the provision of school health services, recruit, compensate, and train health and administrative staff, develop agreements with regional and corporate alliance health plans and other related activities. Grants also would be available to assist in meeting the cost of furnishing health services that are not covered under the bill's comprehensive benefit package or elsewhere, the cost of furnishing enabling services, recruiting, training, and compensating personnel, providing outreach services to at-risk youth and to parents, providing linkage of individuals to health plans, community health services, and social services, and carrying out other activities deemed appropriate by the Secretary. Loans and loan guarantees also would be available with regard to the capital costs incurred in developing these projects.

TITLE IV — MEDICARE AND MEDICAID

States would have the option of integrating all or portions of the Medicare-eligible population in a state into the alliance system. Medicare enrollees would enroll in an alliance health plan in states that elect this option. Individuals enrolled in a health plan of an organization with a Medicare risk-sharing contract before the individual is eligible for Medicare would have the option of remaining enrolled with the organization after the individual is Medicare-eligible.

There are various open enrollment and related provisions designed to encourage managed care under Medicare. Increased information would be available from the Secretary to Medicare beneficiaries concerning capitation plans and Medicare supplemental policies. Special outlier payments could be made to eligible organizations with Medicare risk-sharing contracts.

The bill would provide Medicare coverage of the services of advanced practice nurses. The current Medicare peer review program would be repealed. Payment for Part B services could be made only on an assignment basis. The Secretary would take steps to consolidate the administration of Parts A and B. In doing so the Secretary would contract with a single entity that combines the fiscal intermediary and carrier functions in each area except where the Secretary finds that special regional or national contracts are appropriate. Current requirements for peer review organization precertification of certain surgical procedures would be repealed.

The Secretary could not implement a change in the Medicare billing system and the system for processing of Medicare claims within six months of a previous change. Some changes would be made in the Medicare antifraud and abuse provisions, including modification of the physician self-referral provisions.

The Uniformed Services Health plan and plans and facilities of the Veterans Affairs Department would be considered as eligible organizations under Medicare. The Secretary would provide payments to such plans on behalf of any individuals entitled to Medicare benefits who are enrolled in such a plan.

There are several amendments to the Medicare program designed to create savings. The update for inpatient hospital services would be reduced as would the adjustment for indirect medical education costs and for capital-related costs for inpatient hospital services. Savings would result from changes in the payment adjustments to be made to disproportionate share hospitals. Limits would be placed on increases in the physicians' fee schedule. Limits would be placed on payment for physicians' services furnished by high-cost hospital medical staffs. High-cost hospital medical staffs would be those with a hospital-specific per admission relative value in excess of the allowable average per admission relative value applicable to the medical staff.

The bill includes the procedures for determining the allowable per-admission relative values. Generally, the allowable per-admission relative value would be considered to be excessive if it is equal to 125 percent in the first two years, and 120 percent thereafter, of the 1996 hospital-specific per admission relative value for all hospital medical staffs. The hospital-specific per-admission relative value for a hospital, other than a teaching hospital, would equal the average per-admission relative value for each physician's service furnished to inpatients of the hospital by the hospital's medical staff during 1996.

In order to encourage physicians to provide primary care, the practice expense relative value units applicable to primary care services would be increased by 10 percent. Adjustments would be made in other payment factors to further encourage primary care.

Competitive bidding would be required for the furnishing of certain services including magnetic resonance imaging tests and computerized axial tomography scans, oxygen and oxygen equipment, enteral and parenteral nutrients, supplies, and equipment, clinical diagnostic laboratory tests, and other items and services for which the Secretary determines that the use of competitive acquisition will be appropriate and cost-effective.

A complex system of payment limits would be implemented with regard to health maintenance organizations and comprehensive medical plans with Medicare risk-sharing contracts. There would be a reduction in the routine cost limits for home health services. A 10 percent copayment would be imposed with regard to home health visits provided after an individual has been discharged from a hospital for more than 30 days.

Use of centers of excellence would be expanded with specific direction to use a competitive process to contract with these centers for cataract surgery. Payment would be made to such centers for cataract surgery and related services, coronary artery bypass surgery and related services, and those other services agreed upon by the Secretary and a center.

Medicaid plans would not be required to provide payment for benefits covered by the bill's comprehensive benefit package. Some income and resource-related expansions would be made in eligibility for Medicaid nursing home benefits.

States could receive special payments if they develop integrated long term care programs. The integrated programs would provide a continuum of care covering nursing facility services, home- and community-based services, home and community care for functionally disabled elderly individuals, and community supported living arrangements services. Eligibility for these services essentially would be limited to individuals with incomes that do not exceed the federal poverty line.

The bill would require states to ensure that nursing facility residents are informed of the range of home- and community-based services for which assistance is available. A special program would be created for poverty level children with special needs.

A Medicaid Commission would be established. It would study the possible use of a block grant program to give the states greater flexibility in targeting and delivering needed services. The Commission also would study whether, and if so how, to integrate the long term care services program and the home- and community-based services program with the services covered under the comprehensive benefit package of the bill. The Commission also would study other aspects of improving the long term care aspects of the Medicaid program.

TITLE V — QUALITY AND CONSUMER PROTECTION

□ **Quality Management Program:** The National Board would establish and oversee a performance-based program of quality management and improvement designed to enhance the quality, appropriateness, and effectiveness of health care services and access to those services. A National Quality Management Council would administer the program.

The Council would develop a set of national measures of quality performance. The national measures would be selected to provide information with regard to access, appropriateness, outcomes, health promotion, prevention, and consumer satisfaction. The bill outlines the criteria to be used in developing the measures. The Council would conduct periodic surveys of health care consumers to gather information concerning access, use of health services, health outcomes, and patient satisfaction.

In subject matter areas with respect to which the Council determines that sufficient information and consensus exist, the Council would recommend that the Board establish goals for performance by health plans and health care providers on a subset of the set of national measures of quality performance. The Council also would evaluate the impact of this health reform legislation on the quality of health services and access to those services.

Alliances annually would publish performance reports concerning each health plan offered in the alliance.

□ **Practice Guidelines:** The Council would direct the Administrator for Health Care Policy and Research to develop and periodically review and update clinically relevant guidelines that could be used by health care providers to assist in determining how diseases, disorders, and other health conditions can most effectively and appropriately be prevented, diagnosed, treated, and managed clinically. The methods to be used, and elements to be included, in developing these guidelines are specified.

□ **Health Care Quality Research:** The Administrator for Health Care Policy and Research would support research directly related to the performance measures identified in the bill. The Council would establish priorities with regard to this research and recommend research projects. Emphasis would be placed on research involving diseases, disorders, and health conditions as to which there is the highest level of uncertainty concerning treatment, there is the widest variation in practice patterns, the costs associated with prevention, diagnosis, treatment, or clinical management are significant, or the rate of incidence or prevalence is high for the population as a whole or for particular subpopulations.

The Board would establish and oversee regional professional foundations to develop programs in lifetime learning for health professionals, foster collaboration among health plans and providers to improve the quality of primary and specialized health care, disseminate information, develop innovative patient education systems, and apply for and conduct health care quality research.

A National Quality Consortium would undertake to support continuing education programs for health professionals and advise on matters related to health care quality research.

□ **Other Quality Provisions:** The bill would exempt from certification requirements clinical laboratories that perform simple laboratory procedures with an insignificant risk of error. Regional and corporate alliances would be required to disseminate various information related to quality and access, ensure that performance and quality standards are continually improved, and conduct educational programs to assist consumers in using quality and other information in choosing health plans. Health plans would have to measure and disclose performance on quality measures.

□ **Health Information Systems:** The National Board would develop and implement a health information system. The system would include data on: enrollment and disenrollment in health plans; clinical encounters and other items and services provided by health care providers; administrative and financial transactions and activities of participating states, alliances, health plans, providers, and others in order to determine compliance with the requirements of the bill; the characteristics of regional alliances and of corporate alliances; the terms of agreements between alliances and health plans; utilization management by health plans; grievances filed against alliances and health plans; and other similar information.

The Board would oversee the establishment of an electronic data network consisting of regional centers to collect, compile, and transmit information. Each eligible individual, employer, health plan, and health care provider would be given a unique identifier number. Information to be included on each individual's health security card is spelled out. The Board would provide technical assistance to the states and other entities participating in the program with respect to the establishment and operation of automated health information systems. Health information privacy standards would be developed. Federal legislation to provide a comprehensive scheme of federal privacy protection for individually identifiable health information would be required. A National Privacy and Health Data Advisory Council would be established.

□ **Health Plan Claims Procedures:** Health plans would have to provide approval or disapproval of completed claims within 30 days after submission of the claims. Plans would have to review claim denials in a timely manner. Procedures would be in place for urgent requests for plan preauthorization.

The bill contains provisions for review by regional alliance complaint review offices of grievances based on acts or practices of health plans. Administrative procedures for these and other reviews are outlined.

States would establish early resolution programs to assist in the mediation of grievances and other disputes. Procedures for the operation of these programs are included. There are extensive provisions relating to the rights of the parties in enforcing the requirements of the bill.

□ **Medical Malpractice:** Health plans would have to adopt alternate dispute resolution systems to address claims of medical malpractice by providers affiliated with each plan. The alternate dispute resolution mechanisms to be used would be arbitration, mediation, or early offers of settlement.

No action could be brought by an individual unless the individual certifies that he or she has consulted and reviewed the facts of the situation with a qualified medical specialist and the individual includes a written report from the medical specialist indicating that there is a reasonable and meritorious cause for the filing of the action.

Attorneys who represent plaintiffs on a contingency fee basis would be limited to a fee of one-third of the total amount recovered. Awards would be reduced by amounts received by the plaintiff from other sources for the same injury. At the request of any party, defendants would not be required to pay damages in a single, lump sum, but could pay on a periodic basis. There is no threshold limit for implementation of the periodic payment limit.

Funds would be provided for demonstration projects to determine whether substituting liability for medical malpractice on the part of the health plan in which a physician participates for the personal liability of the physician will result in improvements in the quality of care provided, reductions in defensive medical practices, and better risk management.

The Secretary would establish a pilot program to determine the effect of applying practice guidelines in the resolution of medical malpractice liability actions.

□ **Fraud and Abuse:** The Secretary and the Attorney General would establish a program: to coordinate the functions of the Attorney General, the Secretary, and other organizations with respect to the prevention, detection, and control of health care fraud and abuse; to conduct investigations, audits, and similar activities relating to the delivery of and payment for health care in the U.S.; and to facilitate the enforcement of statutes applicable to health care fraud and abuse.

In carrying out this program, the Secretary and Attorney General would coordinate with all applicable law enforcement agencies and with health alliances and health plans. An all-payer health care fraud and abuse control account would be established in the Treasury. Funds from fines and other civil penalties would be placed into the account. The funds would be used to help cover the costs of prosecuting health care matters, conducting investigations, conducting audits, and conducting inspections and evaluations.

The fraud and abuse provisions of the Social Security Act would apply to all payers. Certain modifications, including provisions that are more strict, would be made in those provisions.

TITLE VI — PREMIUM CAPS, PREMIUM FINANCING, PLAN PAYMENTS

□ **Regional Alliance Inflation Factors:** The National Board annually would publish the inflation factor applicable to each regional alliance for the following year. The regional alliance inflation factor would be the general health care inflation factor for the year adjusted to take into account material changes in the demographic and socio-economic characteristics of the population of alliance eligible individuals, reduced by the percentage adjustment provided with respect to the regional alliance based on previous excess expenditures, and, for the year 2001, increased by a factor the Board determines to reflect the ratio of the actuarial value of the increase in benefits provided in that year under the comprehensive benefit package to the actuarial value of the benefits that would have been in the package without regard to the increase.

For years 1996-1999, the general health care inflation factor would be the increase in the consumer price index plus 1.5 percentage points for 1996, 1 percentage point for 1997, .5 percentage point for 1998, and 0 percentage points for 1999. The Board would submit to Congress recommendations as to what the general health care inflation factor should be for years after 1999. If Congress fails to enact a law specifying the general health care inflation factor, the Board would compute the factor. In such an event, the factor would be 1 plus the following: the percentage change in the consumer price index for the year; the average annual percentage change in the population during the three previous years; and the average annual percentage change in the real, per capita gross domestic product for the three previous years.

The Board would develop methods to adjust the regional alliance inflation factor to reflect material changes in the demographic characteristics and health status of regional alliance eligible individuals in comparison with the average change for such individuals residing in the U.S.

□ **Baseline Premium Target:** The Board would establish a national per capita baseline premium target equal to the national per capita current coverage health expenditures updated on an annual basis. The average per capita current coverage health expenditures would equal total current health care expenditures covered by the program divided by the estimated population in the U.S. of regional alliance eligible individuals.

The Board annually would determine a per capita premium target for each regional alliance. The target for each alliance would equal the national per capita baseline premium target updated by the regional alliance inflation factor, as determined above, and, for the initial determination, adjusted by the adjustment factor for each alliance.

The adjustment factor for each alliance would take into consideration information on variations in premiums across states and across alliance areas within a state, information on variations in per capita health spending by state, information on variations across states in per capita spending under Medicare and in spending among health alliance areas in a state under Medicare, and area rating factors commonly used by actuaries.

□ **Initial Bidding and Negotiation:** Regional alliances annually would receive bids from each health plan seeking to participate in the program in the alliance area. Following receipt of the bids, the state could negotiate with health plans. Plans could resubmit bids, but only could submit bids that do not exceed the earlier bid, as a result of these negotiations. The final bid would be considered to be the accepted bid.

Each year each alliance would submit to the Board a report that discloses: information regarding the final bids; for the first year, an estimate of the enrollment likely in each plan and, in succeeding years, the actual distribution of enrollment; and limitations on capacity of regional alliance health plans.

For each regional alliance, the Board would determine a weighted average accepted bid for each year. This determination would be based on information on accepted bids for the year and would take into account the information on enrollment distribution. The Board would notify each alliance if the weighted average accepted bid for the alliance is greater than the regional alliance per capita premium target for the alliance. In such cases the Board also would notify the alliance of the reduced weighted average accepted bid for the alliance.

If such notice is provided to an alliance, the Board would notify the alliance and each noncomplying health plan of any plan reduction for the plan and the opportunity to voluntarily reduce the accepted bid in order to avoid the reduction. Procedures for determining the plan reduction follow.

States could elect to assume responsibility for containment of health care expenditures consistent with these provisions of the bill. For states that so elect, if the Board determines that the statewide weighted average of the reduced weighted average accepted bids is less that the statewide weighted average of the regional alliance per capita premium targets for the year, then the amount of the state maintenance of effort payments, as described later in the bill, would be reduced for the following year.

□ **Advisory Commission:** An advisory commission on regional variations in health expenditures would be established. The commission would examine methods of eliminating variation in regional alliance per capita premium targets due to variation in practice patterns when the variation is not due to other factors such as health care input prices and demographic factors. The commission also would examine methods of reducing variation in federal and state payments under the supplemental security income and aid to families with dependent children programs and in other programs.

The recommendations of the advisory commission would be submitted to the Board which would forward detailed recommendations to the Congress. Procedures are outlined for Congressional consideration of these recommendations.

□ **Payment Reductions:** In order to assure that payments to regional alliance health plans by a regional alliance are consistent with the applicable per capita target for the alliance, noncomplying health plans would be subject to a reduction in plan payment. A noncomplying alliance would be one for which the weighted average accepted bid exceeds the regional alliance per capita target for the year. A noncomplying plan would mean a plan offered through a noncomplying alliance if the final accepted bid for the year exceeds the maximum complying bid for the year.

The amount of the plan payment reduction would be the alliance wide reduction percentage of the excess bid amount. The alliance wide reduction percentage for any noncomplying alliance would be the amount by which the weighted average accepted bid for the alliance exceeds the regional alliance per capita target for the alliance divided by the sum, for noncomplying plans offered by the alliance, of the plan proportions of alliance excess bid amount. This is based on the excess bid amount multiplied by the plan enrollment proportion, as compared to enrollment in the alliance, for the plan.

□ **Provider Payment Reduction:** Each health plan would include, as part of its contract with any participating provider, a provision that if the plan is a noncomplying plan in any year, payments to the provider would be reduced by the applicable network reduction percentage. The contract could not include any other provision the state determines otherwise varies the payments to providers because of, or in relation to, a plan payment reduction. The plan reduction percentage, with respect to network providers of a noncomplying plan would be the plan payment reduction amount divided by the final accepted bid for the plan for the year.

The Board could adjust this amount to take into account any estimated increase in volume of services provided that may reasonably occur as a consequence of applying a reduction in payment. This increase could be computed differently for different classes of providers or services or different types of health plans.

Payments for non network providers of noncomplying plans also would be reduced in a similar manner.

□ **Corporate Alliance Expenditures:** The Board would develop a methodology for calculating an annual per capita expenditure equivalent for amounts paid for coverage for the comprehensive benefit package within a corporate alliance. Corporate alliances could petition the Secretary for an adjustment of the inflation adjustment that would otherwise apply to compensate for material changes in the demographic characteristics of the eligible individuals receiving coverage through the alliance.

If a corporate alliance has two excess years in a three year period the Secretary of Labor would terminate the corporate alliance and employers that were corporate alliance employers would become regional alliance employers. An excess year would be one in which the rate of increase for the corporate alliance exceeds the national corporate alliance inflation factor for the year. The national corporate alliance inflation factor for a year would be the average of the general health care inflation factors, as defined earlier, for each of the three previous years.

□ **Single Payer States:** In the case of statewide single payer states, the Board would compute a statewide per capita premium target amount for each year in the same manner as a regional alliance per capita premium target would be determined.

□ **Monitoring:** The Secretary would establish a program to monitor prices and expenditures in the health care system in the U.S. The Secretary periodically would report to the President on the rate of increase in expenditures in each sector of the health care system and how such rates compare with the rate of overall increase in health care spending and rate of increase in the consumer price index.

□ **Family Premium Payments:** Each family enrolled in a health plan would be responsible for payment of the family share of premium. The family share for families enrolled in regional alliances would consist of the regional alliance premium with respect to the class of enrollment and 20 percent of the family shortfall add-on. The premium charged by a regional alliance for families would equal the final accepted bid for the plan multiplied by the uniform per capita conversion factor for the alliance and further multiplied by the premium class factor established by the Board for the class.

The family collection shortfall add-on is the amount that would be the weighted average premium for the alliance, class, and year, if the per capita collection shortfall amount were substituted for the reduced weighted average accepted bid for the alliance. The per capita shortfall amount essentially is the amount which the alliance identifies as owed to the alliance and is not likely to be collected divided by the estimated number of alliance eligible individuals.

Certain credits and discounts also would be permitted in finally determining the family share premium for regional alliance health plans. Special provisions establish the family share premium for enrollees of corporate alliance health plans.

Family obligations for premiums would be limited based on income. For example, the payment obligations for families with adjusted incomes below $40,000 could not exceed 3.9 percent of adjusted income. There are further specifications of the manner in which premium amounts for enrollees in special circumstances would be determined.

□ **Employer Premium Payments:** Employers would pay a premium to the regional alliance that provides health coverage to a qualifying employee. The premium for family enrollment would equal the employer's monthly premium for the class of family enrollment involved multiplied by the number of full time equivalent employees enrolled in that class. The employer premium basically would equal 80 percent of the weighted average premium for the regional alliance and class of enrollment for each enrolled individual or family.

For small employers the employer contribution would be limited based on the number of employees and the average annual wages per full-time employee. For example, an employer with fewer than 25 employees and an average individual wage of up to $12,000 would not pay more than 3.5 percent of the employer's wages. If the average wage for such an employer were between $21,000 and $24,000, premiums could not exceed 7.1 percent of wages. For employers of between 50 and 75 employees, the percentages for the same wage categories would be 5.3 and 7.9 respectively. The percentage of wages limit for all other employers would be 7.9 percent. Other adjustments could be made with regard to employer contributions, including reductions because of excess risk presented by the health risk status of employees and add-ons for premium collection shortfalls.

Self-employed individuals would be considered to be employers and therefore subject to the provisions of the bill. The premium payment for corporate alliance employers would equal 80 percent of the weighted average monthly premium of the health plans offered by the corporate alliance.

□ **Payment to Regional Alliance Health Plans:** Payments to health plans would be determined as a blended plan per capita payment amount consisting of three components multiplied by any applicable adjustment factor. The first component would be the plan bid component which would consist of the final accepted bid of the plan multiplied by the plan bid proportion. The second component would be the aid to families with dependent children component for the alliance. This would consist of the AFDC per capita premium amount, as determined later in the bill, multiplied by the AFDC proportion.

The third component would be the supplemental security income component consisting of the SSI per capita premium amount multiplied by the SSI proportion.

TITLE VII — REVENUE PROVISIONS

□ **Tobacco Excise Tax:** Substantial increases would be made in the tax on tobacco products. As an example, the tax on cigarettes would increase from $12 per thousand to $49.50 per thousand. The tax on cigars would increase from about one cent per thousand to just over 38 cents per thousand. Similar increases would be imposed with regard to cigarette papers, cigarette tubes, smokeless tobacco, and pipe tobacco. A new tax of $12.50 per pound would be imposed on roll-your-own tobacco.

□ **Assessment on Corporate Alliance Employers:** Every corporate alliance employer would pay an assessment equal to one percent of the employer's payroll.

□ **Recapture of Health Subsidies:** High income individuals would pay a recapture amount based on Medicare Part B payments and reductions received by the individual under the credits authorized for enrollees. The threshold amount for imposition of these recapture payments would be $90,000 for individuals, $115,000 in the case of joint returns, and zero in the case of married taxpayers who do not file jointly and who do not live apart.

□ **Other Revenue Provisions:** The net earnings of any individual who is a two percent shareholder of an S corporation and who materially participates in the activities of the corporation would include the individual's pro rata share of the taxable income or loss of the corporation from service-related businesses carried on by the corporation.

Medicare coverage, and the hospital insurance tax, would be extended to all state and local government employees.

□ **Employer Provided Health Care:** The gross income of an employee would include employer provided health coverage except to the extent that the coverage consists of the comprehensive health benefits authorized by the bill or consists of permitted coverage. Certain examples of permitted coverage are provided.

The bill would prohibit inclusion of health benefits in employer sponsored cafeteria plans. Self-employed individuals could deduct 100 percent of the expenses of health coverage for themselves and their families to the extent that the covered health benefits consist of those included in the program's comprehensive benefit package.

□ **Other Provisions:** The bill would strengthen requirements for the funding of retiree health benefit plans and would require coordination of the bill's health program with existing requirements for continuation of health benefits for employees who leave their employer. Ultimately, the continuation of benefits requirements would be repealed.

In order for hospitals and other entities that provide health care services to qualify as charitable entities, they would have to assess the health care needs of their communities and develop a plan to meet those needs. Special rules would apply to health maintenance organizations, both with regard to their possible status as charitable organizations and with regard to the classification of health insurance offered by such organizations.

Entities that issue accident and health insurance contracts or the reinsurance of risks undertaken by other insurance companies under such contracts, operate as health maintenance organizations, or enter into arrangements under which fixed payments or premiums are received as consideration for the organization's agreement to provide or arrange for health care services and the fixed payments or premiums do not vary depending on the amount of health care services provided would be treated for tax purposes, unless otherwise exempt, as an insurance company other than a life insurance company. The bill includes special transition rules for Blue Cross and Blue Shield organizations.

Regional alliances would be treated as tax exempt organizations. Qualified long term care services would be treated as medical care for tax purposes. Long term care insurance would be treated in the same manner as accident and health insurance. Death benefits under life insurance policies that are paid prior to death to a terminally ill individual would not be taxable but would be treated as a benefit paid on death. Special rules would apply to the companies that offer such accelerated death benefits.

A tax credit would be authorized for qualified primary health services providers who serve in a shortage area. Such service would have to be completed within the first 60 months that the individual becomes a qualified primary care provider. Service could not be through obligations under the National Health Service Corps program. The credit would be $1,000 for each month of service by a physician and $500 for each month of service by a nonphysician.

When expensing medical equipment, the maximum aggregate cost which could be taken into account for any taxable year could not exceed $17,500. The aggregate cost that could be taken into account would be increased by the lesser of the cost of health care property placed in service during the taxable year or $10,000. Health care property is defined as property: which is medical equipment used in the screening, monitoring, observation, diagnosis, or treatment of patients in a laboratory, medical or hospital environment; which is owned and used by a physician in the active conduct of the physician's full-time trade or business of providing health services in a health professional shortage area, and substantially all the use of which is in the shortage area.

A tax credit would be authorized for personal assistance expenses required by employed individuals. The credit could be for up to fifty percent of such expenses, or a lower percentage based on income.

TITLE VIII — FEDERAL GOVERNMENT PROGRAMS

□ **Military Health Plans:** The Secretary of Defense could establish one or more Uniformed Services Health Plans in order to provide health care services to members of the uniformed services on active duty for a period of more than 30 days. The benefits also would be available to the families of such individuals. Such a plan could rely upon the use of facilities of the uniformed services for the provision of health care to enrollees. Agreements also could be entered into with civilian health facilities. The benefits of such plans would be those included in the bill's comprehensive benefits package as well as those benefits the individual would be entitled to receive under the uniformed services program.

If such a plan is available, all members of a uniformed service on active duty for more than 30 days would be required to enroll in the plan. The Secretary would make premium payments to health alliances for coverage of members who are not covered by a uniformed services health plan.

Similar provisions would apply to veterans who are eligible for benefits from the Department of Veterans Affairs.

The Federal Employee Health Benefits Plan would be terminated. Federal employees, and the federal government, would be treated as employees and an employer with regard to the requirements of the bill. Special rules would apply with regard to coverage provided to Indians.

There would be certain limitations on the application of the Employee Retirement Income Security Act, ERISA, with regard to alliance health plans.

Added funds would be provided under the supplemental food program for Women, Infants, and Children, WIC.

TITLE IX — AGGREGATE GOVERNMENT PAYMENTS

□ **State Payments:** Essentially states would be required to maintain their payments relating to non-cash assistance recipients.

States would have to contribute toward the premium costs for health plan coverage of individuals who are eligible for aid to families with dependent children, for supplemental security income payments, and for Medicaid.

□ **Federal Payments:** The federal government would pay to each regional alliance an amount equal to the federal medical assistance percentage for each state of 95 percent of the premium amounts paid by the state. The federal payments would be capped with regard to any alliance. Loans could be made to regional alliances to cover any period of temporary cash-flow shortfall attributable to estimation discrepancies, administrative error, or the timing of the receipt of amounts owed and payments required.

TITLE X — COORDINATION OF WORKERS COMPENSATION

Health plans that provide services to enrollees through participating providers would enter into contracts and arrangements to provide or arrange for the provision of workers compensation services to such enrollees in return for payment from the workers compensation carrier. States would coordinate access to specialized workers compensation programs on behalf of health plans. The Secretary of Labor would report on the impact of these provisions on the premium rates charged to employers for workers compensation insurance.

Demonstration projects with respect to treatment of work-related injuries and illnesses would be authorized. Protocols for the appropriate treatment of work-related conditions would be developed. Methods would be developed for providing payment by workers compensation carriers to health plans of a per case, capitated payment for the treatment of specified work-related injuries and illnesses.

Requirements similar to those described above for workers compensation plans also would apply to automobile insurance medical benefits.

A Commission on Integration of Health Benefits would be created to study the feasibility and appropriateness of transferring financial responsibility for all medical benefits, including those currently covered under workers compensation and automobile insurance, to health plans.

TITLE XI — TRANSITIONAL INSURANCE REFORM

The provisions of this title would be administered in a manner to assure the maintenance of current health care coverage and benefits during the period between enactment of the Health Security Act and the dates its provisions are implemented. The title includes enforcement authority for the Secretary, including the authority to impose civil money penalties for failure to comply with the bill's requirements.

The bill would impose requirements for the preservation of current coverage. It would restrict health insurance premium increases during the transition period. It would protect against discrimination of coverage due to preexisting conditions and would limit the ability of self-insured plans to reduce benefits. The bill would create a national transitional health insurance risk pool to assure access to health care coverage, during the transitional period, for individuals who are unable to secure such coverage because of their health status.

TITLE XII — TEMPORARY EMPLOYER ASSESSMENT

Every employer with base period retiree health costs would pay an assessment equal to 50 percent of the greater of the adjusted base period retiree health costs of the employer for the calendar year or the amount by which the employer's applicable retiree health costs for the calendar year were reduced by reason of enactment of this bill. This special assessment would apply to calendar years 1998 through 2000.